NEUROLOGIC EMERGENCIES

2ND EDITION

NEUROLOGIC EMERGENCIES
A SYMPTOM-ORIENTED APPROACH

GREGORY L. HENRY, MD
Clinical Professor of Emergency Medicine
The University of Michigan Medical School
Ann Arbor, Michigan

NEAL LITTLE, MD
Clinical Assistant Professor of Emergency Medicine
The University of Michigan Medical School
Ann Arbor, Michigan

ANDY JAGODA, MD
Professor and Vice Chair of Emergency Medicine
Residency Director
Mount Sinai School of Medicine
New York, New York

THOMAS R. PELLEGRINO, MD
Professor and Chair
Department of Neurology
Eastern Virginia Medical School
Norfolk, Virginia

McGRAW-HILL

New York   Chicago   San Francisco
Lisbon   London   Madrid   Mexico City   Milan
New Delhi   San Juan   Seoul   Singapore
Sydney   Toronto

The **McGraw·Hill** Companies

1 2 3 4 5 6 7 8 9 0 DOC/DOC 0 9 8 7 6 5 4 3

ISBN 0-07-140292-6

This book was set in Times Roman by Circle Graphics, Inc.
The editors were Andrea Seils and Regina Y. Brown.
The production supervisor was Catherine H. Saggese.
The interior text designer was Marsha Cohen/Parallelogram.
The index was prepared by Edwin Durbin.
RR Donnelley was the printer and binder.

This book is printed on acid-free paper.

Library of Congress Cataloging-in-Publication Data
Neurologic emergencies: a symptom-oriented approach /
Gregory L. Henry . . . [et al.].—2nd ed.
      p. ; cm.
    Includes bibliographical references and index.
    ISBN 0-07-140292-6
      1. Neurological emergencies. I. Henry, Gregory L.
    [DNLM: 1. Nervous System Diseases—diagnosis. 2. Diagnosis,
    Differential. 3. Emergencies. 4. Evidence-Based Medicine.
    WL 141 N48374 2003]
    RC350.7 .H398 2003
    616.8′0425—dc21

2002028824

CONTENTS

A valid reason is needed for a second edition of anything. After all, is there something we didn't tell you the first time around? There is ample reason to present a new edition of *Neurologic Emergencies: A Symptom-Oriented Approach*. The scientific world moves forward, although the basics of neuroanatomy, neurologic history taking, and examination remain the same. There have been significant changes over the intervening years as to what truly constitutes a "cost-effective" neurologic evaluation from both a history and physical examination standpoint. How much of what we do is predicated on actual knowledge and understanding versus a ritualized genuflection to the great men of the past? Do we act because we are told and trained to do so or because we actually understand the basis of what we are doing? Do we really need to formally test the 12th cranial nerve in a patient who is speaking clearly? What are the key historical features that make a clinical difference in working up a headache?

Two underlying situations will drive health care in the foreseeable future. First, a growing number of elderly patients with complex medical problems and confusing drug interactions will become the norm. Second will be both the implicit and explicit pressure on the intelligent physician to act in a stewardship role to get maximum value out of both professional time and expensive testing modalities. The days of the knee-jerk head CT may thankfully be drawing to a close. Additionally, the actual armamentarium of lab tests and radiologic studies has expanded exponentially since the first edition of this book. Moving from point A, the patient's complaint, to point B, effective therapy, in the most cost-efficient manner is becoming the real issue in health care. Proper test selection is imperative. There is no reason to do two preliminary studies prior to the one that will actually answer the question. This is where tradition and science truly engage in a "battle royal" on how to move the patient from initial diagnosis to disposition.

A third reason for a new edition to the book is to address the issue of management. The emergency department is the interface between the expensive world of inpatient care and less intense outpatient evaluation and management. As competition for bed space intensifies, the emergency physician will need to make certain that only those patients who truly need hospitalization are admitted.

What has not changed since the first edition and what remains the core of this book is one simple concept: patients don't come to the doctor with diseases, they come with complaints. This work is still symptom-based. "Doctor, I'm weak, Doctor, I'm dizzy, Doctor, I've got a headache" are complaints that will be voiced millions of times this year in emergency departments across the country. A logical approach to rapid investigation and treatment is still required to ensure a smoothly running emergency department. The delicate balance between trivializing a patient's complaints and participating in diagnostic overkill is still the most important basic skill an emergency physician can have. A better understanding of this balancing act continues to be the true function of this book.

ACKNOWLEDGMENTS

The authors wish to express their heartfelt thanks to Mary Jo Wagner, MD, FACEP, for all her efforts in proofreading this work and for her intelligent and insightful criticism of its content. The work is stronger due to her involvement. Dr. Wagner is the Director of the Emergency Medicine Residency Program at Saginaw Cooperative Hospitals, Inc. and Associate Professor of Emergency Medicine at Michigan State University College of Human Medicine.

1

A REVIEW OF BASIC NEUROANATOMY

"The charm of neurology, above all other branches of practical medicine, lies in the way it forces us into daily contact with principles. A knowledge of the structure and functions of the nervous system is necessary to explain the simplest phenomena of disease; this can be only obtained by thinking scientifically."

—Sir Henry Head

Neuroanatomy is frequently considered by medical students to be one of the least enjoyable and most technically intricate disciplines that they must study. The amount of neuroanatomy necessary to practice good clinical medicine, however, is limited. Basic principles apply to each of the various nervous system modalities that can be tested. Mastery of these simple principles and a fundamental understanding of the overall organization of the nervous system allows for accurate localization of disease entities. This chapter attempts to review the basic anatomic concepts necessary to evaluate the historical and physical findings most often seen with acute neurologic problems.

Basic ORGANIZATION OF THE NERVOUS SYSTEM

The human nervous system is composed of carefully integrated units that are involved with informing the organism about what is happening within the body and the world around it. The nervous system processes the information and sends out orders to various end organs to adjust to internal and external environmental changes. The central nervous system consists of the brain and the spinal cord. It is completely encased within the skull and spinal column, thereby having bony protection for its vital structures. The major areas of the brain include the cerebral cortex, subcortical structures, brainstem, and cerebellum[1] (Fig. 1-1). The cerebral hemispheres are separated by the medial longitudinal fissure but are connected at their base by the fibrous corpus callosum, which provides a pathway that allows the two halves of the cerebrum to communicate with each other[1] (Fig. 1-2). Both the right and left cortex are further subdivided into four lobes. The frontal lobe is the most anterior of the segments. Although anatomically the right and left frontal lobes appear the same, they have distinctly different functions. In nearly all right-handed individuals and in at least 50% of left-handed individuals, left-hemisphere dominance provides that the areas for initiation of speech and language lie in the frontal lobe on the left side of the brain.[2]

Initiation of voluntary motor acts begins in the frontal lobes in the respective motor strips.[3] Personality, problem-solving abilities, and reasoning seem to be primarily based in the frontal lobes.[3] Essentially much of what is considered to be personality is also in the frontal lobes. Spontaneity of thoughts and ideas, although not precisely pinned down to one area, is certainly the most affected by lesions in the frontal lobes.[4]

Lying immediately adjacent to and posterior to the frontal lobes are the parietal lobes. Parietal lobes form a principal receiving area for sensory information as well as information from other parts of the body. The parietal lobes are particularly involved in recognition of self with regard to body image and position.[1] Spatial orientation and three-dimensional understanding of objects are parietal lobe functions.[1] The occipital lobes lie most posteriorly on the cerebral cortex. In the occipital lobes, the optic tracts terminate and vision comes to cognition.[5]

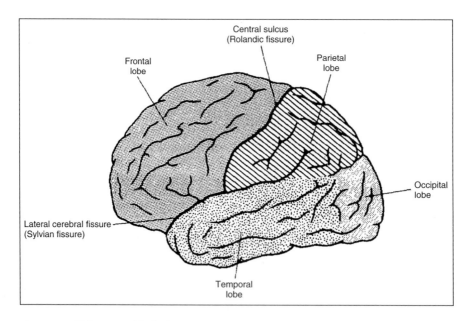

FIGURE 1-1 Major areas of the brain.

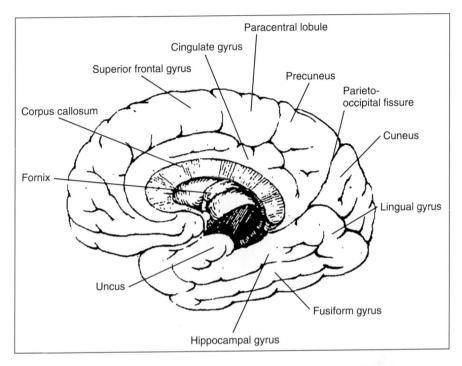

FIGURE 1-2 Medial view of the right cerebral hemisphere. (From Chud J. *Correlative Neuroanatomy and Functional Neurology,* 14th ed. Los Altos, CA: Lange, 1970, p 3, with permission.)

The temporal lobes lie immediately below the frontal and parietal lobes, separated from them by the lateral (Sylvian) fissure. The temporal lobes are basically involved in receiving and monitoring auditory information.[1]

Moving inwardly from the cortex are deeper structures—the basal ganglia and the thalamic structures (Fig. 1-3). The basal ganglia are a group of nuclei that lie between the cortex and the internal capsule.[1] The various elements of the basal ganglia constitute the extrapyramidal tracts, which help to control motor movements.[3]

Medial to the internal capsule are the various thalamic structures (Fig. 1-4). This region includes the thalamus proper, the epithalamus, the subthalamus, and the hypothalamus. The parts of the thalamus surround the third ventricle and form a core of the brain. The nuclei of the thalamus perform a variety of functions, including monitoring homeostasis and relaying information to specific cortical areas.

The hypothalamus, which forms the floor and part of the ventral-lateral walls of the third ventricle, has a close association with the optic chiasm. It is also connected through both nuclei and arterial circulation to the pituitary gland.[1] Regulation of appetite and body temperature is strongly influenced by hypothalamic nuclei.[1] The autonomic nervous system receives substantial input from the hypothalamus. Stimulation of the rostral portions of the hypothalamus, on the other hand, causes excitation of the sympathetic system.[1]

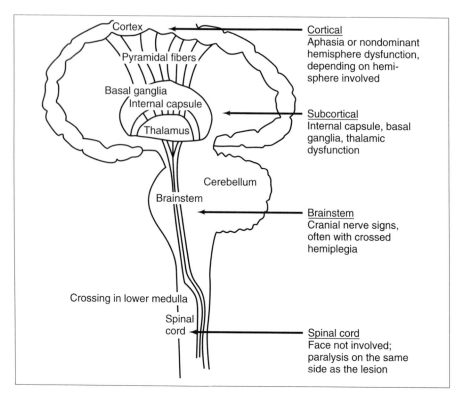

FIGURE 1-3   Motor pathway in the central nervous system.   (From Werner H, Levill L. *Neurology for the House Officer*. New York: Med-Com, 1974, with permission.)

The thalamus, which is the dorsal portion of the diencephalon, serves as the principal relay station for impulses of all types sent to the cerebral cortex. Many impulses come to cognition at the level of the thalamus, although precise localization and integration of this material require cortical interpretation.[1]

The most dorsal portion of the diencephalon is the epithalamus. The epithalamus forms the pineal body and multiple other lesser known structures as well as the roof of the third ventricle. The exact functions of the various areas of the epithalamus are still controversial. It is felt that the pineal body has a secretory function associated with growth and development of the body.[1] Other areas of the epithalamus are related to olfactory nuclei and may be involved with sensory reflexes.[5]

The space within the skull is divided into an anterior, a middle, and a posterior fossa. The cerebral cortex, the subcortex, the basal ganglion, and the majority of the thalamic structures are considered to be anterior and middle fossa elements. Lying below the tentorium cerebelli is the posterior fossa, where the cerebellum and most of the brainstem are located.[5] The brainstem is composed of the midbrain, pons, and medulla. These distinct anatomic regions are interconnected with multiple tracts, making their physiologic function an interrelated process (Fig. 1-5).[5] Cranial nerves III through XII are outgrowths of the brainstem, and their nuclei are located within these

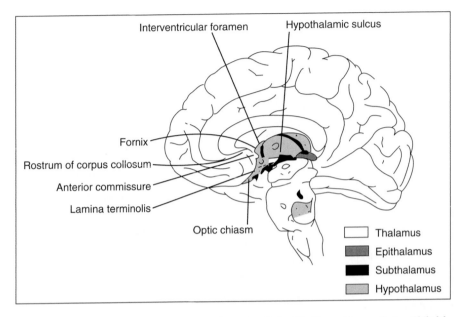

FIGURE 1-4 Thalamus and related structures.   (From Dunkerley GB. *Human Nervous System*. Philadelphia: Davis, 1975, p 94, with permission.)

regions.[1] The brainstem also functions as a conduit carrying information down to the spinal cord and sending information from the spinal cord to nuclei in the thalamus.

The brainstem proceeds caudally to become the spinal cord. The spinal cord runs from the medulla to the first lumbar vertebra.[1] Although literally dozens of tracts have been identified (Fig. 1-6), only three are of major importance for clinical purposes. These tracts include the dorsal columns, the descending motor pathways, and the ascending lateral spinal thalamic tracts.[3] The dorsal columns carry vibration and position sense from the spinal cord to the brainstem, where the tracts cross and ascend to the thalamus and eventually to the sensory cortex. The lateral spinal thalamic tracts cross immediately after entering the spinal cord, ascend directly to the contralateral thalamus, and are then projected to the cerebral cortex. The lateral spinal thalamic tracts carry pain and temperature sensation. The lateral cortical spinal tract, or descending motor pathway, crosses in the medulla and carries motor information to the spinal cord and then eventually to the muscles through the peripheral nerves.

Lying in the posterior fossa directly behind the brainstem is the cerebellum. The cerebellum can be thought of as having a central midline, or vermis, region and large lateral hemispheres. Cerebellar pathways cross immediately and then recross so that they give their input to the ipsilateral side of the body. The midline cerebellar structures basically control and coordinate musculature involved with central midline functioning. The muscles most involved are those controlling the central core of the body with regard to sitting and standing and posturing of the neck and back. The lateral floculonodular lobes exert their controlling influences on the finer motor coordination of the extremities (Table 1-1).[5]

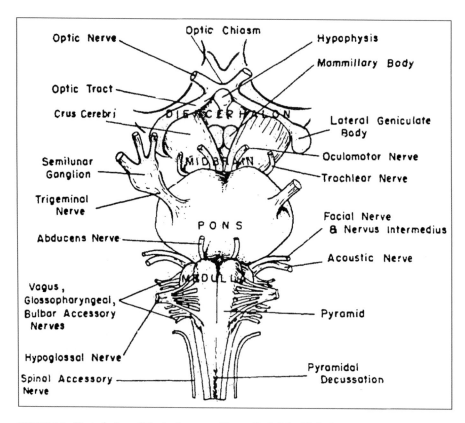

FIGURE 1-5   Ventral view of the brainstem.   (From Clark RG. *Clinical Neuroanatomy and Neurophysiology,* 5th ed. Philadelphia: Davis, 1975, p 51, with permission.)

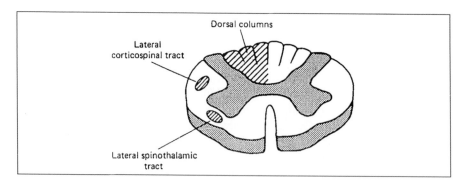

FIGURE 1-6   Spinal cord.

TABLE 1-1 ——————————
CROSSINGS IN THE NERVOUS SYSTEM

Pathway	Function	Crosses	Interpretation
Pyramidal tract	Motor	Lower medulla	Lesion below crossing gives ipsilateral signs
Spinothalamic tract	Pain and temperature (body)	On entry to spinal cord	Lesion is always contralateral to pain and temperature loss (except face)
Spinal tract of fifth nerve	Pain and temperature (face)	Midpons (runs throughout medulla)	If lesion is in medulla or lower pons, ipsilateral loss; above midpons, contralateral loss
Dorsal spinal columns	Position and vibration	Lower medulla	Lesion below crossing gives ipsilateral signs
Cerebellar tracts	Coordination of movement	Crosses twice (on entry to cerebellum and in midbrain)	Because of "double crossing" lesions of cerebellum or cerebellar, tracts usually produce signs and symptoms ipsilateral to lesion
Gaze fibers	Coordinates lateral gaze	Midpons	
Cranial nerves	Cranial nerves	Just above cranial nerve nuclei	Lesion is ipsilateral when cranial nerve nuclei are involved

All the elements of the central nervous system are bathed in cerebrospinal fluid (CSF). This fluid, an utrafiltrate of blood (Fig. 1-7), is made in the choroid plexus of the lateral ventricles.[1] CSF proceeds down through the third ventricle and then through the aqueduct of Sylvius and exits the fourth ventricle through the foramen of Luschka and Magendie to fill the subarachnoid space encompassing the entire brain and spinal cord. Resorption of CSF takes place through the arachnoid granulations along the superior sagittal sinus system. The normal adult nervous system has approximately 130 mL of CSF. The normal production of CSF is about 500 mL/day, or a rate sufficient to replace itself some three to four times over in a 24-hour period.[6]

The elements of the nervous system outside the bony protection of the skull and spinal cord constitute the peripheral nervous system. The cranial and spinal nerves with their associated ganglia are the elements of the peripheral nervous system. Cranial nerves vary considerably in the type of fibers they carry. Some are purely motor, such as the innervation of the extraocular movements of the eyes. Most, however, have mixed functions, carrying both sensory and motor fibers.[1]

The motor fibers of peripheral nerves are divided into somatic fibers that terminate in skeletal muscle and autonomic motor fibers, which innervate smooth muscle, cardiac muscle, and various glands.[1] All spinal nerve roots are mixed nerves carrying both motor and sensory elements[1] (Fig. 1-8).

Once outside the central nervous system, peripheral nerves recombine in the cervical and lumbosacral regions to form intricate plexi. These recombined nerve trunks then subdivide to form specific peripheral nerves.[7]

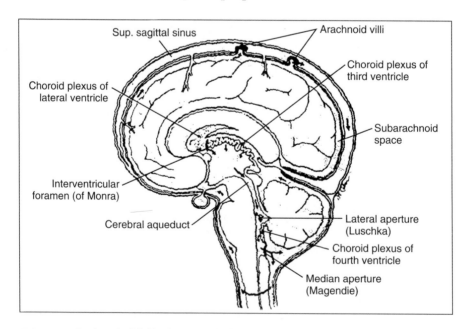

FIGURE 1-7 Cerebrospinal fluid. (From Dunkerley GB. *Human Nervous System*. Philadelphia: Davis, 1975, p 94, with permission.)

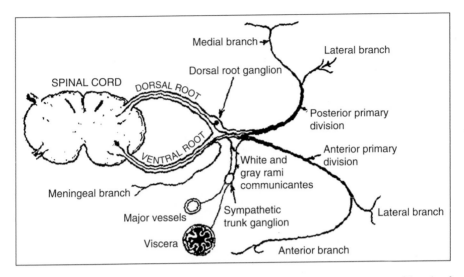

FIGURE 1-8   Peripheral nerve organization.   (From Chusid J. *Correlative Neuroanatomy and Functional Neurology,* 14th ed. Los Altos, CA: Lange, 1970, p 113, with permission.)

FUNCTIONAL NEUROANATOMY

Speech

Human verbal output requires careful integration of multiple areas of the nervous system (Fig. 1-9). Language is formulated in the frontal lobes. Specific motor direction is given by Broca's area in the motor region.[8] This information is then conveyed through the corticobulbar tracts to the various brainstem nuclei, which innervate the muscles involved in moving the teeth, lips, tongue, and palate to form speech. Careful integration of these movements is provided by cerebellar tracts.[3]

The principal areas for receiving, interpreting, and initiating speech are all located around the sylvian and rolandic fissures.[8] These areas are principally supplied by the middle cerebral artery. Wernicke's area, which lies in the primary auditory cortex of the temporal lobe, receives speech and forms a monitoring function.[8] It is then connected to the angular gyrus in the parietal lobe, which interprets and integrates auditory stimuli and connects it to other areas of the brain for interpretation. The arcuate fasciculus then connects these posterior speech areas to Broca's area in the motor strip.[1] From Broca's area, specific motor commands are sent out to be translated into actual speech.

Although the total integration of speech is complex, there are general concepts that can be expressed. One has difficulty in testing speech if there is a hearing abnormality. If this is suspected, hearing should be tested to make sure that deafness is not part of the difficulties in the speech process. Basic understanding of speech and production of speech are dominant hemisphere functions. Problems in

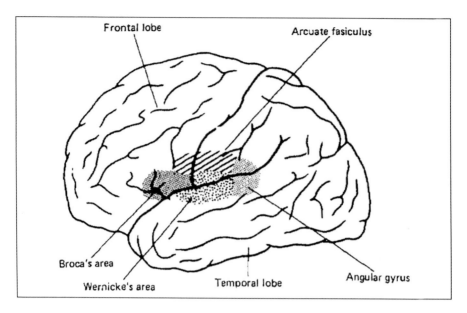

FIGURE 1-9   Cortical speech centers.

either understanding speech, translating that understanding into actions, or word finding are all generally lumped under the aphasic dysphasic syndromes.

The terminology in abnormalities of speech is often confusing. The term *aphasia* should be reserved for a lack or absence of speech. *Dysphasia* is a term used to indicate any disorders of speech involving understanding thought or word finding. The term *Broca's aphasia* is often synonymous with expressive aphasia and is a motor problem. These patients understand what is being said to them and asked of them but have difficulty initiating the motor aspects of speech. *Wernicke's aphasia* is a receptive type of aphasia, in which patients can produce speech and often produce a meaningless or gibberish type speech because they have difficulty in processing incoming information and cannot monitor their own speech patterns. *Nominal aphasia* is the term used when patients have difficulty in finding specific words. Patients suffering from this problem may have difficulty naming the parts of a watch or the specific parts of a pen and yet understand how the instrument should be used. These are often secondary word-association areas, which are usually in the dominant hemisphere. Conductive aphasia generally involves the arcuate fasciculus. Such patients will be able to listen intently and may be able to initiate speech, but they have considerable difficulty in repetition of speech, with preserved comprehension and output.

There are variants of the various speech abnormalities. *Transcortical sensory aphasia* is a Wernicke's type aphasia with preserved repetition. *Transcortical motor aphasia* is a Broca's type aphasia with preserved repetition but inability to initiate one's own speech.

Dysphonia should not be confused with dysphasia or aphasia. This is a disturbance of voice production and may reflect either vocal cord pathology or an abnormality of nerve supply via the vagus nerve. Dysphonia on occasion can be a manifestation of a severe psychological disturbance.

Dysarthria is again a separate entity from dysphasia or dysphonia. A dysarthria is a motor coordination abnormality in which the various motor outputs through the vocal cords, larynx, palate, tongue, and lips lack a synchronized activity. Therefore, dysarthria can reflect difficulties at a multitude of levels.

Lesions of the upper motor neuron type and cerebellar lesions disturb the integration process of speech and tend to produce disturbances in rhythm and symmetry of articulation. Lesions of one or several of the cranial nerves tend to produce characteristic distortions of certain parts of speech. Cerebellar type speech may be anatomic but is generally biochemical. The speech of the intoxicated patient is the classic example of dysarthric speech involving cerebellar coordination (Fig. 1-9).

Motor Pathways

Voluntary motor activity is initiated from the cerebral cortex and proceeds through the internal capsule to enter the brainstem (Fig. 1-10). Motor commands that pass to the various brainstem nuclei travel in the corticobulbar tracts. Motor information that is to proceed farther down the spinal cord to the rest of the body travels in the companion lateral corticospinal tract.[1] Motor commands for brainstem nuclei basically cross at the level of those nuclei.[1] All other motor information for the rest of the body crosses at the lower end of the medulla in the area of the motor decussation.[1]

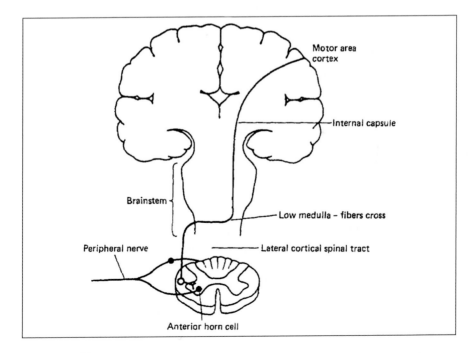

FIGURE 1-10 Motor system.

In the spinal cord, lateral corticospinal tract fibers synapse with specific motor fibers at appropriate levels.

Motor impulses then exit the spinal cord through the anterior spinal roots to enter the peripheral nerves. Finally, motor activity is completed when the peripheral nerve forms a junction with the muscle. The peripheral nerve stimulates this nerve-muscle junction, causing skeletal muscle contraction. The cerebellum exerts its influence on the ipsilateral motor tract. The function of the cerebellum is to continuously adjust, coordinate, and refine motor movements in a smooth and integrated pattern.[3]

Sensory System

Sensory modalities are usually divided into dorsal-column functions and lateral-spinal-thalamic-tract functions. The dorsal columns receive sensory information from the dorsal root ganglia of the peripheral nerves (Fig. 1-11). This information then ascends the spinal cord ipsilaterally until it reaches the medulla and the level of the sensory decussation. At the level of the lower medulla, this sensory information crosses and ascends through the medial lemniscus to the thalamus.

Lateral-spinal-thalamic-tract modalities, which include pain and temperature, enter the spinal cord through the dorsal root ganglion and immediately cross to the contralateral side of the cord and ascend in the contralateral spinal thalamic tract.[5] These fibers then proceed up through the brainstem without further crossing to enter the thalamus.

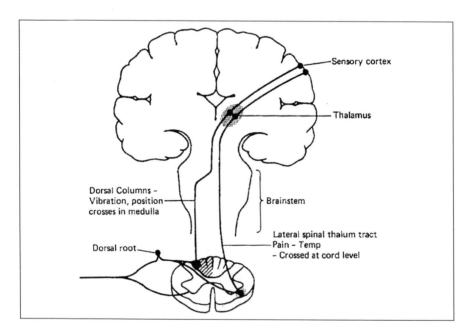

FIGURE 1-11   Sensory system.

Sensation about the face, which is slightly more complex, is handled through the fifth cranial nerve. Pain and temperature sensation from the face enter the brainstem in the midbrain and form the spinal root of the trigeminal nerve. The fibers then descend through the pons and medulla in the spinal tract of V, cross to the opposite side, and ascend with other pain and temperature fibers of the body.[3] Lesions in the upper pons will thus affect both facial and body fibers from the same side of the body. Lesions in the lateral part of the medulla or lower pons that damage the spinal tract of the trigeminal nerve and the lateral spinal thalamic tract will cause alternating analgesia, that is, loss of pain and temperature on the same side of the face and the opposite side of the body. This alternating analgesia is pathognomonic for a brainstem lesion.[4]

Awareness of true touch and pain takes place at the level of the thalamus. Precise localization and integration of sensory information requires cortical localization. It is with the aid of cortical centers that precise localization of a stimulus can be made. Intricate sensory tasks such as graphesthesia (recognition of numbers written in the hands) and stereognosis (identification of objects placed in the hands) require extensive cortical evaluation.

Dermatomes are the topographical representation of the various nerve routes. If pathology is at the level of the nerve route before it has a chance to recombine to form a plexus or a specific peripheral nerve, the area of abnormality will relate to the specific nerve route distribution. Cutaneous or peripheral nerve form patterns are based on combining multiple nerve routes with various alignments (Fig. 1-12).

Vision

The visual pathways are divided into three distinct regions (Fig. 1-13). Vision from the retina to the area of the optic chiasm is carried in a single optic nerve. At the level of the optic chiasm, the optic nerves divide to form the optic tracts. Here the left visual world from each eye and the right visual world from each eye join together to form optic tracts. Light stimulus then passes to the lateral geniculate body, where a superior optic tract and an inferior optic tract proceed posteriorly to terminate in the occipital cortex.

Blindness in one eye represents disease anywhere along the visual axis from the front of the cornea up until the optic chiasm. Optic chiasm lesions usually include pituitary tumors or infarctions and involve the temporal fibers from each eye. This produces the classic bitemporal hemianopsia. An asymmetric bitemporal hemianopsia usually implies that the chiasmal lesion is not perfectly symmetric but still denotes a lesion at that level.[1]

Optic chiasm lesions include pituitary tumors or infarctions and involve the nasal fibers from each eye. An entire optic tract may be involved, producing homonymous hemianopsia. The optic tracts divide quickly, sending a superior branch through the parietal lobe and an inferior branch through the temporal lobe. Lesions of a specific branch result in a quadrantanopia.[1]

The pupils are complex neurologic structures that receive influences from both the autonomic nervous system and the visual reflex arcs. Light stimulus is

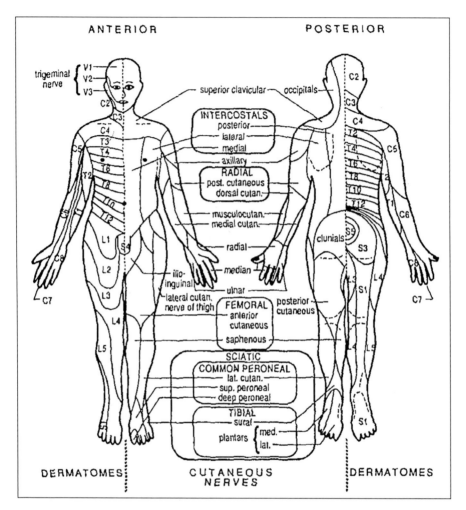

FIGURE 1-12   Dermatomes and peripheral nerve territories.   (From Patton HD, et al. *Introduction to Basic Neurology*. Philadelphia: WB Saunders, 1976, with permission.)

received through cranial nerve II and is passed to midbrain nuclei, which will control pupillary dilation. The pupillary response is affected by fibers proximal to the lateral geniculate bodies or by lesions to the third-nerve parasympathetic fibers themselves[9] (Fig. 1-14).

The anatomy of extraocular movements is important to understand because it serves as the basis for examining the brainstem. In awake patients, voluntary eye movements are under the control of the frontal eye poles. These are centers in each frontal lobe that initiate voluntary eye control.[9] Information is passed through the subcortical structures and descending motor pathways to pontine gaze centers (Fig. 1-15).

Coordination of the eye movements themselves is then carried out through the medial longitudinal fasciculus, which lies in the center of the brainstem. This tract

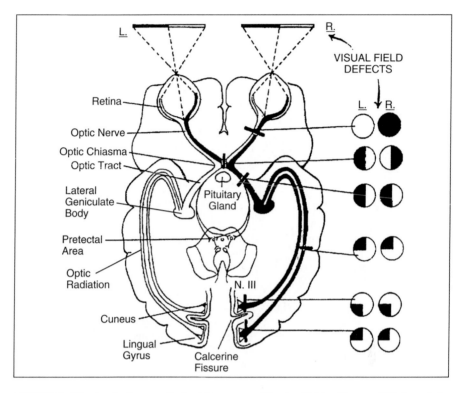

FIGURE 1-13 The visual pathway. On the right are maps of the visual fields with areas of blindness darkened to show the effects of injuries in various locations. (From Clark RG. *Clinical Neuroanatomy and Neurophysiology,* 5th ed. Philadelphia: Davis, 1975, p 113, with permission.)

connects the third, fourth, and sixth cranial nerve nuclei, so that conjugate movement of the eyes takes place. There is a constant input to the pontine gaze centers from each frontal eye pole. Ocular tracking and pursuit movements are coordinated by the posterior visual centers located in the occipital lobes. Once the frontal eye poles have locked onto an object, smooth pursuit is thus ensured by posterior cortical centers sending information to the brainstem.[10]

The Autonomic Nervous System

The autonomic nervous system is made up of the sympathetic and the parasympathetic nervous systems. Sympathetic fibers arise from the thoracic and lumbar regions and synapse in the autonomic chain ganglia. Fibers of the parasympathetic system are from brainstem nuclei and the sacral cord levels. They synapse directly on nuclei of the organ systems involved (Fig. 1-16).

The sympathetic system is the alarm system of the body. Stimulation produces tachycardia, dilation of the bronchi, release of adrenalin, decrease in bowel activity, and inhibition of micturition, as well as increased sweating and dilation of the

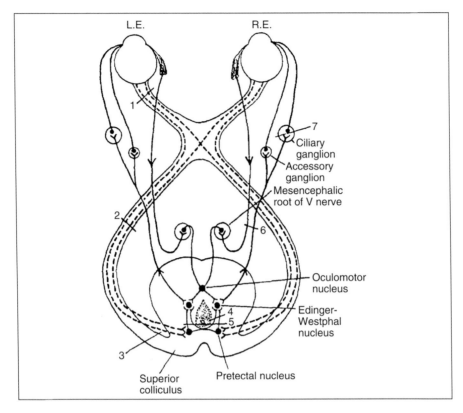

L.E.   R.E.

7
Ciliary
ganglion
Accessory
ganglion
Mesencephalic
root of V nerve

Oculomotor
nucleus

Edinger-
Westphal
nucleus

Superior   Pretectal nucleus
colliculus

FIGURE 1-14   Pupillary pathways.   (From Chusid J. *Correlative Neuroanatomy and Functional Neurology*, 14th ed. Los Altos, CA: Lange, 1970, p 280, with permission.)

pupils. Stimulation of the parasympathetic system causes quite the opposite effects. Stimulation here produces bradycardia, constriction of the bronchi, and increased salivation and lacrimation, as well as increased bowel motility and constriction of the pupils.

The effects of the autonomic nervous system are vast and complex and are frequently blended with other systems of the body. On a purely neurologic basis, with the exception of some very isolated lesions, the autonomic nervous system findings are often difficult to separate out from other systems of the body. Except for their effects on vital signs, these systems are not usually tested in the emergency department.

Innervation of the Bladder

Motor control of the urinary bladder is divided into two parts. Control of the external sphincters is under voluntary control and is mediated through the pudendal nerve supplied by the SI and S2 nerve roots (Fig. 1-17). Internal sphincter control and contraction of the detrusor muscle of the bladder is primarily regulated by the

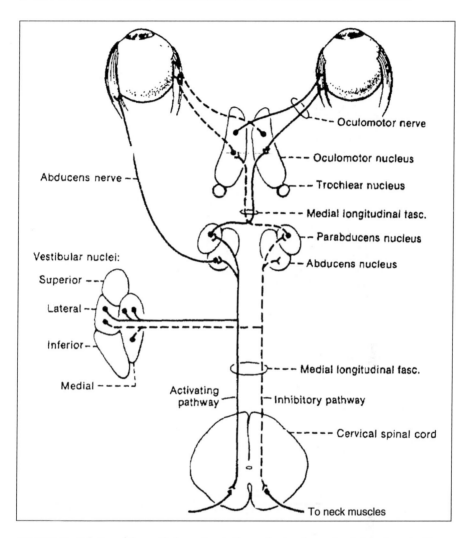

FIGURE 1-15 Relation of the vestibular system to the mechanism for conjugate lateral gaze. (From DeJong RN. *The Neurological Examination,* 4th ed. New York: Harper & Row, 1979, p 148, with permission.)

parasympathetic nervous system originating in sacral roots SI, S2, and S4. These parasympathetic fibers terminate on ganglia located in the wall of the bladder itself. Stimulation of parasympathetic fibers causes emptying of the bladder by contraction of the detrusor muscle and relaxation of the internal sphincter muscle.[11]

The sympathetic nervous system plays a minor role in bladder function.[11] Sympathetic supply to the bladder comes through the sympathetic chain ganglion supplied by upper lumbar segments. Postganglionic fibers then proceed to enter the wall of the bladder and the internal sphincter. The precise actions of the sympathetic nerves with regards to the detrusor muscle are unknown. A loss of sympathetic supply

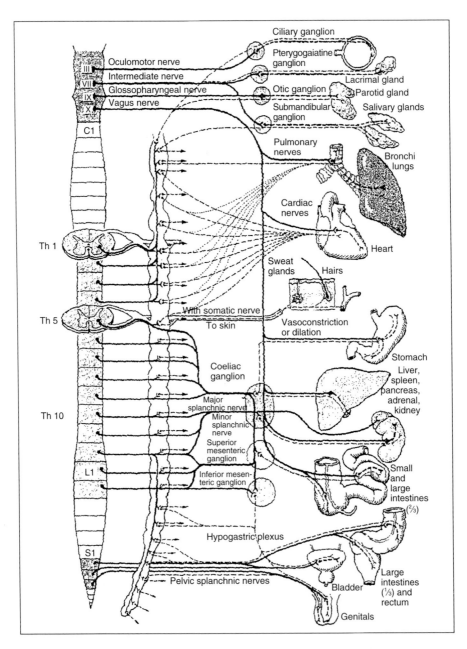

FIGURE 1-16 The peripheral autonomic nervous system. (From Duss P. *Topical Diagnosis in Neurology*, 3rd ed. New York: Thieme, 1998, p 214, with permission.)

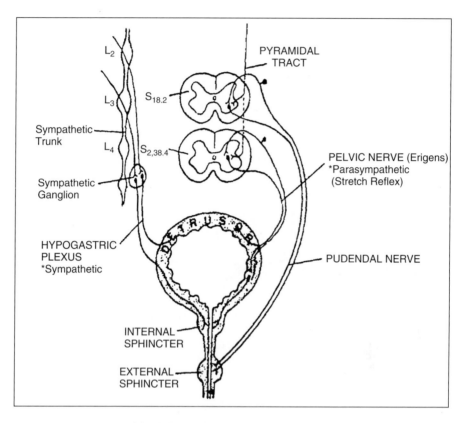

FIGURE 1-17 Innervation of the bladder. (From Clark RG. *Clinical Neuroanatomy and Neurophysiology,* 5th ed. Philadelphia: Davis, 1975, p 125, with permission.)

to the bladder does not measurably affect its function. In the absence of central inhibition and control of the external sphincter muscles, reflex emptying of the bladder occurs with either increased pressure in the wall of the bladder or with stimulation of skin over the lower extremities.[11]

Vascular Anatomy

The arterial supply to the brain and spinal cord can be divided into an anterior and posterior circulation[3] (Figs. 1-18 and 1-19). The anterior circulation is the portion of the vascular network supplied by the carotid arteries. The anterior cerebral arteries are joined at their base by the anterior communicating artery. The anterior cerebrals upon reaching the genu of the corpus collosum turn dorsally along its medial surface, supplying blood to posterior portions of the frontal and parietal lobes, including areas of the motor cortex.[3] Motor fibers particularly concerned with the lower extremities as well as sensory fibers to the lower extremities are usually supplied by branches of the anterior cerebral artery.

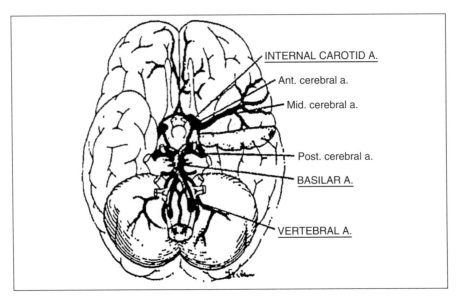

FIGURE 1-18   Arterial circulation of the brain.   (From Dunkerley GB. *Human Nervous System.* Philadelphia: Davis, 1975, p 187, with permission.)

The middle cerebral artery is the terminal extension of the carotid artery. Its branches supply the largest areas of the frontal, parietal, upper occipital, and temporal lobes.[3] Its more medial branches, the lenticulostriate arteries, supply blood to the internal capsule and basal ganglion structures. The anterior circulation is connected to the posterior circulation through the posterior communicating arteries. These arteries are extremely variable in size and configuration and may represent a very poor collateral source of circulation.

The most inferior portions of the cerebral cortex (the cerebellum, the brainstem, and the spinal cord) are supplied by the posterior circulation (Figs. 1-19, 1-20, and 1-21).[12] This circulatory system is made up of the two vertebral arteries, which quickly combine to form the basilar artery. Because of the difference in types of structures supplied, posterior circulation problems are much more likely to result in bilateral symptomatology. They are also more likely to affect consciousness, equilibrium, balance, and coordination of muscle movements.[12]

SUMMARY

Functional neuroanatomy should be the basis on which evaluation of all neurologic symptomatology rests. Careful integration of the patient's complaints and meticulous neurologic examination should pinpoint the anatomic location of the vast majority of neurologic problems.

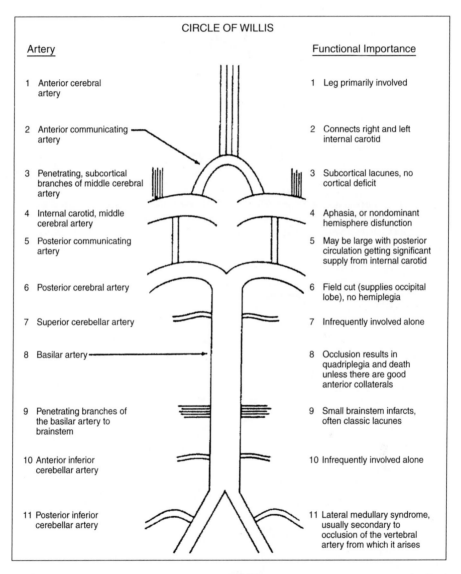

FIGURE 1-19 Arterial circulation of the brain. (From Weiner H, Levitt L. *Neurology for the House Officer*. New York: Med-Com, 1974, p 141, with permission.)

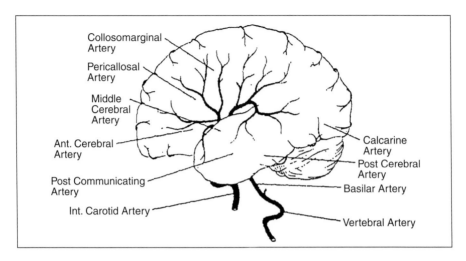

FIGURE 1-20   Left lateral view of the principle arteries of the cerebrum.   The anterior cerebral and the posterior cerebral arteries, on the medial surface, are seen as if projected through the substance of the brain. (From Clark RG. *Neuroanatomy and Neurophysiology,* 5th ed. Philadelphia: Davis, 1975, p 156, with permission.)

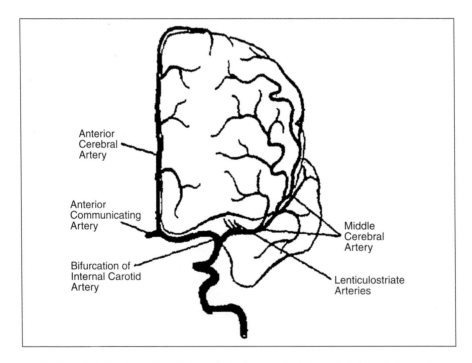

FIGURE 1-21   Anterior view of the anterior and middle cerebral arteries of the left hemisphere.   (From Clark RG. *Clinical Neuroanatomy and Neurophysiology,* 5th ed. Philadelphia: Davis, 1975, p 156, with permission.)

REFERENCES

1. Duus P. *Topical Diagnosis in Neurology,* 3rd ed. New York: Thieme, 1998.
2. Geschwend N. The organization of language and the brain. *Science* 1970;170:940.
3. Crosby E, Humphrey T, Lauer E. *Correlative Anatomy of the Nervous System.* New York: MacMillan, 1962.
4. Simpson J, Magee K. *Clinical Evaluation of the Nervous System.* Ann Arbor, MI: Overbeck, 1970.
5. House E, Pansky B. *Functional Approach to Neuroanatomy,* 2nd ed. New York: McGraw-Hill, 1967.
6. Roos KL. Cerebral spinal fluid. In: Joint R, Griggs R, eds. *Baker's Clinical Neurology.* Philadelphia: Lippincott Williams & Wilkins, 2000.
7. Chusid J. *Correlative Neuroanatomy and Functional Anatomy.* Los Altos, CA: Lange, 1970.
8. Geschwend N. Language and the brain, *Sci Am* 1972;226:76–83.
9. Haerera A. *DeJong's The Neurological Examination,* 5th ed. New York: Lippincott-Raven, 1992.
10. Bender M, Randolph S, Stacy C. Neurology of the visual and oculomotor systems. In: Joint R, Griggs R, eds. *Baker's Clinical Neurology.* Philadelphia: Lippincott Williams & Wilkins, 2000.
11. Low P, et al. Clinical autonomic disorders. In: Joint R, Griggs R, eds. *Baker's Clinical Neurology.* Philadelphia: Lippincott Williams & Wilkins, 1998.
12. Toole J, Cole M: Ischemic cerebrovascular disease. In: Joint R, Griggs R, eds. *Baker's Clinical Neurology.* Philadelphia: Lippincott Williams & Wilkins, 1998.

2

EVALUATION OF A NEUROLOGIC COMPLAINT

BASIC PRINCIPLES

Evaluation of the patient with an acute neurologic complaint requires a carefully selected history and physical examination. In the emergency department or outpatient setting, the time does not exist for the classical evaluation. Patients must be seen expeditiously and decisions made rapidly. The goal of the emergency neurologic evaluation is to identify rapidly progressive or life-threatening disease that cannot wait for more leisurely evaluation. No one examines everything every time. The neurologic examination needs to be focused. When time is limited, the three key items in a neurologic examination are as follows: hear them talk, watch them walk, and look at their eyes. These three simple acts evaluate most of the nervous system and will be the guide to a more detailed evaluation. If the physician can keep these three basic principles in mind, the vast majority of diseases with physical manifestations will be detected.

Little work has been done to prioritize the elements of the neurologic examination. The fundamental question as to what should and should not be included for each neurologic complaint has not been fully delineated. Increased patient loads are causing physicians to ask pertinent questions as to the value of certain neurologic testing. This chapter will focus on what are the most and least productive parts of the neurologic exam.

Most of the neurologic evaluation is done by simple observation. There are four major ways in which the nervous system can manifest pathology. Ablative or deficiency problems present with a lack of ability of the nervous system to perform a specific function. This may mean destruction or functional impairment of specific nervous system tracks. Inability to move an extremity following a hemispheric infarct is an example. An irritative phenomenon indicates that a specific tract is intact but that an overabundance of impulses or abnormal impulses are being conveyed. The most graphic example of the irritative phenomenon is the major motor seizure. Release syndromes indicate that the nervous system has lost the ability to coordinate or control and temper various activities once they have been initiated. The hyperreflexia and spasticity seen in upper motor neuron lesions or the motor rebound phenomena of cerebellar disease are illustrative of the release phenomena. Compensation phenomena are seen throughout the nervous system. The body adjusts its approach to solving specific problems by compensating for deficits. The head tilt seen in ocular nerve palsies or the circumduction of a paretic limb are examples of the compensation phenomena.

Careful observation of these four major manifestations of nervous-system disease through careful history and during physical examination is important to making diagnoses (Table 2-1).

HISTORY

The unusual historical features important in understanding all disease are required in the neurologic history. Manner of onset, duration of the symptoms, and exacerbating or mitigating factors can be elicited. Current concomitant illnesses, medications, and previous such episodes are also important aspects of history taking.[1]

TABLE 2-1
SUMMARY OF NERVOUS SYSTEM RESPONSE TO DISEASE

Disease	Type of Loss	Example
Ablative	Interruption of nervous tract or inability to initiate a specific activity	Paralysis following a cerebral vascular lesion
Irritative phenomena	Overabundance or abnormal nervous system discharge	Major motor seizure
Release phenomena	Inability to control initiated activities	Hyperreflexia and spasticity
Compensation	Integration of various other nervous system functions to adjust for other nervous system deficits	Circumduction of a paralyzed limb

Certain general concepts about neurologic disease can be stated. The pace of onset and progression of symptoms help delineate the disease process involved.

1 *Rapid onset:* Vascular disease generally presents with a rapid onset, and the maximum deficit is reached almost immediately.[2] A major hemorrhage or infarct may give a very large functional deficit, which tends to improve with time. Multiple small infarctions also give a rapid onset of a more minor neurologic symptomatology; with each new infarct, they progress to involve even wider areas. The transient ischemic attack should be considered the forerunner of stroke.[2,3] These episodes present with maximal deficit early and then clear without any neurologic residual within a short period.

2 *Slow onset—variable course:* Degenerative disease and neoplasms are disease entities that generally follow a mildly undulating but downhill course. They are usually not composed of sudden changes or shifts and tend to be unrelenting in their symptomatology.

3 *Variable onset—changing rapidly from symptomatic to asymptomatic:* In multiple sclerosis an extremely variable course is the rule. Multiple, anatomically unrelated areas with varied symptomatology and fluctuating examinations should suggest multiple sclerosis.[4,5]

4 *Rapidly reversible diffuse process:* Transient reversible neurologic diseases are those that involve the central nervous system through affecting the supply of oxygen or nutrients or involving chemical substances that may depress or alter neurologic function. These diseases, such as toxic ingestions, hypoglycemia, renal failure, and so on, provide generally diffuse nonfocal alterations of the nervous system that improve with resolution of the underlying problem. In the case of hypoglycemia, focal findings are common and may represent a false localizing sign.

In the ambulatory setting, the history taking must be specifically directed toward the chief complaint of the patient (Table 2-2). It is important that for each chief complaint, pertinent positives and negatives important to the differential diagnosis be obtained from the patient (Table 2-3).

TABLE 2-2 ————————————————————————————
SUMMARY TIME COURSE OF NEUROLOGIC PROBLEMS

Time Course	Neurologic Diseases
Seconds to minutes	Vascular
Minutes to hours	Metabolic
Hours to days	Metabolic or infection
Days to weeks	Infection; tumor; compressive masses
Months to years	Slow tumors or degenerative disease

TABLE 2-3

SPECIFIC HISTORICAL FEATURES IN NEUROLOGIC DISEASE

Chief Complaint	Historical Features
Coma or altered mental status	History taken from family and friends, etc.; trauma, drugs, alcohol, seizure history, kidney disease, heart disease, previous episodes
Stroke (acute lateralized deficit)	General neurologic history; area of maximum deficit; time course; previous episodes; cardiovascular disease; diabetes; drug usage
Seizures	History obtained from witnesses; the current antiepileptic medications, other medication and drug usage; other metabolic diseases; present length of time unconsciousness; approximate rate and pattern of recovery; presence of single or multiple seizures; history of trauma or other underlying conditions
Headaches	Basic headache history; current mode of onset; location, duration, pulsations; associated weakness, numbness, visual problems, nausea, vomiting; relationship to food intake; time of year; activity loss of consciousness; trauma; medications
Minor head trauma	Nature and type of trauma, loss of consciousness, specific focal symptoms, generalized systemic symptoms
Dizziness	Rate of onset, duration, exacerbating factors; presence of sensation of movement, presence of sensation of fainting; visual, auditory changes; nausea, vomiting; drug history, medications; current illnesses
Syncope	General medical conditions; medications and drug usage; activity at the time of syncopal episode; length of loss of consciousness; presence or absence of seizure activity; presence of pulses; heart rate during the episode; previous episodes
Double vision, blindness	General medical conditions; current medications, drugs or concomitant neurologic disease; bilateral or unilateral change in vision; type of loss (i.e., peripheral, central, total); patient's usual visual status; trauma; current infection; other related neurologic symptomatology; pain

Physical examination

The nervous system can be altered by pathology in any organ system of the body. The foundation of the proper neurologic examination is the good physical examination.[5]

Vital Signs

Appropriate vital signs are important. The nervous system can be dramatically altered by inadequate cardiac output from arrhythmias or shock. Likewise, hypertension in extremes can severely alter neurologic function. Extremes of temperature, either hyperthermia or hypothermia, can markedly affect mental status and general nervous system functioning. Arrhythmias may be associated with and the result of acute vascular events of the nervous system.

General Physical

An examination of a neurologic complaint may require attention to selected parts of the general physical examination. Examination of the head and neck, paying particular attention to bruises and palpable areas of tenderness or deformity, is important in cases of suspected trauma. Cardiac examination may be extremely useful in the patient complaining of intermittent weakness, dizziness, or focal deficits. General examination of the limbs and trunk may give clues about the possibility of trauma or underlying disease. Lateral tongue biting, when present, has a high association with a major motor seizure having recently taken place.[6]

Neurologic examination

The emergency neurologic examination may not be the same as the examination performed in a neurologist's office. The point is for the physician to get to the underlying diagnosis in the most judicious manner. Modifications of the neurologic examination will be required depending on the chief complaint of the patient. The basic underlying examination points (hear them talk, watch them walk, look at their eyes) is still valid. It forms the core of the neurologic examination.

Mental Status

Mental status examination is generally carried out while the history is being obtained. A full formal mental status examination is usually not required in the ambulatory setting. The manner in which a patient understands and answers questions and is concerned and involved with his or her own chief complaint is the best general assessment of mental status.[7,8]

When a more complete detailed mental status is required, a common system to follow is based on the mnemonic Jim A. Motsig:

J *Judgment*—Tested by problem solving and situational analysis, i.e., "How would you find your way if lost in a city?"

I *Intelligence*—Based on patient's previous level of education and functioning, i.e., choice of words, general vocabulary, problem-solving ability.

M *Memory*—Three types: instantaneous memory, or ability to repeat back something said within the past minute; short-term memory, remembrance of events that have taken place within the past few hours or days; and past memory, what is remembered from patient's more remote past.

A *Affect*—Patients' basic response to the disease process. Are they extremely indifferent to a severe functional deficit or are they inappropriately upset and anguished over essentially no problem?

M *Mood*—Is the patient appropriately angry or sad in the context of surrounding events?

O *Orientation*—To time, person, place.

T *Thought processes and content*—What are the thoughts preoccupying the patients? Do they have unusual or bizarre delusions about their disease process?

S *Speech*—Presence of aphasia, dysphagia, dysarthrias, and so on. Rate and cadence of speech are important.

I *Insight*—Does the patient have any understanding of his or her disease process and its relation to the situation?

G *Grooming*—Can the patient dress him or herself appropriately and care for the body in an appropriate manner?

The key to mental status examination is in evaluating the story the patient is telling. Orientation to time and place as well as being able to relate the historical events of the illness are the core to understanding the patient. If there is one area of mental status that stands out above all others in importance, it is speech and language. Not only does speech test the inventory of cortical function with regard to language, but also incoordination of such output may be detected as dysarthrias. In testing memory it is good to remember that different types of memory require different parts of the brain. Past, remote memory may be well maintained and yet the patients who have transient global amnesia may have little understanding of what has happened over the last few days. Likewise, patients can have excellent memory of their past life and yet cannot remember three objects assigned to them to recall over a period of 5 minutes. Such lapses may indicate an inability to form or imprint new memory. General level of wakefulness, speed and smoothness of speech, and participation and involvement with their own health care should be the guide for the clinician in knowing when further mental status checking is required. In no other area is expansion or contraction of the examination as important as in mental status.

The goal of mental status testing is to detect rapidly whether a complex evaluation is required. Excellent tests of general functioning, besides just listening to the patient talk, include simple yet sensitive indicators of patient performance. The first of these is three-object retention. Simply retaining the memory of three dissimilar objects over the period of the evaluation is a good general indicator of the patient's cortical function. An excellent combination test is one that involves three separate parts: right-left orientation, crossing the midline of the body, and movement without the aid of vision. The patient is asked to remember three separate commands and not to begin them until all parts have been given. The patient is then asked to close the eyes, take the right thumb and touch the left ear, and then stick out the tongue. This deceptively simple maneuver tests multiple areas of the cortex. In general, a patient who can perform a three-part test with crossing the midline motor activities, without the use of visual input, has reasonable alertness and mental status functioning.

In patients who seem to perform basic tests well, the use of double linked but unrelated questions can be useful in sorting out fine and more subtle cortical problems. If patients are asked a question such as "do you walk to work or carry your lunch?" they must recognize that these two questions are unrelated. If they are unable to do so, more detailed mental status testing may be required.

In patients with bizarre thought disorders, the actual neurologic functioning in terms of speech, memory retention, and so on may be quite good and yet thinking may be deranged. A provocative question such as "do helicopters eat their young?" will occasionally provoke very bizarre responses from patients suffering from major thought disorders. It may be useful to ask patients about major psychotic symptoms. If it is suggested that the patient is hearing voices, it is perfectly reasonable to ask about this. Any crisis that is precipitated is better handled at that time rather than allowing the condition to go undiagnosed and untreated. Agitated patients in psychotic states frequently wish to discuss the symptoms that are troubling them.[8]

Assessment of speech is essential in the evaluation of a patient's mental process. It is important to remember that speech is divided among its reception, understanding, initiation, and mechanical production. Lesions along any part of these pathways can cause problems. Whether we are conscious of it or not, we test speech on every human being with whom we speak. Speech has a cadence and a rhythm. Abnormalities in rhythmic flow of speech should be noted. Rate of speech and word-finding ability are also essential elements of the communication process.

In testing speech, it is important to understand that the patient may have a hearing difficulty. If the patient does not initially respond, asking the questions in a louder, more direct voice or with the patient having a full view of the examiner's lips may increase the responsiveness. Asking simple yes/no questions and expanding to more complex commands is the technique to be used if the patient seems to have communication difficulties. The spontaneity of speech is also important. For a patient who is carrying on normal conversation with well-articulated speech, it is generally unnecessary to test any other specific areas. Fluent speech generally means that the motor system is in tact. Unusually paraphasic or meaningless speech can be indicative of a Wernicke's type aphasia. Assessment of the aphasias/dysphagias is outlined in Figure 2-1.

Dysphonia is an abnormality in the actual production of the volume of speech. If this seems to be a problem, one can ask the patient to cough. Assuming that the laryngeal mechanisms are normal, a normal coughing sound should be produced. A cough that lacks an explosive start, occasionally referred to as a bovine cough, can be found with vocal cord paralysis. If the patient is asked to sustain a sound by saying the letter "E" for a long period and cannot do this, the possibility of myasthenia exists. Further testing for myasthenia gravis may be required.

Dysarthrias are problems in the actual motor coordination of speech. Repeating difficult phrases (Peter Piper picked a peck of pickled peppers) may be extremely difficult for a patient who cannot coordinate motor movements. The rhythm of such speech is usually abnormal, and slurring of words is common. Such dysarthria can be either a chemical problem, such as that induced by alcohol intoxication, or part of the involvement of diseases such as multiple sclerosis or hereditary ataxias. Delayed speech with difficulty in word formation as well as articulation can be seen in extraparaneural dysarthria and in a disease such as Parkinson's. Figure 2-2 outlines the evaluation of dysarthria.

Cranial Nerves

For a summary of cranial nerve evaluation, see Table 2-4.

I. Olfactory nerve: Extremely difficult to test in an emergency department or outpatient setting; usually not of value in making a specific diagnosis.[9] Testing of this system is so complex that it is to be considered a research level process and is rarely helpful in the clinical setting.

II. Optic nerve: Examined with visual acuity, funduscopy, and pupillary response. The second cranial nerve is actually an extension of the brain, and the optic nerve head is the only place in the body where the brain is directly visible. It is tested by the amount of light received in areas of the visual fields in which the light is sensed. The light reflex, both directly and consensually, may be tested. Areas of vision are tested through confrontational field testing. Such testing is done with simultaneous finger movement in the four principal quadrants of vision, which is usually sufficient (see Chap. 8).[1,10] Confrontation testing of visual fields is only required when a cortical lesion is suspected or a specific complaint of partial visual loss is voiced by the patient.

III. Oculomotor nerve: Parasympathetic fibers tested through the pupillary reflex arc in conjunction with the second cranial nerve. Somatic motor function is checked by extraocular movements in conjunction with nerves IV and VI (see Fig. 8-1).[1,10] All extraoccular muscles, except for the superial oblique and lateral rectus, are intervated by cranial nerve III.

IV, VI. Trochlear and abducens nerves respectively: Cranial nerves IV and VI are tested in conjunction with cranial nerve III during the extraocular movements of

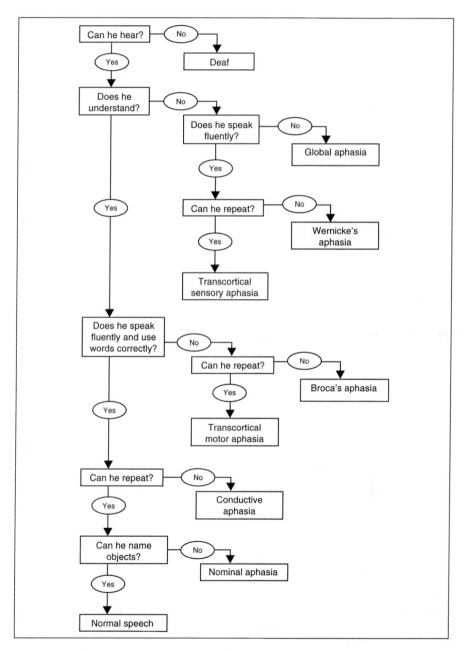

FIGURE 2-1 Flow chart for aphasia. (Adapted from Fuller G, Gale M. *Neurological Examination Made Easy,* 2nd ed. London: Churchill Livingstone, 1999, with permission.)

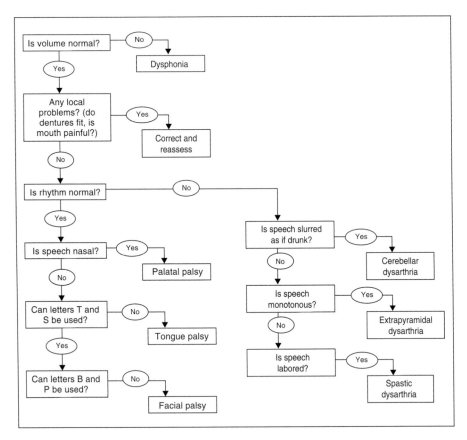

FIGURE 2-2   Flow chart for dysarthria.   (Adapted from Fuller G, Gale M. *Neurological Examination Made Easy,* 2nd ed. London: Churchill Livingstone, 1999, with permission.)

the eyes (Fig. 2-3). Cranial nerve IV innervates only the superior oblique muscles and thus aids in pulling the eye medially and downward. The sixth cranial nerve innervates only the lateral rectus muscle and is involved in all abduction movements of the eye. All other extraocular muscles are innervated by the third cranial nerve (see Fig. 8-1).

V. Trigeminal nerve: Motor tested by assessing strength of the masseter and ptery-goid muscles of the jaw. The masseter muscle is tested by forceful closing of the jaw. The pterygoid muscles are tested by side-to-side movement of the jaw. The sensory limb of the fifth cranial nerve is tested with fine touch to the face and the corneal reflex (Fig. 2-4).[10,11] When postnuclear pathology is suspected, all three divisions of the nerve need to be tested.

VII. Facial nerve: The motor function is tested by observing movement of facial musculature. Facial innervation has both crossed and uncrossed fibers except for the lower portion around the mouth. Therefore, lesions to the seventh nerve fibers

TABLE 2-4 —————————————————————————————————

SUMMARY OF SCREENING CRANIAL NERVE EXAMINATION

Nerve	Testing	Comments
Cranial nerve I: olfactory nerve	None	An advance made, not routine
Cranial nerve II: optic nerve	Pupils, gross visual fields	Field testing only if history suggestive of cortical lesion visual complaint
Cranial nerve III: oculomotor nerve	Extraocular movements	Best rapid test of the brainstem
Cranial nerve IV: trochlear nerve		
Cranial nerve VI: abduceris nerve		
Cranial nerve V: trigeminal nerve	Facial sensation— mastication muscles	Three divisions of the nerve
Cranial nerve VII: facial nerve	Facial muscles	Other division of VII *not* generally tested
Cranial nerve VIII: auditory nerve	Gross hearing— tuning fork tests	Finer tests of hearing not done unless symptoms related to hearing or brainstem
Cranial nerve IX: glossopharyngeal nerve	Stimulated swallowing	If patient is swallowing normally and handling secretions
Cranial nerve X: vagus		
Cranial nerve XI: accessory nerve	Shoulder shrug— sternocleidomastoid function	Rarely tested unless brainstem complaint
Cranial nerve XII: hypoglossal nerve	Tongue strength	No formal testing unless abnormal speech or brainstem complaint

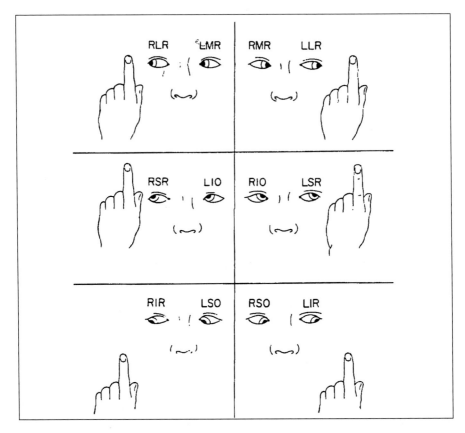

Abbreviation	Muscle	Nerve
LR	lateral rectus	6th CN
SO	system oblique	4th CN
IO	inferior oblique	3rd CN
MR	medial rectus	3rd CN
SR	superior rectus	3rd CN
IR	inferior rectus	3rd CN

FIGURE 2-3   Extraocular movement testing.   (From Simpson J, Magee K. *Clinical Evaluation of the Nervous System.* Ann Arbor, MI: Overbeck, 1970, with permission.)

above the seventh nerve nucleus will result in only minimal facial dysfunction. Lesions to the seventh nerve that affect the actual nerve distal to the nucleus will result in an entire hemiparesis of the face.

VIII. Acoustic nerve: Tested by assessing gross speech reception threshold and discrimination of sounds. Tuning-fork tests are utilized to determine the location of a hearing deficit within the ear, acoustic nerve, or central nervous system.

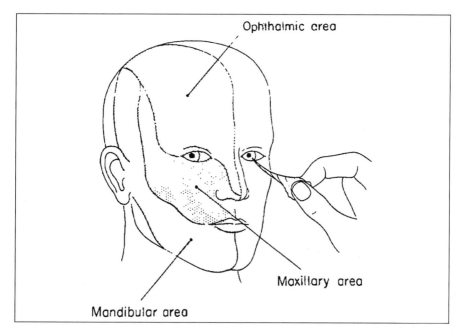

FIGURE 2-4   Sensory areas, trigeminal nerve.   (From Simpson J, Magee K. *Clinical Evaluation of the Nervous System.* Ann Arbor, MI: Overbeck, 1970, with permission.)

The Weber test determines lateralization of sound. It is performed by striking a tuning fork and placing it in the center of the top of the head. If the sound lateralizes to one specific side, this is the side with the conduction deficit. The Rinne test compares air conduction with bone conduction.[1] This test is performed by striking the tuning fork and then placing it on the *mastoid* bone behind the ear and comparing it with the sound heard by just placing the tuning fork near the auditory canal itself. If bone conduction is greater than ear conduction, the patient has a conductive hearing loss. Unless there is a specific brainstem- or hearing-related complaint, formal testing of hearing is not generally required.

IX, X, and XI.   Glossopharyngeal, vagus, and accessory cranial nerves, respectively: Are not generally tested on the screening neurologic examination because of a lack of lateralization and specificity. A patient who is speaking and swallowing normally and does not have a brainstem type of complaint does not need individual testing of these nerves.[5] These nerves are usually specifically tested only if there are other indications of brainstem or posterior fossa involvement.

XII.   Hypoglossal nerve: Formally check by examining for deviation of the tongue on voluntary protrusion. The tongue deviates toward the side of the weakness or involvement.[1,10] A patient who is speaking normally does not have a 12th nerve lesion and does not require formal testing. On rare occasions, local disease may mimic a 12th nerve lesion.[12,13]

Motor System

Cerebellum, Gait, and Station

The motor system is best checked through observation.[1,14] General bulk of the musculature is noted along with any abnormal motor movements. Both gross movements, such as chorea and tremors, are recorded as well as fine muscle fasciculations. The best test for the motor system is to observe the patient using musculature for normal activities. Walking on the heels and toes is an excellent test for strength in the lower extremities. Hand grip, dorsiflexion of the wrist, and abduction of the arms at the shoulders are all excellent tests for upper limb strength.

An extremely sensitive but nonspecific test for involvement of the motor system is pronator drift.[1] Patients are asked to extend their arms in front of them with the palms upward and then to close their eyes and maintain this position. There are four possible responses to a pronator drift test. If, when the eyes are closed, the arms remain outstretched without any deviation for 10 seconds, the test should be considered normal. This would indicate no difference in the outflow tracts of the two major motor tracts.

In the event of involvement of the motor tract and without the aid of the visual system to correct imbalances, the limb on the affected side will slowly drift downward, and the hand will begin to pronate. This can be an extremely subtle check on the motor system and is positive much earlier than confrontational strength testing. The third possible response is observed when one arm will elevate and the fingers will seem to move in a searching manner in space. This is generally not a motor system problem. It represents a lack of spatial orientation when the patient is forced to maintain a stationary position and is due to the lack of compensating visual input and almost always to a lesion in the parietal lobe.

The fourth possible response on a pronator drift test is that of impersistence. This is typically seen in older patients with frontal lobe disease. If they are asked to extend the arms and then close the eyes they have difficulty maintaining this for any length of time without visual input. It can be extremely frustrating to the examiner, who may initially confuse this with noncooperation. Motor impersistence is associated with frontal lobe disease.

Strength in the motor system should be graded on a 0 to 5 scale with 0 being no flicker of movement and 5 being normal strength. The best test of both coordination and strength is to watch the patient walk or complete some other motor activity.[1]

Tone in the motor system is best tested passively.[13] Arms at the elbows and legs at the knees can simply be put through a range of motion without assistance from the patient. Hesitations and cog-wheel-type limitations with generally increased tone or spasm may be noted.

Specific tests for cerebellar coordination include finger-nose testing of the upper extremities and heel-shin testing in the lower extremities. These movements test the lateral hemispheres of the cerebellum. Midline cerebellar structures are tested by having patients sit on the bed or stand and see if they can maintain their position without using their arms or assistance from the examiner. Tandom walking, i.e., heel-to-toe walking, is also an excellent test of central or midline cerebellar functions. Rapid alternating movement testing can be added to sharpen or check equivocal findings on the screening test.[1]

An important differential point in evaluating the motor system is to decide whether the lesion is upper motor neuron or lower motor neuron in nature. Upper motor neuron lesions refer to involvement of the nervous system centrally from the cortex to synaptic connections with the anterior horn cell in the spinal cord. The lower motor neuron refers to the neuron that proceeds from the spinal cord through the peripheral nerve to the muscle proper. The important differences between upper and lower motor neuron lesions are summarized in Table 2-5.

Sensory Abilities

Sensory testing is the least accurate and generally least reproducible portion of the neurologic examination.[14] It is totally dependent on the responses of the patient. Both dorsal column and lateral spinal thalamic tract functions should be tested.

TABLE 2-5

DIFFERENTIATION BETWEEN UPPER AND LOWER MOTOR NEURON WEAKNESS

Parameter	Upper Motor Neuron[a]	Lower Motor Neuron[b]
Type and distribution of weakness	Lesions in brain: "pyramidal distribution," i.e., distal, especially hand muscles, and weaker extensors in arm and weaker flexors in legs Lesions in cord: variable, depending on location	Depends on which lower motor neurons involved: which segments, roots, or nerves
Tone	Spasticity: greater in flexors in arms and extensors in legs	Flaccidity
Bulk	Slight atrophy of disuse only	Atrophy may be marked
Associated reflexes	Accentuated reflexes; Babinski sign present	Absent or diminished; no Babinski sign
Fasciculations	No	Possible

[a] Synonyms: pyramidal tract, corticospinal tract, corticobulbar tract.
[b] Synonyms: anterior horn cell, ventral horn cell, somatic motor portions of cranial nerves, final common pathway.

Dorsal column functions include vibration and position sense, which are checked by use of the tuning fork or by the graded movement of the joints of the extremities. It is important to record how far proximally one must move on a patient's extremities for them to properly identify sensory modalities.

Lateral spinal thalamic tract functions include temperature and pin sensation, which are likewise checked by moving from distal to proximal areas along the extremities and then up the trunk of the body. If a patient can feel a sensation distally, more proximal testing is unnecessary unless a specific area of numbness is mentioned by the patient. It should be remembered that the innervation of the legs is not from the most distal segments of the spinal cord. The most distal spinal cord segments innervate the anus and genitalia of the patient. Examination in this area tests the most distal portions of the spinal cord. Distal segments are usually not tested unless there is a specific complaint relative to these areas or a lower spinal cord or if a cauda equina lesion is suspected.

If a patient expresses concern over a specific area of sensory loss, it is generally wise to have the area delineated by the patient and then to test the limits specifically. A sensory level may be found in patients who have a spinal cord injury.

In the emergency department, it is important to recognize specific patterns of sensory loss. Lesions involving the specific nerve roots and peripheral nerves must be separated from central nervous system involvement (Fig. 2-5). Table 2-6 summarizes these specific sensory patterns.

Cortical localization and interpretation of sensation can be tested by looking for extinction of double simultaneous stimuli (DSS). A sensitive indicator for parietal lobe dysfunction is when two stimuli given to two opposite sides of the body at the exact same time cannot be distinguished. The appreciation of stimuli presented on symmetrically opposite areas of the body requires normal parietal lobe function.

If only one stimulus is perceived, the parietal cortex on the opposite side from the nonperceived stimulus may be involved. Such parietal extinction also holds true for visual stimuli. Appreciation of fingers in the various visual fields presented separately but denied when presented simultaneously is pathognomonic for visual extinction from parietal lobe disease.

The Romberg test represents input from a combination of systems. With the feet together, the arms to the sides, and the eyes open, the Romberg test evaluates the cerebellar integration of visual, sensory, and vestibular inputs with respect to orientation in space. If the patient is steady with eyes open, the systems must basically be intact. If the patient then becomes unsteady with the eyes closed, then position sense from the extremities is not reaching the central nervous system. This is not a cerebellar problem but a dorsal column or peripheral nerve sensory problem.[10]

REFLEXES

Tendon reflexes are only of importance when compared side to side and between the upper and lower extremities and lesions above and below the foramen magnum. Tendon reflexes are usually checked at the ankles, knees, forearms, and elbows. The ab-

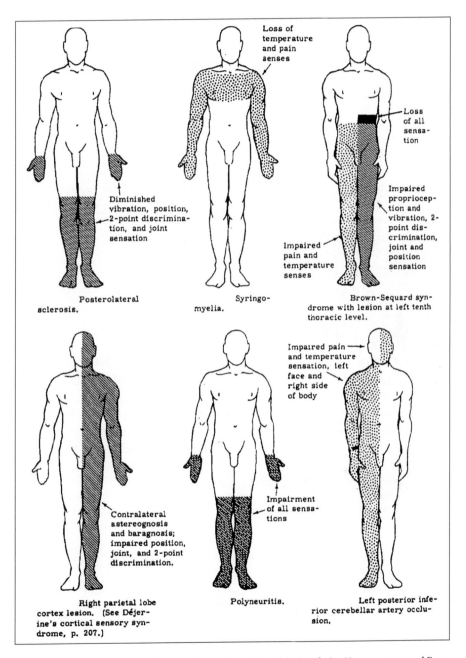

FIGURE 2-5   Principle patterns of sensory loss.   (From Chusid J. *Correlative Neuroanatomy and Functional Neurology,* 14th ed. Los Altos, CA: Lange, 1970, with permission.)

TABLE 2-6

ANATOMIC CORRELATES OF SENSORY LOSS PATTERNS

Pattern of Loss	Anatomic Location
Specific dermatomal segment	Involvement of isolated nerve root or roots
Specific peripheral nerve	Structural lesion involving isolated peripheral nerve or vascular compromise to the nerve
Diminished vibration and position in the limbs	Lesion of the dorsal columns in the spinal cord
Loss of temperature and pain across or in the arms and shoulders in a capelike distribution	Central cord syndrome: trauma or syringomyelia; developmental
Loss of all sensation below a specific vertebral level	Complete spinal cord transection
Loss of vibration and proprioception on one side; loss of pain and temperature on the opposite side of the body below a specific level	Brown-Sequard syndrome with hemisection of the spinal cord
Complete loss of sensation on one side of the body including head neck, trunk, and extremities	Central nervous system located, above the upper brainstem and internal capsule region
Loss of all sensory modalities on distal limbs	Peripheral neuropathy of the arms and legs from any cause
Impairment of sensory modality on one side of the face and the opposite side of the neck and body	Involvement of uncrossed facial fibers and crossed body fibers in the middle to lower brainstem or multiple lesions

solute level of any reflex is not as important as is the symmetry or asymmetry found. Reflexes are usually graded on a 0 to 4+ basis. 4+ reflexes indicate clonus or some type of sustained uninhibited reflex function. Zero reflexes indicate that the reflex simply cannot be elicited. In examining tendon reflexes, it may be necessary to divert the patient's attention if there is any suspicion that concentration is affecting the results (Table 2-7).

Regressive reflexes indicate some degree of inhibition of the central nervous system on reflex activities. A positive Babinski's sign is nonspecific but denotes some decreased influence from the upper motor neuron. Regressive reflexes in the head and neck area include snouting, sucking, rooting, and so on. The presence of these reflexes

TABLE 2-7 —————

PRIMARY REFLEXES

Reflex	Roots Involved	Muscles Involved
Jaw jerk	Fifth cranial nerve	Masseter and pterygoids
Ankle jerk	S1–S2	Gastrocnemius
Knee jerk	L3–L4	Quadriceps
Biceps	C5–C6	Biceps
Brachioradialis	C5–C6	Brachioradialis
Triceps	C7–C8	Triceps

usually indicates long-standing cortical disease and lack of frontal lobe inhibition of these more primitive reflex activities.[7]

AUTONOMIC NERVOUS SYSTEM

Testing the autonomic nervous system is extremely complex and is usually not required. Certain autonomic functions with regard to vision are covered under the chapter on pupillary abnormalities, but the overall functioning of the autonomic nervous system requires multiple inputs. Therefore, blood pressure, pulse, general vascular tone, sweating, and so on are all affected by multiple systems and various forms of pathology. Proper testing of the autonomic nervous system can be done on a nonemergent basis with a series of stress maneuvers.[15]

EXAMINATION MODIFICATIONS FOR SPECIFIC COMPLAINTS

Just as the neurologic history has important information that can be obtained relevant to each specific chief complaint, the physical exam may be modified to accommodate individual symptoms. Pertinent neurologic exam modifications based on the patient's presenting complaint are summarized in Table 2-8.

Specific examination protocols have been developed to enhance communication and reproduce ability between various examiners over time. The two that are currently being used are the Glasgow Coma Scale (Table 2-9) and the National Institutes of Health Stroke Scale (Table 2-10). The Glasgow Coma Scale has limitations at the higher end of neurologic performance. There can be patients with scores of 15 (the highest possible on the scale) who are not neurologically normal. It is, however, a standardized way of following patient conditions and is useful in statistical analysis of the head-injured patients.

The National Institutes of Health Stroke Scale is used in decision making for the giving of thrombolytic therapy to stroke patients. Examinations both before and after CT scanning are compared as a part of current inclusion criteria (see stroke discussion in Chap. 4).

TABLE 2-8

NEUROLOGIC EXAMINATION FOR SPECIFIC
CHIEF COMPLAINTS

Presenting Signs; Symptoms	Additional Examinations to Be Considered
Confusion; delirium	Formal mental status testing; aphasia; regressive reflexes
Flat affect	Evaluation of thought content and pathologic reflexes (snouting, sucking, grasping)
Blurred, dimmed, or absent vision	Visual acuity and light perception; funduscopic exam; slit lamp and swinging flashlight exam (see Marcus Gunn pupil, Chap. 8); visual fields, optokinetic nystagmus; intraocular pressure red glass testing
Headache	Careful palpation of head and neck structures for meningismus and funduscopic evaluation
Focal weakness	Systemic testing of nerve roots and/or peripheral nerve involved in the area of motor and sensory loss and hemispheric testing
Nonfocal weakness	Test for muscle fatigue including lid lag and pronator drift and stress tolerance
Dizziness	Orthostatic vital signs, positional testing: Nylen-Barany test and cardiac examination
Stupor, coma	Best level of consciousness, respiratory pattern; Doll's eye movements or caloric testing; pupillary responses, motor responses, and posturing; decorticate, decerebrate, flaccid
Neurotrauma	Coma: go directly to coma protocol Awake: perform limited examination until cervical spine properly evaluated Most important: check for bilaterality of motor functioning, level of consciousness, and attentiveness
Back pain without direct trauma	Straight leg raising sign, anal tone, or perianal sensation

TABLE 2-9 ——————————————————————
THE GLASGOW COMA SCALE FOR ALL AGE GROUPS

Score	4 yr to Adult	Child < 4 yr	Infant
Eye opening			
4	Spontaneous	Spontaneous	Spontaneous
3	To speech	To speech	To speech
2	To pain	To pain	To pain
1	No response	No response	No response
Verbal response			
5	Alert and oriented	Oriented, social, speaks, interacts	Coos, babbles
4	Disoriented conversation	Confused speech, disoriented, consolable, aware	Irritable cry
3	Speaking but nonsensical	Inappropriate words, inconsolable, unaware	Cries to pain
2	Moans or unintelligible sounds	Incomprehensible, agitated, restless, unaware	Moans to pain
1	No response	No response	No response
Motor response			
6	Follows commands	Normal, spontaneous movements	Normal, spontaneous movements
5	Localizes pain	Localizes pain	Withdraws to touch
4	Movement or withdrawal to pain	Withdraws to pain	Withdraws to pain
3	Decorticate flexion	Decorticate flexion	Decorticate flexion
2	Decerebrate extension	Decerebrate extension	Decerebrate extension
1	No response	No response	No response

Summary

The directed neurologic examination can be both effort and time efficient. Concentrating on simple indicators of mental status, motor activity, and upper cranial nerves will produce the greatest benefit for time spent by the examiner. The neurologic exam needs to be modified based on the patient's presenting complaints and various positive findings in the examination itself.

TABLE 2-10 — NATIONAL INSTITUTES OF HEALTH STROKE SCALE

Category	Patient Response	Score
1a. Level of consciousness (LOC)	Alert	0
	Drowsy	1
	Stuporous	2
	Coma	3
1b. LOC questions	Answers both correctly	0
	Answers one correctly	1
	Answers none correctly	2
1c. LOC commands	Obeys both correctly	0
	Obeys one correctly	1
	Obeys none correctly	2
2. Best gaze	Normal	0
	Partial gaze palsy	1
	Forced deviation	2
3. Best visual	No visual loss	0
	Partial hemianopsia	1
	Complete hemianopsia	2
4. Facial palsy	Normal	0
	Minor facial weakness	1
	Partial facial weakness	2
	No facial movement	3
5. Best motor arm	No drift after 10 sec	0
	Drift	1
	Cannot resist gravity	2
	No effort against gravity	3
6. Best motor leg	No drift after 5 sec	0
	Drift	1
	Cannot resist gravity	2
	No effort against gravity	3
7. Limb ataxia	Absent	0
	Present in upper or lower extremities	1
	Present in both upper and lower extremities	2
8. Sensory	Normal	0
	Partial loss	1
	Dense loss	2
9. Neglect	No neglect	0
	Partial neglect	1
	Complete neglect	2
10. Dysarthria	Normal articulation	0
	Mild to moderate dysarthria	1
	Near unintelligible or worse	2
11. Best language	No aphasia	0
	Mild to moderate aphasia	1
	Severe aphasia	2
	Mute	3

REFERENCES

1. Fuller G. *Neurological Examination Made Easy,* 2nd ed. Edinburgh: Churchill Livingstone, 2000

2. Acheson J, Hutchinson EC. The natural history of focal cerebral vascular disease. *Q J Med* 1971;50:15.

3. National Institute of Neurologic Cerebrovascular Disease and Stroke. A classification and outline of cerebral vascular diseases. Ad hoc committee report. *Stroke* 1976;6:594–616.

4. Bannister R, Brain W. *Brain and Bannisters' Clinical Neurology,* 7th ed. New York: Oxford University Press, 1992.

5. Henry G. Emergency neurological examination. In: Tintinalli J, ed. *A Study Guide in Emergency Medicine,* 4th ed. New York: McGraw-Hill, 1996, p 1005.

6. Benbadissr A, et al. Value of tongue biting in the diagnosis of seizures. *Arch Intern Med* 1995;2:2346.

7. Denny-Brown D. *Handbook of Neurological Examination and Case Recording.* Cambridge, MA: Harvard University Press, 1965.

8. Mungas D. In-office mental status testing: a practical guide. *Geriatrics* 1991;446:54–58, 63, 66.

9. Werner W, Goetz C, eds. *Neurology for the Non-neurologist.* New York: Harper & Row, 1981.

10. Haerer A, DeJong RN. *The Neurologic Examination,* 5th ed. New York: Lippincott-Raven, 1992.

11. Shunklande WE. The trigeminal nerve. Part I: An overview. *Cranio* 2000;218:238–248.

12. Silvester KC, Barnes S. Adenoidcystic carcinoma of the tongue presenting as a hypoglossal nerve palsy. *Br J Oral Maxillofac Surg* 1990;28:122–124.

13. Felix JK, Schwartz RH, Myers GJ. Isolated hypoglossal nerve paralysis following influenza vaccination. *Am J Dis Child* 1976;130:82–83.

14. Simpson J, Magee K. *Clinical Evaluation of the Neurosystem.* Ann Arbor, MI: Overbeck, 1970.

15. Ravits JM. Autonomic nervous system testing. *Muscle Nerve* 1997;20:919–937.

3
ALTERED STATES
OF CONSCIOUSNESS
AND COMA

The maintenance of consciousness is the most important function of the central nervous system. Alterations of consciousness are common, accounting for 5% of emergency department visits in a recent large survey.[1] Despite its obvious importance, and despite the frequency of its clinical disorders, *consciousness* is difficult to define. A practical operational definition is that consciousness is a meaningful awareness of one's self and one's environment. It is important to recognize that an individual's state of conscious awareness cannot be directly observed; physicians *infer* the quality and content of a patient's consciousness by observing his or her capacity to respond to internal and external stimuli. As a result, physicians may easily be misled in their assessment of patients' mental function. Some movements or "responses" by patients may imply conscious awareness where none exists; conversely, the absence of some responses may imply impaired consciousness in a patient who is actually fully awake and aware.

Conscious awareness depends on the integrated function of large portions of the brain and brainstem; any alteration of consciousness is a highly sensitive indicator of disordered brain function. Because of the sensitivity of consciousness to alterations of CNS function, even relatively benign and reversible processes such as drug intoxication or postictal confusion following a seizure may cause major alterations of consciousness. Alterations of consciousness are often the earliest signs of evolving brain lesions; early recognition and treatment of such processes may provide an opportunity for intervention before permanent injury occurs. The task of the acute care physician is to promptly recognize and evaluate alterations of mental function and to distinguish relatively benign from more malignant processes. The importance of the clinical assessment cannot be overemphasized; in a recent series, the correct diagnosis was made in over 50% of patients from the history and physical examination.[1]

Early recognition and management of malignant processes affords the best hope for a good outcome, and early recognition of benign processes can avoid the expense and the potential risks of unnecessary diagnostic and treatment measures.

DEFINITIONS AND TERMS

As a clinical discipline, neurology is well known for the apparent mystery of its methods and for the obscurity of its terminology. This is especially true as regards the assessment of consciousness and its variations. For practical purposes, consciousness may be considered to have two components, arousal and "content." Arousal is roughly synonymous with "wakefulness" and implies the ability to perceive external or internal stimuli; content refers to the capacity to process stimuli and to make a coherent response. Clinical disorders of consciousness may involve disorders of either arousal, or content, or both.

Disorders of Arousal

Patients with disorders of arousal appear to be asleep. Sleep, of course, is a normal condition of diminished arousal from which an individual can be aroused to full consciousness.

Lethargy is a condition from which an individual can be aroused with stimulation. When awakened, the patient displays less than normal awareness of him- or herself or the environment. Left undisturbed, the patient will once again fall asleep.

Stupor is a condition of diminished awareness from which the individual can be aroused only with vigorous stimulation; even when most fully aroused, the patient is unable to interact in a meaningful way with the environment or the examiner. Such patients may groan to noxious stimuli or utter a few words but cannot carry on a meaningful conversation or respond appropriately to questions or commands.

Coma is a condition of diminished awareness from which the patient cannot be aroused, even with vigorous stimulation. Responses, if any, to noxious stimulation, tend to be stereotyped or reflexive, without evidence of any meaning or purpose.

Obtundation is a term often used to refer generally to any condition of reduced awareness; it is too imprecise as to be of practical use in clinical settings.

It should be evident that there is no clear distinction among the states of lethargy, stupor, and coma; rather, these conditions overlap and patients will often move from one state to the other as their clinical condition evolves. Because of the imprecision of all these terms, they are best avoided by clinicians; it is far more useful to specify what specific stimuli were required to arouse the patient and what level of function the patient was able to achieve once aroused.

Disorders of Content

Patients with disorders of content appear to be awake and may even appear to be hypervigilant. Despite their apparent alertness, they are impaired in their ability to think coherently or to respond appropriately to their environment.

The *vegetative state* is characterized by the presence of arousal responses mediated by brainstem reflexes, but without any conscious awareness. It is not commonly confronted in the acute care setting. It most often occurs in individuals with severe brain injury who survive their initial insult; such patients present initially with unresponsive coma and subsequently recover their basic brainstem reflexes but do not regain conscious awareness. These patients may exhibit arousal responses to external stimulation (eye opening, pupillary light reflexes, reflex eye movements, and so on), but they have no purposeful responses to questions or commands. They do not orient toward the examiner or follow a visual target; there is no sign of conscious awareness. A vegetative state is termed *persistent* if it persists for 1 month after the initial insult and *permanent* if it persists for 3 months after a metabolic or hypoxic-ischemic insult or 1 year after traumatic injury.[2]

Dementia is characterized by impairment of memory and of the ability to think logically and coherently; affected patients gradually lose the ability to respond appropriately to their surroundings. The process is typically gradual in onset and progression rather than acute or subacute as in delirium (see below). Patients are usually awake and alert and may respond appropriately to simple stimuli, such as noxious or painful stimuli, smiles or greetings, and so forth, but they are unable to respond in a meaningful way to more complex stimuli. Patients with profound dementia may be virtually mute and immobile, unable to respond at all although apparently awake. Such very profound dementia may occur either as the consequence of severe acute brain injury or at the end of a progressive disorder such as Alzheimer's disease.

Delirium is characterized by impairment of the ability to think logically and clearly and to respond appropriately to internal or external stimuli. Delirium is a common problem occurring in as many as 10% of elderly patients in the acute care setting, but it is frequently overlooked.[3,4] The onset is often quite abrupt, and the patient's level of arousal may vary from minute to minute from mild lethargy through dramatic agitation and hypervigilance. Patients may be calm and quiet, or wildly agitated and combative, with markedly increased sympathetic tone e.g., fever, tachycardia, and sweating. These patients are frequently highly distractible and may appear to be responding to multiple internal and external stimuli; auditory and visual hallucinations are frequent. It is particularly likely to occur in elderly patients, in patients with other medical problems, and in other individuals with previously compromised mental function (such as Alzheimer's disease or other dementias).[5,6]

Disorders That May Mimic Impaired Consciousness or Coma

There are several conditions in which patients with normal mental status may be misdiagnosed as having impaired consciousness or even coma. It is important that these conditions be correctly identified to prevent unnecessary diagnostic studies and to permit appropriate treatment.

The *locked-in state* is a rare condition that may occur in patients with lesions affecting the ventral pons. The descending motor tracts are interrupted, leaving the patient without any voluntary motor function of the face, the pharynx, or the body. Because the lesion is below the midbrain centers for control of vertical eye movements and eye opening, these movements are preserved, but lateral eye movements are absent or severely impaired. Because of bilateral facial paralysis, patients are unable to close their eyes. Thus these individuals are unable to speak or to make any movement other than to move their eyes upward. Their state may be easily mistaken for coma, but they nonetheless may be fully alert to all that is going on around them (including the casual remarks of their physicians and other caregivers). The clue to the diagnosis is the presence of spontaneous eye-opening in an apparently unconscious patient; the ability of the patient to gaze upward on command confirms the diagnosis. A similar situation may occur (minus the vertical eye movements) in patients treated with neuromuscular blocking agents. When there is any doubt about the matter, it is best to behave as if all patients are fully awake and alert.

Occasionally patients present with apparent unresponsiveness to external stimulation (including even noxious or painful stimulation). This is termed *psychogenic unresponsiveness.* They may appear to be awake or asleep; despite their apparent lack of any conscious or voluntary responses, careful examination reveals normal reflex responses (such as pursuit eye movements, nystagmus on caloric testing, protective reflexes), which suggest conscious awareness. Often such patients will forcefully resist attempts to open their eyes and they may actively resist examination. Recognition of this rare syndrome requires an alert and astute physician. Although psychogenic unresponsiveness may occasionally be the result of deliberate malingering, it more often indicates a profound psychologic disturbance (see Chap. 10). It is essential for physicians to recall that these patients are awake and alert, and to carefully avoid insensitive or inappropriate remarks, which may vastly complicate both diagnosis and treatment.[7]

PATHOPHYSIOLOGY OF ALTERED CONSCIOUSNESS

Maintenance of normal conscious awareness requires the integrated function of the ascending reticular activating system (ARAS) in the upper brainstem and the cerebral hemispheres. Accordingly, substantial alteration of consciousness implies pathology affecting either the ARAS or *both* cerebral hemispheres. Either structural lesions or toxic or metabolic derangements may affect these structures and result in impairment or loss of consciousness. Figures 3-1 and 3-2 illustrate a variety of structural lesions affecting the brainstem and cerebral hemispheres, some affecting consciousness and some not. Note that brainstem lesions causing coma are generally limited to those affecting the midline structures of the upper pons or the midbrain; lesions confined to the lower pons or the medulla, or unilateral lesions, are unlikely to result in coma. Unilateral structural lesions of the cerebral hemispheres, even if quite large, do not generally cause coma; conversely, even relatively small bilateral lesions of the hemispheres (e.g., bilateral thalamic lesions) may result in coma.

Disorders of the ARAS

The ARAS is a complex system of nuclei and fiber tracts extending from the cervical spinal cord through the brainstem to the thalami. The portions of the ARAS

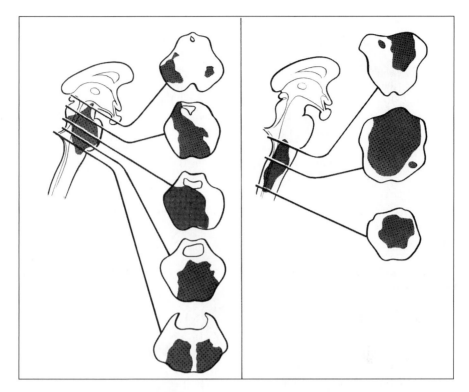

FIGURE 3-1   Brain lesions not causing sustained coma.   (From Plum F, Posner JB. *The Diagnosis of Stupor and Coma,* 3rd ed. Philadelphia: FA Davis, 1982, with permission.)

in the upper pons and the midbrain are primarily responsible for maintaining the cerebral hemispheres and cortex in a state of readiness to respond to and process internal or external stimuli. During sleep, the cerebral cortex is unresponsive to stimulation; the ARAS maintains surveillance of internal and external environment and can arouse the cortex as necessary. Disorders of arousal, therefore, imply either failure of the ARAS or inability of the cortex to respond to stimulation. The ARAS may be affected directly by intrinsic or toxic/metabolic processes, or indirectly by lesions in the supratentorial or infratentorial compartments.

Intrinsic Lesions

Because of its relatively small size, the ARAS may be affected by small structural lesions intrinsic to the brainstem such as ischemic stroke or hemorrhage. Head trauma may produce shearing or torsional forces of the upper brainstem resulting directly in failure of the ARAS.

Toxic/Metabolic Lesions

Although the ARAS is relatively resistant to toxic and metabolic insults, severe derangements may result in ARAS failure. Examples include severe hypothermia, severe drug intoxication, or severe hypoxia or ischemia.

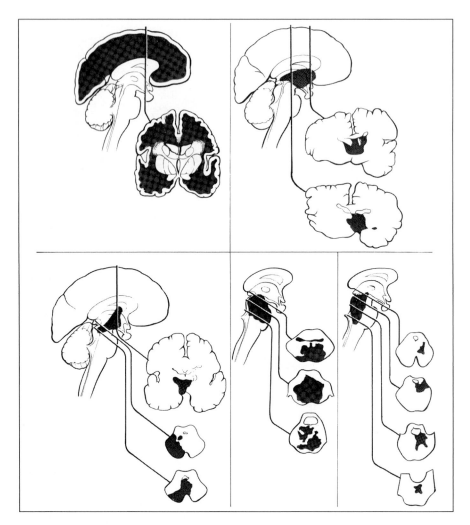

FIGURE 3-2   Brain lesions causing sustained coma.   (From Plum F, Posner JB. *The Diagnosis of Stupor and Coma,* 3rd ed. Philadelphia: FA Davis, 1982, with permission.)

Supratentorial lesions include mass lesions such as epidural or subdural hematomas, intracerebral hematomas, infectious lesions (such as brain abcesses), cerebral edema from stroke, encephalitis, trauma, or severe metabolic insults, hydrocephalus, tumors, and so on. Mass lesions may result in herniation of the supratentorial contents downward through the tentorium with compression of the ARAS.

Infratentorial lesions affecting the cerebellum can result in expanding mass lesions in the posterior fossa with direct compression of the upper brainstem and even upward herniation of the posterior fossa through the tentorium. Less commonly, the same process may result from abcesses, tumors, and other lesions affecting the cerebellum or posterior fossa (Figure 3-3).

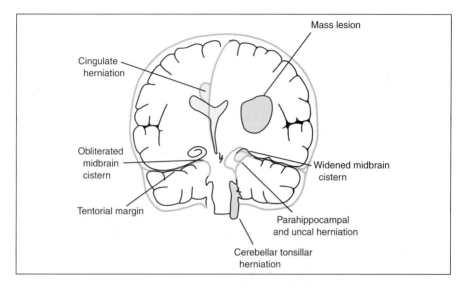

FIGURE 3-3 Brain herniations between dural compartments. Transfalcial, uncalparahippocampal, and cerebellar herniations are shown. (From Victor M, Ropper AH. *Adams and Victor's Principles of Neurology,* 7th ed. New York: McGraw-Hill, 2000, p 376, with permission.)

Disorders of the Cerebral Hemispheres

As has already been noted, profound alterations of consciousness do not generally result from focal or unilateral lesions of the cerebral hemispheres unless both hemispheres are affected. In clinical practice, this most commonly occurs as the result of toxic or metabolic processes that affect the brain diffusely. Other potential causes include infection, seizure activity, or increased intracranial pressure.

Toxic-metabolic encephalopathies may result from an enormous array of potential causes. Perfusion failure (cardiac arrest or severe hypotension), profound hypoxemia, hypo- or hyperglycemia, renal or hepatic failure, electrolyte abnormalities, and intoxication with licit or illicit drugs may all result in impairment or loss of consciousness. The clinical picture may range from mild confusion through frank delirium, or from mild lethargy through frank coma. A similar clinical picture may result from intracranial infections (meningitis and encephalitis), or subarachnoid hemorrhage.

Seizures may cause impairment or loss of consciousness; when motor or behavioral phenomena are present, seizures are easily recognized. However, seizures may be unaccompanied by any abnormal movements or only by very subtle movements that can be easily overlooked. Either generalized or partial seizures may be followed by a postictal period of diminished consciousness that may persist for many hours.

Increased intracranial pressure may result from a variety of causes. Obstruction of the normal pathways of cerebrospinal fluid (CSF) drainage by mass lesions, blood, or other causes may lead to acute hydrocephalus. Cerebral edema may result from infection, electrolyte abnormalities, trauma, and other causes. Mass lesions (e.g., intracerebral hemorrhages, tumor, subdural or epidural hematomas) may all cause increases in intracranial pressure with diminished consciousness or coma. Diminished consciousness is more likely to result from acute increases in intracranial pressure; in chronic disorders such as idiopathic intracranial hypertension (pseudotumor cerebri) or slowly growing mass lesions, even very large increases in intracranial pressure may not affect consciousness.

INITIAL ASSESSMENT AND MANAGEMENT

The usual stepwise approach to a clinical problem is to obtain a history first, then to conduct a physical examination and any necessary laboratory and imaging studies, and finally to make a diagnosis and initiate treatment. The patient in coma, or with severely altered mental status, presents special problems; an adequate history is frequently unobtainable and the physical examination may be very limited. The urgency of the clinical situation may require that initial treatment be started before a definite diagnosis has been established; instead, diagnostic assessment and empiric treatment must be done simultaneously. Even so, it is essential that diagnosis and treatment be carried out in as systematic and organized a fashion as possible. The initial assessment of patients with impaired consciousness should seek to accomplish several goals urgently:

1. Recognize and manage immediately life-threatening conditions.
2. Establish the patient's current level of consciousness and neurologic function.
3. Establish a differential diagnosis of the likely causes of the patient's condition.
4. Initiate treatment and definitive diagnostic study.

Assessment of Vital Signs

The first step, of course, is to assess and manage the patient's vital functions—the classic "ABCs" of emergency medical care; this includes an immediate serum glucose determination.

Adequate oxygenation and ventilation are priorities. The airway should be secured, by intubation if needed, both to ensure adequate oxygenation and to prevent aspiration. Although observation of the pattern of respiration is of limited practical value in localizing lesions causing alterations or loss of consciousness, the respiratory pattern should be observed, whenever possible, prior to any intervention. The presence of spontaneous respiration implies at least some preservation of brainstem function. Rhythmic regular respiration (e.g., Cheyne-Stokes respiration, spontaneous hyperventilation) implies intact brainstem function. Lesions of the pons may result in *apneustic breathing,* characterized by a prolonged pause (*inspiratory cramp*) after each inspiration. An irregular or chaotic pattern (*Biot's breathing*) implies a lesion at the lower pons or medulla and warns of impending respiratory failure.[5]

Adequate perfusion should be ensured. Shock should be managed aggressively, and cardiac arrythmias should be monitored and treated as indicated. Hyper- and hypotension should be considered to have a nonneurologic cause until proved otherwise. In general, acute hypertension should not be treated urgently unless there is some other indication for such treatment (e.g., myocardial ischemia), or if true hypertensive encephalopathy is the likely diagnosis (p. 74).

A rectal temperature should be obtained. Very high or very low temperatures may be either the cause of the patient's obtundation or the result of some other process. Very high temperatures may result from sepsis, from heat stroke, or from the neuroleptic malignant syndrome; very low temperatures may result from overwhelming sepsis or from environmental exposure. Vital signs be should be monitored closely and reviewed regularly by the physician.

Obtaining the History

Depending on the clinical situation, obtaining a history may have to be deferred until after initial assessment and stabilization of the patient. It is important to remember, however, that even a very limited clinical history may vastly simplify the process of diagnosis. Although the patient is often unable to supply any history, witnesses may be able to describe the onset and progression of the patient's clinical symptoms. They may be aware of recent or chronic medical illnesses such as AIDS, diabetes, or heart disease, or of previous episodes of altered consciousness. Specific questions about alcohol or drug use, or possible recent trauma, should be asked. Witnesses should be assured that all information is confidential and will not be shared with law enforcement officers, family members or friends, or others without due process. Wallet cards, pill bottles, or medical alert tags may all yield helpful information.

Empiric Management

Intravenous access should be established and blood drawn for laboratory studies. It is common practice to give thiamine 100 mg, glucose 25 to 50 mg, and naloxone 0.8 to 1.6 mg on an empiric basis to virtually all patients with altered mental status. Naloxone may precipitate acute narcotic withdrawal, and the physician may suddenly be confronted with a severely agitated or delirious patient, therefore careful titration is recommend. Any or all can be omitted if the available history or initial data (such as a normal or elevated blood glucose level) make it clear that they are unnecessary. It is important that any patient potentially at risk for nutritional deficiency (alcoholics or other substance abusers, severely debilitated patients, homeless persons, and others) be given thiamine when being given glucose.

Seizures, if present, should be controlled (see Chap. 11).

Neurologic Examination

Once the vital functions are secured, a brief neurologic examination should be done to assess the patient's actual level of function, to begin the process of diagnosis, and to establish a baseline against which subsequent examinations can be compared. The neurologic examination of patients with impaired consciousness must be tailored to the patient's ability to cooperate. A useful initial neurologic examination can be carried out in only a few minutes if the physician concentrates on the essentials; a more detailed examination, if needed, can be accomplished later.

Assessment of Mental Status

The first step is to assess the patient's actual level of consciousness. The patient should be observed carefully for any spontaneous movements. Does he or she maintain a normal supine posture? Are the eyes open or closed? (If the eyes are open, the patient may be awake, even if unresponsive.) The patient should be addressed (by name if known) and the response observed. If the patient responds to voice, the ability to respond appropriately to questions or commands should be assessed. If there is no response to voice, response to touch and finally to noxious or painful stimuli should be assessed. Note that a noxious stimulus need not be painful. Gentle pressure on the sternum, the clavicles, or other bony prominences will often suffice. If more painful stimuli are required, vigorous pressure on the same areas is appropriate. It is important to avoid any risk of actual injury to the patient; twisting nipples, squeezing testicles, and other potentially dangerous maneuvers should not be used. In patients with suspected cervical spinal cord injury, some stimulus above the neck (such as firm pressure on the mastoid process or over the supraorbital notch) should be tried. The specific stimuli used and the exact character of the patient's responses should be recorded. Note any sign of purposeful responses and also note whether responses are bilateral or limited to one side. Note any posturing or any change in pulse, blood pressure, or respiration in response to stimulation. Vague terms such as "lethargy," "stupor," and so forth convey too little information and should be avoided.

In patients with a history of head trauma, the Glasgow Coma Scale is widely used to assess the patient's level of function (see Chap. 2 and Chap. 9).

Examination of the Eyes

The important functions of those parts of the upper brainstem most concerned with maintaining consciousness can be reliably assessed by a careful examination of the eyes. Intact function of the pupils, eyelids, and eye movements implies intact function of the relevant portions of the upper brainstem and ARAS and suggests that the alteration of consciousness or mentation is probably due to a lesion affecting the cerebral hemispheres.

Fundus Examination

The presence of papilledema suggests raised intracranial pressure of at least several hours' duration or longer; unfortunately, the absence of papilledema does not indicate normal intracranial pressure. Likewise, spontaneous venous pulsations, when present, imply normal pressure; the absence of such pulsations is of no diagnostic significance. Note that venous pulsations, even if present, are frequently difficult to see. Subhyaloid hemorrhages may be seen in patients with subarachnoid hemorrhage. There may be signs of chronic hypertension or diabetes, but these are of little help in the acute situation.

Pupils

The size, shape, reactivity, and symmetry of the pupils should be assessed and recorded. Any apparent abnormality of pupil function must be interpreted in the context of the entire clinical history and examination. Abnormalities of pupil function can result from recent or remote eye surgery or trauma, topical or systemic medications or toxins, or other acquired conditions, rather than from disorders of the nervous system.

The *size* of the pupils is regulated by inputs from both the sympathetic and parasympathetic nervous systems. Pupillary constriction is controlled by parasympathetic fibers that originate from the Edinger-Westphal nuclei located in the midbrain in close association with the ARAS. Failure of the pupils to react to light may indicate a lesion affecting the Edinger-Westphal nuclei, the parasympathetic fibers that travel in association with the third (oculomotor) nerve, or cholinergic neuromuscular junctions in the iris (Figure 3-4). Dilation of the pupils is controlled by

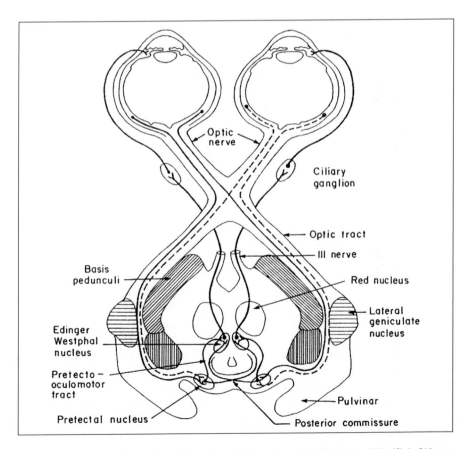

FIGURE 3-4   Diagram of the pupillary light reflex.   (Adapted from Walsh FB, Hoyt WF. *Clinical Neuro-Ophthalmology,* 3rd ed. Baltimore: Williams & Wilkins, 1969, with permission.)

the sympathetic pathway that begins in the hypothalamus and extends through the cervical spinal cord to the upper thoracic cord (T1level). The fibers then follow the sympathetic chain to the superior cervical ganglion and then the carotid artery to the orbit. Failure of the pupils to dilate properly in the presence of dim light (e.g., Horner's syndrome) can indicate a lesion anywhere along this extended sympathetic pathway.

The size of the pupils can be affected by a wide variety of drugs and toxins, as well as by structural lesions affecting various parts of the nervous system. Abnormalities of pupil size or function without other focal abnormalities on neurologic examination should strongly suggest drug or toxic effects on the pupils; both intraocular and systemic drugs can affect pupil size. Table 3-1 gives a partial list of drugs and toxins affecting pupillary size. Structural lesions of the brain, brainstem, or cranial nerves causing abnormalities of pupillary function will virtually always be associated with other abnormalities on neurologic examination.

Pupil Reactivity

The pupils will normally constrict abruptly when stimulated with bright light (the light reaction) or when presented with a nearby visual target (accommodation). The light reaction is very resistant to drugs and toxins; absence of any response to light usually indicates a structural lesion affecting the midbrain tegmentum. (Potent topical cycloplegic drugs may also completely block the light reaction.) Lesions of the cerebral hemispheres will not affect the light reflex. The reflex may be very difficult to see in patients with very small pupils—a magnifying lens (such as a high-plus lens on the ophthalmoscope) may be used to look for any reaction. *Any constriction* is significant and indicates that the parasympathetic pathway is anatomically intact.

The accommodation reflex cannot be assessed in an unconscious patient. In patients with psychogenic unresponsiveness, sudden presentation of a nearby visual stimulus, such as suddenly holding a mirror in front of the patient, may elicit an accommodation reflex; this indicates intact vision (and preserved consciousness!).

Pupil Symmetry

Drugs or toxins affecting pupillary function can be expected to affect both sides equally (unless a topical agent has been used in only one eye). Some asymmetry of the pupils (usually <1 mm) may be seen in normal persons, but such pupils will respond symmetrically to changes in lighting. Asymmetry of the pupillary light reflex strongly suggests a structural lesion. When faced with asymmetric pupils, the clinician must determine which pupil is abnormal. Careful observation of the pupils at different light levels will demonstrate either failure of constriction of the larger pupil, suggesting a third nerve lesion, or failure of dilation of the smaller pupil, suggesting a Horner's syndrome. If the eyes are open, ptosis on the side of the larger pupil suggests a third nerve lesion; ptosis on the side of the smaller pupil indicates Horner's syndrome. If a third nerve lesion is present, abnormal eye movements may also be observed (see below).

TABLE 3-1 —————————————————————————————
DRUGS AND TOXINS THAT AFFECT PUPIL SIZE AND FUNCTION

Drugs and Toxins That May Cause Enlarged Pupils
Anticholinergic agents
  Atropine
  Trihexyphenidyl (Artane)
  Benztropine (Cogentin)
  Scopolamine[a]
  Tropicamide[a]
  Cyclopentolate[a]
  Gentamicin[a]
  Jimson weed, nightshade, other plant toxins
  Botulinum toxin
Adrenergic agents
  Epinephrine
  Phenylephrine
  Ephedrine
  Amphetamine, dextroamphetamine
  Cocaine
  Chlorpheniramine[a]

Drugs and Toxins That May Cause Small Pupils
Cholinergic agents
  Pilocarpine[a]
  Methacholine[a]
  Carbachol[a]
  Physostigmine, neostigmine, pyridostigmine[b]
  Organic phosphate esters (insecticides)[c]
Antiadrenergic agents
  Dibenzyline
  Phentolamine
  Tolazoline
  Guanethidine
  Bretylium
  Monoamine oxidase inhibitors
Other agents
  Opiates and synthetic narcotics

[a] Drugs used primarily as topical agents in ophthalmology. Although not causing coma or altered mental status, they may confuse the physical examination.
[b] Used primarily in the treatment of myasthenia gravis.
[c] Rarely encountered in clinical practice; some of these agents have potential for use in terrorist attacks.

Eye Movements

The control of eye movements is highly complex and depends on the integrated function of multiple areas of the hemispheres and brainstem. Fortunately, the practical clinical assessment of eye movements, particularly in unconscious patients, is usually quite straightforward.

Lateral movement of each eye is controlled by the ipsilateral sixth (abducens) nucleus via the abducens nerve. Medial, upward, and downward movements of each eye are controlled by the ipsilateral third (oculomotor) nucleus via the oculomotor nerve. (The fourth (trochlear) nucleus and nerve can be ignored in this setting.) The individual cranial nerve nuclei are under the control of supranuclear gaze centers, which serve to ensure that both eyes move together in conjugate fashion. Lateral gaze to each side is controlled by the ipsilateral pontine paramedian reticular formation (PPRF), which is adjacent to the sixth nerve nucleus in the pons; output from the PPRF controls the ipsilateral sixth nerve nucleus and, via the medial longitudinal fasciculus (MLF), the contralateral third nerve nucleus. Thus, activation of the PPRF on one side will induce both eyes to turn to that side (Figure 3-5). Vertical eye movements are controlled by accessory oculomotor nuclei in the upper midbrain; when activated, these nuclei induce the third nerve nuclei to turn the eyes upward or downward in coordinated fashion. The anatomy is complex, but understanding it is crucial if the physical examination is to yield useful information.

Review of the relevant neuroanatomy will make it clear that lesions at or above the supranuclear gaze centers (the PPRFs and accessory oculomotor nuclei) will cause *conjugate* disorders of eye movements (both eyes will move together and will be equally impaired). Conversely, a lesion that causes *disconjugate* eye movements must be located below the level of the gaze centers, that is, in the brainstem, affecting either the MLF or the cranial nerve nuclei, or outside the central nervous system (CNS), affecting the cranial nerves or the extraocular muscles. Valuable information can thus be obtained by observation of voluntary eye movements in conscious patients, and by observation of reflex eye movements in unconscious patients.

Voluntary and *pursuit* eye movements result when the supranuclear gaze centers are activated by the cerebral cortex. Voluntary movements are initiated in the frontal eye fields; voluntary activation of one of the frontal eye fields results in deviation of the eyes to the opposite side. Focal seizure activity may also induce deviation of the eyes to the contralateral side. Conversely, injury to one of the frontal lobes (such as an acute stroke) *may* result in deviation of the eyes *toward* the injured side due to the unopposed output of the intact frontal lobe. This sign is not always present; even when it is present initially, it may resolve within a short time. Pursuit movements are controlled by the parietal-occipital areas, but injury to these areas does not produce predictable or reliable localizing signs. Clearly, preservation of voluntary or pursuit eye movements implies intact cortical function and consciousness, even in an otherwise unresponsive patient.

Unconscious patients will sometimes exhibit slow roving eye movements. These may be conjugate or disconjugate; disconjugate movements in this setting do not imply a brainstem or cranial nerve lesion as long as both eyes are moving. It should

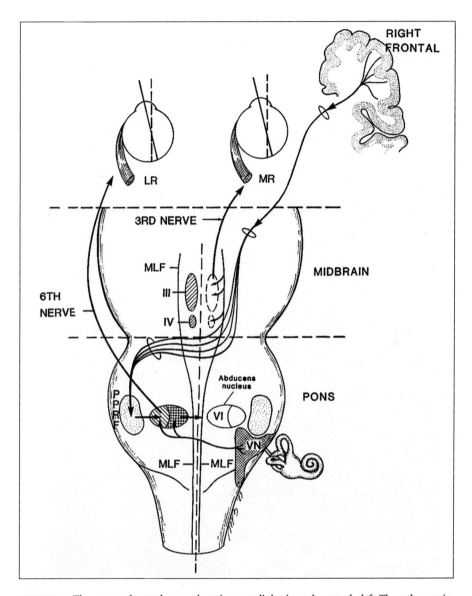

FIGURE 3-5   The supranuclear pathways subserving saccadic horizontal gaze to the left. The pathway originates in the right frontal cortex, descends in the internal capsule, decussates at the level of the rostral pons, and descends to synapse in the left pontine paramedian reticular formation (PPRF). Further connections with the ipsilateral sixth nerve nucleus and contralateral medial longitudinal fasciculus are also indicated. Cranial nerve nuclei III and IV are labeled on the left; the nucleus of VI and vestibular nuclei (VN) are labeled on the right. LR, lateral rectus; MR, medial rectus; MLF, medial longitudinal fasciculus. (From Victor M, Ropper AH. *Adams and Victor's Principles of Neurology,* 7th ed. New York: McGraw-Hill, 2000, p 273, with permission.)

be recalled that these slow roving eye movements *cannot* be mimicked by a conscious patient.

Reflex eye movements can be elicited by maneuvers designed to activate the supranuclear gaze centers. The *oculocephalic (Doll's eye)* reflex is elicited by passively moving the patient's head from side to side or forward and backward and observing any resulting eye movements. *The test is contraindicated if there is any suspicion of a cervical spine injury.* The patient's eyes are held open and the head is turned briskly first to one side and then to the other. The expected response is conjugate deviation of the eyes to the side opposite the direction of head movement. Similar responses (upward and downward movements of the eyes) can be elicited by passive flexion and extension of the neck. The presence of oculocephalic reflexes implies normal function of the brainstem gaze centers and nuclei; failure of the response indicates brainstem failure. A disconjugate response indicates a focal lesion in the brainstem or cranial nerves. Note that the response cannot be obtained in awake patients (Figure 3-6).

If the oculocephalic reflex cannot be obtained, or if the test is contraindicated, the oculovestibular (caloric) reflexes can be tested. If performed with ice water (see below), the test is very painful in the awake patient; ice water should *only* be used to assess brainstem function in patients known to be unconscious. A more gentle version of the test using water only a few degrees below body temperature can be used in awake patients to assess vestibular function. It is unnecessary to perform the test in patients with intact oculocephalic reflexes since it is simply a more vigorous test of the same anatomic systems. The test is performed with the patient supine; if possible the head should be elevated about 30 degrees (though this is not strictly necessary). The ear is then irrigated with 50 to 60 mL of ice-cold water via a small catheter. It is preferable (but not strictly necessary) that the ear be clear of impacted cerumen. A normal response (in a patient with intact brainstem function) is tonic conjugate deviation of the eyes toward the irrigated ear. Absence of any response indicates profound impairment of brainstem function. As with the oculocephalic reflex, a disconjugate response indicates a focal lesion of the brainstem or cranial nerves. Both sides should be tested, with a 5-minute delay between sides (Figure 3-6 and Tables 3-2 and 3-3).

It is important to recognize that failure of these reflexes does not necessarily imply an irreversible process; the reflexes may be abolished by completely reversible profound toxic or metabolic insults (e.g., barbiturate intoxication) or by neuromuscular blockade.

Other Cranial Nerves

Most other tests of cranial nerve function cannot be carried out in unconscious patients. In patients who can be aroused, at least in part, careful examination of facial movements can yield helpful localizing information. Clear, well-articulated speech, even if nonsensical, implies normal lower brainstem function. Conversely, the gag reflex yields little useful information and is not a reliable guide to the patient's ability to swallow safely or to protect the airway from aspiration. The pres-

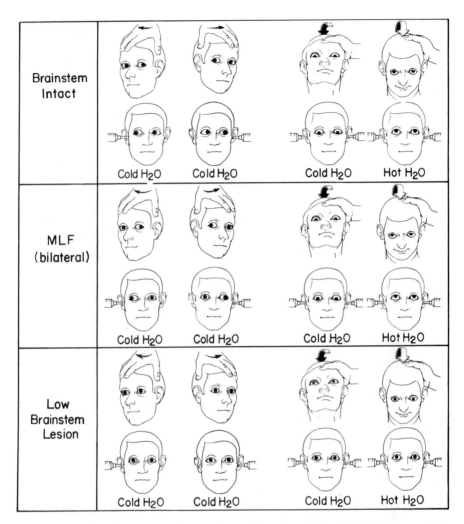

Brainstem Intact				
	Cold H₂O	Cold H₂O	Cold H₂O	Hot H₂O
MLF (bilateral)				
	Cold H₂O	Cold H₂O	Cold H₂O	Hot H₂O
Low Brainstem Lesion				
	Cold H₂O	Cold H₂O	Cold H₂O	Hot H₂O

FIGURE 3-6   Ocular reflexes in unconscious patients.   (From Plum F, Posner JB. *The Diagnosis of Stupor and Coma,* 3rd ed. Philadelphia: FA Davis, 1982, with permission.)

ence of the gag and cough reflexes does suggest some preservation of brainstem function but is otherwise of little diagnostic value.

Motor and Sensory Testing

Standard tests of motor function cannot be carried out in unconscious patients; such tests are of limited value even in patients with less severely impaired consciousness since reliable motor testing requires the full cooperation and effort of the patient.

Patients should be observed carefully for any spontaneous motor activity. Purposeful activity such as rearranging the bedclothes to preserve modesty or to place the limbs in a position of comfort indicates a high level of brain activity, even in an

TABLE 3-2

INTERPRETATION OF OCULOCEPHALIC (DOLL'S EYE) REFLEXES[a]

Stimulus	Response	Interpretation
Lateral rotation of head	Eyes remain conjugate, move opposite to head movement	Normal
	No movement either eye with head moved in either direction	Brainstem lesion Bilateral labyrinth dysfunction Drugs/anesthesia
	Eyes move normally with head turned in one direction, no response when head turned in opposite direction	Unilateral lesion in PPRF (lateral gaze center)
	One eye abducts, opposite eye does not adduct	Third nerve lesion Internuclear ophthalmoplegia
Flexion/extension of the head	Eyes remain conjugate, move opposite to head movement	Normal
	No movement either eye with head moved in either direction	Brainstem lesion Bilateral labyrinth dysfunction Drugs/anesthesia
	No upward movement either eye, normal downward movement	Lesions of dorsal midbrain (Parinaud's syndrome)
	Only one eye moves	Third nerve palsy

[a] Drugs that impair vestibular or oculomotor function (anticholinergics, TCAs, neuromuscular blocking agents, and so on) may impair these responses.
SOURCE: adapted from Berger JR. Clinical approach to stupor and coma. In Bradley WG et al., eds. *Neurology in Clinical Practice*, 2nd ed. Boston: Butterworth-Heinemann, 1996 (with permission).

otherwise unresponsive patient. Rhythmic twitching or jerking movements may indicate seizure activity; random twitching and jerking movements (myoclonus) may indicate a diffuse toxic or metabolic brain injury. Movements of the face but not of the body or extremities may indicate a lesion of the cervical spinal cord. Movement of the arms but not the legs may indicate a low cervical or thoracic spinal cord injury. Movement of only one side of the body may indicate hemiplegia.

Movements in response to stimulation should be observed next. Simple withdrawal of a limb from noxious stimulation indicates intact function at spinal cord

TABLE 3-3 ——————————————————————————

INTERPRETATION OF CALORIC (OCULOVESTIBULAR) TESTING

Stimulus	Response	Interpretation
Cold water in right ear	Nystagmus—slow phase to right, fast phase to left	Normal—brainstem and cortex intact
	No response	Obstructed ear canal, "dead" labyrinth, eighth nerve lesion, brainstem lesion (PPRF)
	Tonic deviation of eyes to right, no nystagmus	Brainstem intact— toxic/metabolic process, structural lesion above brainstem
Cold water in left ear		Responses opposite to above
Warm water in left ear (if no response to cold water in right ear)	Nystagmus—slow phase to right, fast phase to left	Confirms peripheral lesion on right— blocked canal, "dead" labyrinth, eighth nerve lesion—*brainstem and cortex intact*
	Tonic deviation of eyes to right	Confirms peripheral lesion on right (see above)—*brainstem intact*

[a] Drugs that impair vestibular or oculomotor function (anticholinergics, tricyclics, neuromuscular blocking agents, prior use of aminoglycosides) may impair these responses.
SOURCE: adapted from Berger JR. Clinical approach to stupor and coma. In Bradley WG et al., eds. *Neurology in Clinical Practice*, 2nd ed. Boston: Butterworth-Heinemann, 1996 (with permission).

levels, but movement of two or more extremities when only one is stimulated indicates function at upper brainstem levels. Similarly, decorticate or decerebrate posturing indicates preserved function of the upper brainstem. More complex responses such as purposeful attempts to avoid or remove noxious stimulation indicate higher levels of brain function. Patients with catatonia may have increased muscle tone; muscle rigidity may result from poisoning with neuroleptic drugs. Absence of any muscle tone and lack of any response to stimulation suggests a severe brain injury but can be seen as well in patients with cervical spinal cord injuries or with neuromuscular blockade; noxious stimulation above the neck (such as firm pressure on the mastoid processes) should be utilized to be sure there is no response.

Reflexes

Reflex testing is of very limited value in unconscious patients. Asymmetry of reflexes between the two sides, or between the upper and lower limbs, may have limited localizing value. Similarly, the presence or absence of Babinski signs is of little help. Absence of the Babinski sign is of no diagnostic significance, and presence of the sign indicates only an "upper motor neuron" process—virtually a foregone conclusion in an unconscious patient!

General Physical Examination

The general appearance of the patient should be noted. Cachexia may indicate severe malnutrition or a chronic wasting illness such as AIDS, chronic infection, or cancer.

Head and Neck Region

Signs of trauma, such as hematoma over the mastoid processes (Battle's sign), raccoon eyes, and local tenderness and crepitus, all suggest severe neurotrauma and should be sought. Hemorrhage from the nose and ears or discoloration at the base of the skull indicates possible skull fracture. Palpation of the skull may reveal skull fractures or evidence of previous neurosurgical procedures. Palpation of the neck is generally not helpful in the unconscious patient. When in any doubt, it is safer to assume that there may be a cervical spine injury and to take proper precautions until the necessary x-ray studies have been obtained. Even without specific signs of trauma to the head and neck region, evidence of significant trauma to the rest of the body should suggest possible trauma to the central nervous system.

Passive flexion of the neck should be attempted—nuchal rigidity should suggest the presence of meningeal irritation from infection or subarachnoid hemorrhage. As usual, this is contraindicated if there is any suspicion of a cervical spine injury.

Breath

The physician should not assume that coma is due to alcohol merely because the odor of alcohol is detectable. Although high levels of alcohol can produce obtundation or even coma, this should be regarded as a diagnosis of exclusion. The fruity fragrance of acetone can easily be mistaken for alcohol. Rarely, the distinctive odor of anaerobic infection or of *fetor hepaticus* may be detected. A feculent odor suggests bowel obstruction. Cyanide has the distinctive odor of almonds.

Skin

Needle tracks suggest IV drug use or recent treatment with intravenous drugs. Cyanosis suggests hypoxemia, polycythemia, or an abnormal hemoglobin. Pallor may indicate that the patient has inadequate oxygen-carrying capacity due to blood loss or anemia. A "cherry–red" color of the mucous membranes may indicate carbon monoxide poisoning but is not reliably present. Other skin findings such as multiple abscesses, cellulitis, uremic frost, or icterus may point to underlying conditions that affect mental status.

Cardiac Examination

Both tachyarrhythmias and bradyarrhythmias can alter mental status because of decreased cardiac output. Paroxysmal arrhythmias, chronic atrial fibrillation, valvular heart disease, or intracardiac shunts may all predispose to embolization and stroke. Infectious endocarditis is also an important risk factor for stroke. Acute myocardial infarction may reduce cardiac output enough to depress consciousness.

Abdominal Examination

Organomegaly, ascites, bruits, and pulsatile masses should be noted to detect conditions that are causative of altered mental status. Hepatomegaly, ascites, and flank area ecchymoses may be signs of disorders that may cause altered mental status. Pelvic and rectal examinations may be necessary in certain comatose patients in whom there is no obvious cause for abnormal vital signs.

LABORATORY STUDIES AND IMAGING

Laboratory Studies

In general, the use of "routine" laboratory studies is discouraged since such tests rarely yield useful information; it is usually much more efficient to obtain selected tests to answer specific questions. In unconscious patients, however, much of the information usually obtained from the history and physical examination is unavailable, and the clinician is more often forced to rely on a "shotgun" approach to obtaining laboratory data.

A *CBC* is appropriate in most patients; severe anemia, marked leukopenia, or leukocytosis should be noted. Marked reduction in the platelet count may indicate sepsis, disseminated intravascular coagulation (DIC), eclampsia (HELLP syndrome), or alcoholism and implies an increased risk of bleeding. Abnormal clotting studies (*prothrombin time [PT] and partial thromboplastin time [PTT]*) indicate either a coagulopathy or treatment with anticoagulants. Blood *glucose* should be checked, as either marked hypoglycemia or hyperglycemia can result in coma. Serum *electrolytes and osmolality* and *BUN* should be checked. (Note that elevated BUN, unless acute, is usually not associated with profound alteration of consciousness.) In patients with seizures, assays for commonly used anticonvulsants can be helpful in suggesting a preexisting seizure disorder and assessing the adequacy of treatment.

Arterial blood gases allow assessment of the patient's respiratory status; profound hypoxemia or hypercarbia or severe acidemia or alkalemia may be either the cause or the effect of alterations in mental status. A *blood alcohol level* may be helpful in excluding alcohol intoxication but is not very helpful in demonstrating that a patient's condition is *due* to alcohol intoxication. *Urine drug screens* are of little help; these qualitative tests only confirm the presence or absence of a few substances and, even if positive, do not demonstrate that the substance(s) detected is the cause of the patient's symptoms. Once a differential diagnosis is established, further studies may be helpful.

Lumbar puncture can confirm or exclude infectious meningitis or subarachnoid hemorrhage. In unconscious patients, lumbar puncture should be delayed until after a computed tomography (CT) scan has been obtained. If infectious meningitis is suspected, empiric antibiotic treatment should be started immediately and lumbar puncture performed when it is determined to be safe. Lumbar puncture is essential if subarachnoid hemorrhage is suspected and CT scanning is negative.

Electroencephalography (EEG) is rarely indicated on an emergency basis. However, EEG may be diagnostic when nonconvulsive seizure activity is suspected. This may occur in patients who present with status epilepticus; if patients do not begin to recover after their obvious seizures are controlled, continuing nonconvulsive seizures may be present. Occasional patients who present apparently awake but confused may be having continuous nonconvulsive seizures. Finally, urgent EEG should be considered in any patient who has required neuromuscular blockade to facilitate management of seizures, to be sure that the seizure activity is actually stopped.

Imaging Studies

CT scanning of the head is the most important emergency radiographic study in patients with coma or altered consciousness; for most scans obtained in the acute care setting, no contrast material is needed. CT scans can be obtained within minutes, even in minimally cooperative patients, and will reliably detect or exclude many intracranial structural lesions such as epidural and subdural hematomas, intracerebral hemorrhages, abcesses and tumors, acute hydrocephalus, etc. CT will usually (but not always) identify subarachnoid hemorrhage.[8] CT images will also easily identify skull fractures; *plain films of the skull* are rarely needed. CT scans are less sensitive in identifying small lesions in the brainstem and posterior fossa; for these patients, *magnetic resonance imaging (MRI)* is the procedure of choice. MR imaging requires much more time and much more patient cooperation and usually adds little information in the *emergency* evaluation of unconscious patients.

Cervical spine films should be obtained in all patients in whom trauma to the cervical spine cannot be excluded. The neck should be immobilized until the cervical spine has been cleared.

SPECIFIC CAUSES OF COMA AND ALTERED MENTAL STATUS

Coma or altered mental status may result from a wide variety of primary or secondary processes affecting the nervous system. Table 3-4 lists some of the more important clinical problems. Much more extensive lists can be found in the classic text by Plum

TABLE 3-4
COMMON CAUSES OF COMA

Focal Lesions

History of focal signs at onset, focal findings on examination, imaging
studies abnormal

Trauma: epidural or subdural hematomas, intracerebral hemorrhage,
cerebral or brainstem contusion.

Infection: brain abscess (bacterial, fungal, *Toxoplasma*, and so on), focal
encephalitis (herpes simplex)

Stroke: intracerebral hemorrhage, ischemic stroke (large), brainstem
stroke, or hemorrhage

Neoplasm: primary or metastatic, especially if large or multiple, or
associated with significant cerebral edema.

Nonfocal (Diffuse) Lesions

No history of focal signs at onset, no focal findings on examination, imaging
studies normal or nondiagnostic.

Trauma: diffuse neuronal injury, increased intracranial pressure, traumatic
subarachnoid hemorrhage.

Infection: meningitis (especially bacterial), encephalitis

Vascular: spontaneous subarachnoid hemorrhage, hypertensive
encephalopathy

Seizures: convulsive or nonconvulsive, status epilepticus

Toxic/metabolic disorders:

Hypoxemia/global ischemia/hypercarbia

Hypoglycemia/hyperglycemia, ketoacidosis

Electrolyte disorders

Hyponatremia/hypernatremia

Hypercalcemia

Hepatic failure

Renal failure

Thyroid disease: thyroid storm, myxedema coma

Hyperthermia: heat stroke, neuroleptic malignant syndrome

Hypothermia: exposure

Drugs and toxins:

Alcohol intoxication

Opiates and barbiturates

Benzodiazepines and other sedatives and anxiolytics

Antidepressants, phenothiazines, other psychiatric drugs

Anticonvulsants

Multiple illicit drugs

and Posner.[9] Many of these conditions are extremely unlikely to be seen in the acute care setting.

Trauma

Head trauma can cause coma by several different mechanisms, and more than one mechanism may be important in a given patient. *Structural lesions* resulting from head injury include epidural and subdural hematomas, as well as intracerebral or brainstem hemorrhages and contusions. These lesions may cause coma by raising intracranial pressure (ICP), thereby reducing cerebral blood flow, or by compression of the ARAS via herniation syndromes, or by direct injury to the ARAS (as in brainstem hemorrhage). Patients with coma following head injury should be assumed to have raised ICP and be treated accordingly. Hyperventilation will rapidly lower the ICP but may also reduce cerebral blood flow; it should be utilized only when urgently needed and only for as long as necessary to institute other measures.[10] Rapid infusion of mannitol 0.75 to 1.0 mg/kg will also lower ICP, albeit more slowly. Other measures include neuromuscular blockade and CSF drainage (when available). The definitive diagnostic procedure is usually CT scanning. Trauma may also result in *diffuse neuronal injury* with no identifiable structural lesion. The pathophysiology of this process is complex, but there is marked impairment of cerebral blood flow and increases in the levels of extracellular excitatory amino acids, both of which result in ongoing neuronal injury. These patients develop cerebral edema with a marked rise in intracranial pressure, further compromising already tenuous cerebral blood flow. No specific treatment is available and management is controversial; every effort should be made to maintain systemic blood pressure and oxygenation, and neurosurgical consultation should be obtained.

Infection

Acute bacterial meningitis is virtually always fatal unless treated promptly and aggressively. The classical clinical triad is headache, fever, and nuchal rigidity; mental status changes occur early and patients may present in stupor or coma. These patients will not, of course, complain of headache, but nuchal rigidity can be detected even in comatose patients. Treatment should be initiated as soon as possible after the diagnosis is suspected; it is preferable but not mandatory that a lumbar puncture (LP) be obtained prior to beginning treatment, both to confirm the clinical diagnosis and to obtain CSF for bacteriologic studies. There has been endless controversy regarding the need to obtain a CT scan of the brain prior to performing an LP. Although it is widely agreed that the risk of herniation following LP in these patients is actually very low, the practical fact is that most physicians are reluctant to proceed with LP without prior neuroimaging. Accordingly, empiric antibiotic therapy should be initiated immediately and the LP completed as soon as possible thereafter. CSF cultures may remain positive for several hours following the first dose of antibiotics, and assays for bacterial antigens may yield a specific diagnosis even if cultures are negative. Current recommendations are that therapy be initiated with broad-spectrum antibiotic coverage (including coverage for *Listeria*) until antibiotic sensitivities are known.[11,12] Immunosuppressed patients (due to AIDS, chemotherapy, steroid therapy, and so on) may require broader coverage.

Meningitis may be caused by organisms other than bacteria, such as mycobacteria, fungi, spirochetes, and viruses, and by noninfectious processes such as cancer and some drugs. These conditions are loosely grouped under the term *aseptic meningitis*. They tend to be less acute in onset and less fulminant in their course than bacterial meningitis but ultimately may be no less lethal. They are often characterized by a predominance of lymphocytes in the CSF rather than by polymorphonuclear cells (PMNs), but this is not reliable, since PMNs may predominate early in the course. These conditions are therefore often difficult or impossible to distinguish reliably from acute bacterial meningitis, especially in the acute setting. In general, it is better to assume that acute meningitis is bacterial until proved otherwise.

Encephalitis is an acute febrile illness characterized by fever, headache, and altered mental status. Meningeal signs are common but may not be dramatic. Seizures are common and focal neurologic signs may occur. The CSF often shows a lymphocytic pleocytosis but may be normal early in the course. Treatment and prognosis depend on the specific causative organism; although viral infections are the most frequent cause, a similar picture can result from Rocky Mountain spotted fever, erlichiosis, Lyme disease, or leptospirosis and from protozoan diseases such as *Naegleria*.[12] Extensive diagnostic testing is often required to establish a diagnosis. The most common sporadic viral encephalitis in the United States is caused by *Herpes simplex type 1 (HSV)*. The clinical diagnosis may be supported by MRI evidence of an acute inflammatory lesion in the temporal lobes and by characteristic EEG abnormalities. Definitive diagnosis is usually by demonstration of herpesvirus in the CSF by the polymerase chain reaction (PCR). Suspected HSV encephalitis should be treated empirically with IV acyclovir 10 mg/kg q8h. During those months when mosquitoes are active, arthropod-borne encephalitides such as eastern or western equine encephalitis, West Nile encephalitis, and others may be seen.

Stroke

Stroke is discussed in detail in Chapter 4. Acute ischemic stroke is rarely a cause of coma unless the lesion is in the brainstem. Stroke syndromes that present with rapid decline in mental status should suggest intracerebral hemorrhage; CT scanning is diagnostic. Some patients with acute parenchymal hemorrhage, especially in the cerebellum, may benefit from emergency surgery, and neurosurgical consultation should be considered. Ischemic stroke may result in secondary cerebral edema with increased intracranial pressure and herniation, usually over a course of several days; CT scanning is diagnostic. Treatment of these patients is expectant and the prognosis usually bleak.

Seizures

Seizure activity may cause altered mental status or coma by several mechanisms. Many seizures, of course, are followed by a postictal period of altered mental status ranging in duration from minutes to hours or even longer. Often the history will suggest the diagnosis; the patients will show gradual recovery without specific treatment, reassuring the physician that the process is benign and self-limited. More difficult to recognize, and less familiar, are situations in which altered mental status or coma are the result of ongoing seizure activity. In patients with prolonged convulsive status epilepticus, the motor manifestations may gradually wane, leaving the patient comatose but without obvious seizure activity. This may occur as well in patients treated for convulsive status; the convulsive movements may stop, giving the physician the illusion that the seizures have been controlled while the brain seizure activity continues unabated. This is a special problem, of course, in the occasional patients who require neuromuscular blocking agents to facilitate the management of their convulsive seizures. In addition, occasional patients are seen with nonconvulsive complex partial or absence seizures. Very careful observation of these patients will often reveal subtle signs of seizure activity such as intermittent or persistent nystagmus, subtle twitching of the mouth, the face, or the extremities, and so on. Emergency EEG, if available, will confirm the diagnosis. If the diagnosis is strongly suspected and EEG is not available, empiric treatment for status epilepticus is appropriate.

Hypertensive Encephalopathy

Hypertensive encephalopathy (HE) is a fairly unusual condition, more often suspected than confirmed. It occurs as a result of the failure of cerebral vascular autoregulation in the face of sustained severe hypertension, usually with mean arterial blood pressure (MAP) greater than 160 mmHg. Patients develop cerebral edema with raised ICP and petechial hemorrhages. The clinical picture is characterized by altered mental status that may progress to coma, seizures, papilledema, and marked elevation of blood pressure. Focal signs are usually mild and transient. The CT scan may reveal extensive low-density regions in both hemispheres, suggesting bilateral strokes, but these lesions are completely reversible with treatment. HE is a true medical emergency with high mortality if not treated aggressively. The usual treatment is IV nitroprusside to control the blood pressure rapidly, but care must be taken not to lower the blood pressure too far too fast; in the face of increased ICP, excessive lowering of systemic blood pressure may lead to cerebral ischemia.

A safe rule of thumb is to lower the MAP by 25% over the first hour.[13] Use of nitroprusside usually requires an arterial line for continuous measurement of blood pressure; agents such as labetolol may be used if an arterial line is not available.

Toxic and Metabolic Causes of Coma

In most acute care settings, toxic or metabolic disorders are the most common causes of coma and other altered mental states such as acute confusion and delirium. These disorders are generally characterized by absence of focal signs and relative preservation of brainstem function with more profound impairment of cerebral function. Especially in the elderly, acute delirium may complicate virtually any medical condition or may be provoked by a wide variety of drugs and toxins. Accordingly, every effort should be made to obtain a detailed drug history. Family members and others should be asked about any other medications or toxins available in the home that may have been ingested by mistake. The "plastic bag test," in which family members are asked to bring in the entire contents of the family medicine chest in a plastic bag, may be diagnostic. Regardless of the specific cause, the clinical presentations are quite similar and nonspecific. A complete discussion of each cannot be undertaken in this brief review, but some of the more common will be discussed briefly.

Hypoxia

The brain is dependent on a continuing supply of oxygen and metabolic substrates to maintain its intense metabolic activity; even a very brief interruption leads to impaired consciousness or coma. Cerebral hypoxia most commonly results from perfusion failure (see below) but may result as well from impairment of ventilation, impairment of pulmonary gas exchange (pulmonary embolism, severe pneumonia, acute respiratory distress syndrome, pulmonary edema, and so on), or reduced blood oxygen carrying capacity, as in carbon monoxide (CO) poisoning or methemoglobinemia. CO poisoning is not uncommon; the diagnosis is often suggested by the history. A clinical clue is the presence of hypoxemia without cyanosis; the well-known "cherry-red" color of the mucous membranes is uncommon and not reliable. There is no effective treatment for the brain disorder per se in hypoxia; treatment should be directed at the underlying disorder. The prognosis depends on the depth and duration of the cerebral hypoxia.

Ischemia

In addition to requiring a continuing supply of oxygen and nutrients, as noted above, the brain also requires continuous perfusion to remove the toxic by-products of its metabolism. Cerebral ischemia thus delivers a double insult, both depriving the brain of oxygen and substrate and allowing the toxic by-products of anaerobic metabolism to accumulate rapidly. In this setting, permanent neuronal injury may occur within minutes.

Global cerebral ischemia most often results from pump failure (cardiogenic shock, cardiac arrest, and so on) but may also develop as a consequence of profound systemic hypotension of whatever cause. A similar clinical picture may be seen as a consequence of widespread small vessel occlusive disease, such as in disseminated intravascular coagulation, thrombotic thrombocytopenic purpura, and similar conditions. As in the case of cerebral hypoxia, there is no treatment for the brain disorder per se; everything depends on prompt recognition and treatment of the primary problem.

Hypoglycemia and Hyperglycemia

Profound hypoglycemia is a fairly common cause of altered mental status in the acute care setting. Causes include inadequate food intake in patients taking insulin or oral hypoglycemic agents or overdose of these medications. The treatment is rapid replacement of glucose (with thiamine, as indicated). Hyperglycemia, with or without ketoacidosis, is also an important cause of coma. It must be remembered that either hypoglycemia or hyperglycemia may cause seizures (including focal seizures) and focal neurologic deficits mimicking stroke. The appropriate treatment is to normalize the blood sugar; anticonvulsants and stroke treatment protocols are ineffective and not indicated.

Electrolyte Abnormalities

Severe hyponatremia may cause altered mental status or coma. Symptoms usually do not occur unless the serum sodium is <125 mEq/L; seizures and coma usually do not occur unless the serum sodium is <115 mEq/L. The severity of the clinical syndrome depends both on the sodium level and on the rate of decrease of the sodium; even profound hyponatremia may be well tolerated if developed over a long period of time. The treatment of severe hyponatremia remains somewhat controversial, since too rapid correction can have severe consequences, including osmotic demyelination (central pontine myelinolysis). In general, the more acute the hyponatremia, the more rapidly replacement can proceed.[14] Hypernatremia is less commonly encountered and is most often the consequence of dehydration. It may be encountered in patients receiving parenteral feedings, especially if they are also receiving diuretics. It should be considered in chronically debilitated patients, especially the very elderly, with altered mental status. The treatment is rehydration; this should be undertaken with care to avoid the risk of water intoxication. Hypercalcemia is an occasional cause of obtundation and coma, particularly in patients with cancer.

Hepatic and Renal Failure

Either hepatic or renal failure may produce a clinical syndrome characterized by progressive obtundation, asterixis and/or myoclonus, and eventual coma. This clinical syndrome is nonspecific and similar to that seen in a wide variety of other toxic/metabolic encephalopathies. The diagnosis in each case will be based on clinical suspicion and appropriate laboratory studies. It should be remembered that these clinical syndromes are often reversible, so that aggressive evaluation and treatment should be pursued.

Alcohol Intoxication

Ethyl alcohol is the most common intoxicant encountered in the acute care setting. The effects of alcohol are usually transient and no treatment is required. It is essential that the physician not be misled and assume that the presence of alcohol, even at high levels, is necessarily the cause of a given patient's altered mental status. Any of the other causes of altered mental status or coma, including potentially lethal conditions such as intracranial mass lesions, meningitis, and others may easily be present but overlooked in the apparently intoxicated patient. Accordingly, each patient needs careful assessment. Other alcohols such as methanol or ethylene glycol are occasionally used as intoxicants as well. Their presence should be suspected in an apparently intoxicated patient with a significant osmolal gap and negative ethanol level.

Drugs

An enormous number of drugs may cause obtundation and coma, usually, but not necessarily, when taken in overdose. Prescription drugs, over-the-counter drugs, and recreational drugs all may be responsible. Common urine drug screens are qualitative and indicate only that a patient has used a drug recently; such screens do not indicate that any given drug is the cause of the patient's clinical symptoms. Specific assays are available for some agents and may be very helpful. *Opiates* are common offenders; the diagnosis is established by the prompt response to intravenous naloxone. The physician should recall that the duration of action of the offending drug may exceed that of naloxone and that repeated doses may be needed. *Barbiturates* are also common, but no diagnostic or therapeutic antidote is available. It should be recalled that barbiturates per se have no permanent adverse effects on the brain and that even profoundly depressed patients may make a full recovery. *Benzodiazepines* rarely cause coma by themselves but may potentiate other intoxicants; flumazenil will reverse benzodiazepine effects but may provoke acute withdrawal with agitation, delirium, and seizures.

Anticholinergic drugs such as atropine, trihexyphenidyl, and benztropine, as well as agents such as tricyclic antidepressants (e.g., amitriptyline) often cause a severe agitated delirium; patients present with dilated pupils, tachycardia, and hot, dry, flushed skin. ("Mad as a hatter, red as a beet, dry as a bone.") Treatment with physostigmine may result in dramatic, albeit transient, improvement.

With any drug-induced or metabolic encephalopathy, specific treatment depends on the specific cause. Supportive measures include keeping the patient in a quiet and comfortable space; a family member or other person may help to keep the patient calm. Pain should be controlled. Pharmacologic treatment should be avoided if possible. When needed, antipsychotic drugs such as haloperidol and others are probably the drugs of choice. Benzodiazepines are also widely used, but there are few data regarding their effectiveness in this setting.[5]

Summary

The patient with severely altered mental status or coma is a true medical emergency with a high likelihood of death or permanent disability. The physician's immediate actions should be as follows:

1. Assess the patient's vital signs and stabilize if necessary.
2. Determine whether the underlying disorder is structural or diffuse.
3. Initiate emergency treatment.
4. Determine the specific diagnosis.
5. Arrange appropriate consultation and continuing treatment.

The initial emphasis should always be on the rapid identification and management of potentially treatable conditions. It is much less critical if the diagnosis of a self-limited or untreatable condition is missed.

REFERENCES

1. Kanich WS, Brady WJ, Huff SJ. Altered mental status in the emergency department: most efficient diagnostic tools and most frequent causes. *Ann Emerg Med* 2001;37:547.

2. The Multi-Society Task Force on PVS. Medical aspects of the persistent vegetative state. *N Engl J Med* 1994;330:1499–1508, 1572–1579.

3. Hustey FM, Meldon SW. The prevalence and documentation of impaired mental status in elderly emergency department patients. *Ann Emerg Med* 2002;39:248–253.

4. Sanders AB. Missed delirium in older emergency department patients: a quality-of-care problem. *Ann Emerg Med* 2002;39:338–341.

5. American Psychiatric Association Work Group on Delirium. Practice guideline for the treatment of patients with delirium. *Am J Psychiatry* 1999;156(Suppl):1–20.

6. Johnson MH. Assessing confused patients. *J Neurol Neurosurg Psychiatry* 2001; 71(Suppl I):i7.

7. Cartlidge N. States related to or confused with coma. *J Neurol Neurosurg Psychiatry* 2001;71(Suppl I):i18.

8. Edlow JA, Wyer PC. Feedback: computed tomography for subarachnoid hemorrhage—don't throw the baby out with the bathwater [Response]. *Ann Emerg Med* 2001; 37:680–685.

9. Plum F, Posner JB. *The Diagnosis of Stupor and Coma,* 3rd ed. Philadelphia: FA Davis, 1982.

10. Chesnut RM. Guidelines for the management of severe head injury: what we know and what we think we know. *J Trauma* 1997;42(Suppl):S19–S22.

11. Feske SK. Coma and confusional states: emergency diagnosis and management. *Neurol Clin North Am* 1998;16:237.

12. Pruitt AA. Infections of the nervous system. *Neurol Clin North Am* 1998;16:419.

13. Gray RO, Mathews JJ. Hypertension. In: Marx JA, et al., eds. *Rosen's Emergency Medicine: Concepts and Clinical Practice,* 5th ed. St. Louis: Mosby, 2001, pp 1158–1171.

14. Sagar SM. Toxic and metabolic disorders. In: Samuels MA, ed. *Manual of Neurologic Therapeutics,* 6th ed. Philadelphia: Lippincott Williams & Wilkins, 1999, p 327.

4

ACUTE FOCAL NEUROLOGIC DEFICITS

Patients with acute focal neurologic deficits are frequently seen in the acute care setting and can pose difficult challenges to the clinical skills of physicians. These patients are sometimes subjected to a brief and superficial neurologic examination and then sent for a computed tomography (CT) scan of the head in the hope that some diagnosis will be revealed. When, as frequently occurs, the scan is unrevealing, the patient is assigned a tentative but virtually meaningless diagnosis such as "rule out stroke." In the past, when treatment options were limited, this approach, although certainly not elegant, was at least not likely to result in much actual harm to the patient. Now, with potentially beneficial but hazardous treatments available (e.g., thrombolytic therapy for stroke), there are potentially more serious consequences for incorrect or delayed diagnoses, and greater pressure on the acute care physician to make a correct and timely diagnosis.

An *acute neurologic deficit* is one that develops over 24 hours or less. In fact, most such deficits evolve much more rapidly, often over a period of only a few minutes. A *focal* deficit is one that is due to injury or dysfunction in a localized area of the nervous system. The focal nature of the neurologic deficit may not always be immediately apparent; a patient who at first appears to be confused or disoriented (suggesting a diffuse process) may be found on careful evaluation to actually have dysphasia, a disorder of language function caused by a discrete focal lesion. Conversely, a patient who presents with weakness in the lower extremities may be found on careful evaluation to have generalized weakness and decreased reflexes, suggesting a more diffuse process. Clearly, in both examples, the correct diagnosis depends on careful clinical assessment.

CLINICAL ASSESSMENT

The process of clinical diagnosis depends on a clear understanding of what is to be diagnosed. Accordingly, the importance of a clear and adequate history cannot be overemphasized. Failure to obtain an adequate history can easily result in expensive, invasive, potentially hazardous, and ultimately useless investigation of symptoms never actually experienced by the patient. At the same time, necessary and appropriate studies may be omitted. Even with patients who are confused, disoriented, or unconscious (signs usually suggesting a diffuse process), a proper history, obtained from family or other witnesses, may suggest a focal onset to the clinical syndrome.

The most important goal of the history is to obtain an accurate and detailed description of the specific symptoms experienced by the patient. An appropriately detailed history will often suggest the correct diagnosis, or at least sharply limit the number of reasonable diagnoses. For example, pain in the left shoulder and left arm may be due to a cervical radiculopathy, a brachial plexus lesion, a torn rotator cuff, or coronary artery disease (among other possibilities); an adequate history will often distinguish among these. Similarly, a complaint of "dizziness" may actually refer to vertigo, dysequilibrium, impending syncope, or lightheadedness. Each of these symptoms implies a different differential diagnosis, and investigation of any one of them will probably not help in the diagnosis of any of the others. It is helpful to ask about any specific functional impairments; this will often give the physician a much better insight into the patient's complaints than a simple recitation of symptoms. Once the character of the patient's symptoms is clearly understood, the usual questions concerning onset, progression, associated symptoms, etc., should be pursued.

The next step in the clinical assessment is the neurologic examination. This has been discussed in detail in Chapter 2; only a few comments will be added here. The examination should serve to:

1. Clarify the exact nature of the clinical symptoms. For example, is a "weak" leg truly weak, or is it actually numb, clumsy, or stiff? Is the patient with slurred speech truly dysphasic or only dysarthric?
2. Identify clinical findings not recognized by the patient. For example, is a weak leg accompanied by minor weakness in the ipsilateral arm?
3. Localize the anatomic basis for the symptom. For example, is leg weakness accompanied by increased reflexes and an upgoing toe, or by absent reflexes and muscle atrophy?

In many cases, a fairly comprehensive neurologic examination will be needed. A "complete" examination is rarely needed even if it were possible. Still, the examination should be carefully planned as one can easily omit a crucial part of the examination. It is better to be too detailed than to be too superficial. It is particularly important to "examine the complaint," that is, to observe the patient attempting to perform the specific activity that is problematic. A patient with a gait disorder, for example, should be observed while trying to walk and cannot be fully examined while lying supine on a gurney.

At the conclusion of the initial clinical assessment, the physician should be prepared to answer three questions:

1. Are the patient's symptoms probably due to a focal lesion in the nervous system?
2. Where is the lesion?
3. What is (are) the likely cause(s) of the lesion?

Note that the likely location of the lesion must be determined before a differential diagnosis can be suggested. The ability to localize the lesion depends on the reliability of the neurologic examination A brief list of some common clues to localization is given in Table 4-1. The more sophisticated the physician's clinical skills, the more accurate the anatomic diagnosis and the shorter the differential diagnosis is likely to be. Once a differential diagnosis is established, the necessary laboratory and imaging studies can be obtained to confirm the correct diagnosis and to exclude the others. An imaging study of the wrong part of the body (e.g., a CT scan of the head in a patient who has a spinal cord problem) is unlikely to contribute much to diagnostic clarity.

Acute focal neurologic deficits may be due to a wide variety of entities. The most likely causes in a particular patient are determined by the part of the nervous system affected, the time course, and the clinical context. The most common causes of lesions in various parts of the nervous system are discussed below.

ACUTE FOCAL LESIONS OF THE BRAIN AND BRAINSTEM

The most common causes of acute focal lesions affecting the brain and brainstem are listed in Table 4-2.

Stroke

The most common cause of an acute focal lesion affecting the brain, the brainstem, or the cerebellum is stroke. A *stroke* is defined as an acute focal loss of brain function caused by a disruption of brain blood flow. Depending on their mechanism, strokes are classified as either *ischemic* or *hemorrhagic;* most strokes (approximately 85%) are ischemic. The term *stroke* is not ordinarily applied to the more global ischemic injury resulting from profound hypotension, cardiac arrest, and so on. The term *cerebrovascular accident* (CVA), often used as a synonym for stroke, conveys no additional information. *Subarachnoid hemorrhage,* in which bleeding occurs into the subarachnoid space, often from a ruptured aneurysm or other vascular lesion, is not included in this definition of stroke.

Ischemic stroke occurs as a result of partial or complete occlusion of a vessel supplying blood to the brain. Depending on the adequacy of any collateral circulation, the cerebral blood flow (CBF) to the affected region of the brain is reduced. Reduction of CBF below 50% of normal (approx. 20 mL blood/100 g brain tissue/min) results in neuronal dysfunction and the appearance of neurologic deficits. Reduction of CBF below 25% of normal causes metabolic failure and initiates a cascade of events leading to cell death. Current thinking is that an ischemic stroke is charac-

TABLE 4-1
CLUES TO CLINICAL LOCALIZATION

Brain Lesions
Language disorders (aphasias)[a]
Agnosias and apraxias[b]
Visual field defects (affecting both eyes)[c]
Motor deficits, sensory deficits involving the face, arm, and leg on the same
    side of the body (the side opposite the lesion)
Alterations of consciousness, perception, or behavior
"Cortical" sensory impairment—astereognosis, impaired graphesthesia, etc.

Brainstem Lesions
Cranial nerve abnormalities[d]
Alternating hemiplegia—weakness of cranial nerve function on one side and
    of the body on the opposite side

Spinal Cord Lesions
Sensory or motor "levels"
Mixed "upper motor neuron" and "lower motor neuron" signs
Sensory dissociation (impaired pain/temperature sensation on one side of the
    body, impaired vibration/position sense on the opposite side)
Sensory/motor dissociation (impaired pain/temperature sensation on one side
    of the body, impaired motor function on the opposite side)
Early impairment of bladder, bowel, or sexual function

Peripheral Nerve/Root Lesions
Motor impairment, sensory impairment, or both confined to the distribution
    of a single peripheral nerve or nerve root
Pain confined to the distribution of a single peripheral nerve or nerve root

---

[a] Aphasia implies a lesion in the dominant (usually the left) hemisphere. The many subtypes of aphasias
  discussed in textbooks are rarely seen in pure form in clinical practice and are of little localizing value
  in the emergency setting.
[b] These are most often recognized in patients with right parietal lesions (in whom language function is
  preserved).
[c] Vision deficits confined to only one eye are caused by lesions anterior to the optic chiasm on the affected
  side, not by lesions of the brain.
[d] Cranial nerve lesions due to brainstem lesions will virtually always be associated with clinical signs
  affecting other parts of the nervous system (e.g., long tract signs).

---

terized by an *ischemic core*, in which CBF is markedly reduced; permanent neuronal
injury occurs within minutes. The core is surrounded by an *ischemic penumbra*,
a zone of relative reduction of CBF in which permanent neuronal injury may be
delayed for several hours. The goal of acute stroke therapy is to enhance the prospects
for survival of this potentially salvageable tissue, either by restoring adequate perfusion to ischemic tissue before permanent damage occurs, or by enhancing the ability
of brain tissue to withstand ischemic stress.[1]

TABLE 4-2 ————————————————————————————

ETIOLOGIES OF ACUTE FOCAL LESIONS OF
THE BRAIN AND BRAINSTEM

Vascular Disorders
Stroke (ischemic or hemorrhagic)
Transient ischemic attack (TIA)
Migraine
Venous thrombosis

Infectious Disorders
Brain abscess (bacterial, fungal, protozoan, etc.)
Encephalitis (especially herpes simplex)

Mass Lesions
Neoplasms (primary and metastatic)
Epidural/subdural hematomas/empyemas

Metabolic Disorders
Hypoglycemia/hyperglycemia

Seizures
Focal seizures
Postictal (Todd's) paralysis

Inflammatory/Granulomatous Disorders
Multiple sclerosis
Sarcoidosis
Cerebral vasculitis (with or without systemic vasculitis)

Hemorrhagic stroke occurs as a result of leakage of blood from a damaged vessel into the surrounding brain; tissue damage may occur as a result of the physical disruption of brain parenchyma, displacement or distortion of nearby structures (mass effect), brain edema, and raised intracranial pressure. In some cases, an initial ischemic infarction can be complicated by secondary hemorrhage into the infarcted tissue.

It is important to recognize that either vascular occlusion or hemorrhage occur as the final result of some underlying process; effective diagnosis and management require recognition and treatment not only of the stroke syndrome but of the underlying cause as well. Table 4-3 lists some potential causes of stroke. Clearly, many of these diagnoses are not established in the acute care setting.

Clinical Evaluation

In most cases, the clinical diagnosis of stroke is straightforward. The abrupt onset of symptoms consistent with an acute focal brain injury is virtually diagnostic. Often the clinical picture will suggest a lesion in a specific vascular territory, such as the

TABLE 4-3

CAUSES OF STROKE[a]

A. Ischemic Stroke

Vascular Disorders
Atheromatous disease (extracranial or intracranial)
Small-vessel vasculopathy (diabetes, hypertension, lupus, etc)
Primary vascular disease (fibromuscular dysplasia, congenital stenosis or
    atresia, Moya—moya, etc.)
Arterial dissection (spontaneous or traumatic)
Infectious/inflammatory disease (meningitis, granulomatous angiitis, etc.)

Cardiac Disorders
Atrial fibrillation
Myocardial infarction
Valvular heart disease, endocarditis
Cardiomyopathies
Intracardiac shunts (patent foramen ovale, atrial septal defects, etc.)
Atrial myxoma

Hematologic Disorders
Sickle cell disease
Hyperviscosity syndromes
Hypercoaguable states (pregnancy, oral contraceptives, coagulopathies)

B. Hemorrhagic Stroke
Small vessel vasculopathy (hypertension, diabetes, amyloid angiopathy, etc.)
Vascular anomalies (arteriovenous malformation, hemangiomas, etc)
Intracranial aneurysms (including mycotic aneurysms)
Coagulation disorders (primary and iatrogenic)

[a] This list is not intended to be exhaustive, but rather to give the reader some sense of the wide range
   of different disorders that may present with stroke.

middle cerebral artery or one of its branches, the vertebral-basilar system, and other
locations. Strokes in the territory of the middle cerebral arteries will present with
weakness of the contralateral face and arm with less severe weakness of the leg, and
sometimes with a visual field deficit. With left hemisphere lesions, aphasia may be
present as well. Lesions in the anterior cerebral artery territory will usually have
weakness of the contralateral leg with relative sparing of the arm and face, generally without visual field deficits. Lesions of the posterior cerebral arteries will cause
contralateral visual field deficits, usually with minimal motor deficits. Lesions in the
brainstem may cause a variety of cranial nerve signs, especially diplopia, vertigo, and
dysequilibrium, together with unilateral or bilateral motor deficits. Most patients
with stroke will present with one of a small number of common and easily recognized syndromes.

The time of onset of the symptoms should be accurately determined, if possible. This information is critical if the patient is to be considered a possible candidate for thrombolytic therapy (see below). The manner of onset and subsequent evolution of the symptoms may suggest the likely mechanism of the stroke. Abrupt onset, with the deficit reaching its maximum extent within minutes, suggests embolic occlusion of a vessel, the embolus having originated either in a larger proximal vessel or in the heart. Multiple lesions in different arterial distributions also suggest embolism from a central source. A stuttering course suggests progressive occlusion of an extra- or intracranial vessel, or recurrent emboli from a nearby vessel (such as the internal carotid artery). A history of premonitory transient ischemic attacks (TIAs) suggests atheromatous disease of the ipsilateral internal carotid artery. The presence of severe headache at onset, abrupt loss of consciousness, or steady progression of a neurologic deficit should suggest intracerebral hemorrhage.

The clinical context may also suggest the likely mechanism of the stroke. The presence of atrial fibrillation, a history of cardiac valve disease (or replacement), or evidence of recent myocardial infarction should all suggest possible cardiogenic embolism. Strokes in younger patients should suggest inflammatory vasculopathy, a cardiac lesion, arterial dissection, or (rarely) a coagulopathy.

Patients with suspected stroke need an appropriate neurologic examination. It is often helpful to use a structured rating scale such as the National Institutes of Health Stroke Scale (NIHSS) to record the neurologic deficits and grade the severity of the stroke (Table 4-4). The NIHSS is based directly on a structured neurologic examination and yields scores between 0 and 42. Scores over 20 are generally considered to indicate "severe" stroke; however, a patient with an isolated severe aphasia (NIHSS score 2 or 3) may nonetheless have a devastating injury.

Differential Diagnosis

Even in patients with seemingly "obvious" stroke, it is well to recall that there is ample opportunity for diagnostic error. Error rates of 2% to 20% in the clinical diagnosis of stroke have been reported.[2,3] The potential differential diagnosis includes virtually every cause of an acute focal deficit. The most common conditions mistaken for stroke in one series of 411 patients are listed in Table 4-5. Even though many of these conditions may cause symptoms that appear to be acute, the neurologic deficits actually develop over hours or days or longer. Careful questioning may be necessary to extract a reliable history from anxious patients and families, many of whom will have already made their own diagnosis of stroke before coming to the emergency department.

Imaging Studies

CT scanning remains the initial imaging procedure of choice for most patients with suspected stroke. CT scans can usually be performed quickly and without concern for possible implanted metal, pacemakers, infusion pumps, and other devices. In addition, adequate images can usually be obtained even in minimally cooperative patients. Contrast enhancement is usually omitted but should be considered if there is concern about lesions other than stroke, such as neoplasm or infection. CT is

TABLE 4-4

THE NIH STROKE SCALE

Examination Item	Response	Points
1a. Level of consciousness	Alert	0
	Drowsy	1
	Stuporous	2
	Comatose	3
1b. Level of consciousness Ask patient age and current month	Both correct	0
	One correct	1
	Both incorrect	2
1c. Level of consciousness Ask patient to close eyes. Ask patient to make a fist	Both correct	0
	One correct	1
	Both incorrect	2
2. Best gaze	Normal	0
	Partial gaze palsy	1
	Forced deviation of eyes	2
3. Visual fields	Normal	0
	Partial hemianopia	1
	Complete hemianopia	2
	Bilateral hemianopia (cortical blindness)	3
4. Facial weakness	Normal	0
	Minor weakness	1
	Parial weakness	2
	Complete paralysis	3
5–8. Motor function (test all four limbs)	No drift	0
	Drift present	1
	Some effort against gravity	2
	No effort against gravity	3
	No movement	4
	Not testable	9
9. Limb ataxia (Score if present— cannot be scored in a plegic limb or if patient unable to perform.)	Absent	0
	Present in one limb	1
	Present in two limbs	2
10. Sensory (pinprick)	Normal	0
	Partial loss	1
	Complete loss	2

TABLE 4-4

THE NIH STROKE SCALE *(continued)*

Examination Item	Response	Points
11. Best language	No aphasia	0
	Mild/moderate aphasia	1
	Severe aphasia	2
	Mute	3
12. Dysarthria	Normal articulation	0
	Mild/moderate dysarthria	1
	Unintelligible	2
	Untestable	X
13. Neglect/inattention	None	0
	Partial neglect	1
	Complete neglect	2
Total		0–42

The NIH Stroke Scale—Instructions[a]

1a. The examiner must choose a response even if full evaluation is prevented by obstacles such as an ET tube, language barrier, or bandages—note that the level of arousal, not the content of consciousness, is being evaluated.

1b. Score only the first answer to each question—not partial credit for "close" answers. Do not repeat the questions or "coach" the patient. Aphasic or stuporous patients are scored "2." Patients who cannot speak because of physical barriers (e.g., an ET tube) are scored "1."

1c. Test the nonparetic hand. Another suitable one-step command may be used if the hands cannot be tested. Score only the first response. If the patient does not respond to command, the requested movement can be demonstrated by the examiner.

2. Only horizontal movements are tested. Voluntary, pursuit, or oculocephalic reflex movements can be tested, but not caloric responses.

3. Fields can be tested using confrontation, finger counting, or visual threat. Note that visual *fields* are being tested, not vision in each eye; this can be done even in a patient with monocular blindness. Patients who are blind (from any cause) are scored "3."

4. Ask or use pantomime to encourage the patient to show teeth and to close the eyes. Score grimace to noxious stimulus in the patient who cannot respond.

(continued)

TABLE 4-4

THE NIH STROKE SCALE *(continued)*

5 & 6. The limb is placed in the appropriate position—arm extended 90 degrees (patient sitting) or 45 degrees (patient supine); the leg is placed at 30 degrees elevation (patient is supine). Each limb is tested separately. Score drift if the arm drifts downward before 10 seconds or the leg drifts downward before 5 seconds.

7. Use standard finger-nose-finger and heel-shin maneuvers. Ataxia is scored only if out of proportion to weakness—ataxia is not scored if the patient cannot understand or if the tested limb is plegic. Score 9 only for amputation or joint fusion.

8. Use pinprick or other noxious stimulus. Only sensory loss attributable to stroke can be scored (e.g., do not score sensory loss secondary to peripheral neuropathy).

9. Be sure to distinguish true aphasia from dysarthria (#10). Patients in coma are scored as "3."

10. If aphasia is present, any spontaneous speech is scored. Patients who are mute are scored "2." Score "3" only if speech is physically impossible (e.g., intubated patient).

11. Neglect is scored only if clearly present. Note that neglect may not be testable in patients with severe sensory loss; such patients are scored as normal on this item.

[a] This is only a brief summary of the instructions. Use of the scale should be demonstrated by an experienced user or by instructional video to obtain maximum reliability and reproducible results.
[b] Scores of "9" (untestable items) are not included in the final score.

TABLE 4-5

CONDITIONS THAT MIMICKED STROKE IN 411 PATIENTS

Condition	Frequency (%)
Seizure	13 (16.7)
Systemic infection	13 (16.7)
Brain tumor	12 (15.4)
Toxic/metabolic	10 (12.8)
Positional vertigo	5 (6.4)
Cardiac	4 (5.1)
Syncope	4 (5.1)
Other	17 (4.1)

Other conditions included trauma, subdural hematoma, herpes encephalitis, transient global amnesia, dementia, demyelinating disease, cervical spine fracture, myasthenia gravis, parkinsonism, hypertensive encephalopathy, and conversion disorder.

SOURCE: from Libman RB, et al. Conditions that mimic stroke in the emergency department. *Arch Neurol* 1995;52:1119–1122. (with permission) virtually 100% sensitive in detecting intracerebral blood and is highly sensitive for intracranial mass lesions. Unfortunately, CT is not very sensitive for acute ischemic lesions (approximately 30% are detectable at 3 hours and 60% at 24 hours). In patients with large lesions, subtle changes may be evident within hours but are not reliably present. In effect, CT is more helpful in detecting hemorrhage and excluding alternative diagnoses than in confirming the diagnosis of acute stroke.[4] Even "positive" scans must be interpreted with caution, since a lesion detected on the scan may not be the lesion responsible for the patient's symptoms.

There is wide variation in physician skills in the interpretation of CT scans in patients with acute stroke. In a recent study, physicians presented with a series of test scans interpreted approximately 70% of the studies correctly; neurologists and radiologists fared slightly better than emergency physicians. In films with subtle evidence of intracerebral hemorrhage (an absolute contraindication to thrombolytic therapy; see below), the error rates were as high as 43%. The authors suggest that specific training may be needed if physicians are to use such scans to make treatment decisions.[5]

Magnetic resonance imaging (MRI) is more sensitive than CT in detecting acute ischemic lesions. Although modern MRI systems can obtain images within minutes, the usefulness of MRI is limited by technical considerations. MRI cannot be performed on patients with implanted pacemakers or similar devices, or on patients with ferromagnetic metals in the body. Although technically possible, MRI is more difficult in patients who require mechanical ventilation. MRI imaging requires that the patient remain very still throughout the examination, and the technique may be impossible in confused, aphasic, or agitated patients. Finally, effective MRI requires the immediate availability of equipment and staff, as well as physicians experienced in the interpretation of the images. Despite these limitations, the use of MRI in acute stroke patients is likely to become more widespread, especially as new and more powerful techniques are developed that may directly affect acute treatment decisions. Diffusion- and perfusion-weighted imaging can allow accurate identification of the core and penumbra regions of acute strokes; these techniques may permit rapid identification of patients likely to benefit from thrombolytic therapy (see below).[6–8] MR angiography can provide rapid noninvasive imaging of vascular occlusions and may help select patients who are candidates for intraarterial thrombolytic therapy. MR technology is developing rapidly, and regular consultation with radiologists should be obtained so that stroke patients can receive the benefits of the most up-to-date imaging studies. At present, these approaches are still being evaluated, and their ultimate usefulness in the acute setting is uncertain.

Atheromatous disease of the extracranial and intracranial carotid and vertebral-basilar arterial systems are important causes of stroke. Other vascular disorders such as fibromuscular dysplasia, congenital anomalies, or vasculitis may be important in some patients. *Vascular imaging studies* may provide important information regarding the cause of a stroke or TIA (see below) and may help suggest appropriate treatment to reduce the risk of recurrent stroke. At this time, these studies are of little help in guiding the initial management of the patient with a completed stroke. Techniques available for vascular imaging include ultrasound (extracranial and transcranial), MR angiography, CT angiography, and contrast angiography, among others. The advantages and limitations of these studies are beyond the scope of this discussion; not all studies are easily available in all practice settings. Local availability, expertise, and experience will guide the choice of the most appropriate studies until more definitive comparison data become available.

In patients with suspected cardiogenic embolism, transthoracic and transesophageal ultrasound examinations may be helpful in identifying the source of emboli and in guiding treatment decisions.

Laboratory Studies

The diagnosis of stroke depends largely on the clinical assessment and on the imaging studies. Laboratory studies may help to elucidate the likely cause of the stroke and may be helpful in guiding therapy. The current American Heart Association Guideline suggests that an electrocardiogram (ECG), chest x-ray, complete blood count (CBC) with platelet count, coagulation studies (plasma thromboplastin [PT] and partial thromboplastin time [PTT]), electrolytes, and glucose should be obtained.[9] A *stat* blood glucose should be obtained to rule out severe hypo- or hyperglycemia, either of which may cause acute focal symptoms mimicking stroke or may require treatment (see below). Prolonged ECG monitoring may be helpful in detecting paroxysmal arrhythmias such as atrial fibrillation. Other laboratory studies may be ordered depending on the clinical setting.

Lumbar puncture is usually not indicated, but it may be required in patients with suspected subarachnoid hemorrhage or in patients with suspected meningeal disease (such as infection, tumor infiltration, granulomatous disease, and other conditions).

Electroencephalography (EEG) is rarely indicated, but it may be useful in patients in whom ongoing nonconvulsive seizure activity is suspected.

Acute Stroke Management

Thrombolytic Therapy

The approach to the treatment of acute stroke changed dramatically with publication of a clinical trial of recombinant tissue plasminogen activator (tPA) by the National Institute of Neurological Disorders and Stroke (NINDS) rt-PA Stroke Study Group in 1995.[10] Since then there has been a virtual avalanche of publications regarding the potential risks, benefits, and appropriate use of such treatment. A detailed review of this extensive literature is beyond the scope of this discussion, but the current state of the art can be summarized.

The NINDS trial results demonstrated that treatment with tPA of acute ischemic stroke within 3 hours of symptom onset resulted in a modest improvement in patient outcome. There was an absolute increase of 11% to 13% (relative increase 24% to 35%) in the proportion of patients with normal or near-normal neurologic function at 3 months after stroke compared with placebo-treated controls. This modest benefit did come at a substantial price, however, 6.4% of treated patients had symptomatic intracerebral hemorrhage (with 50% mortality), versus only 0.6% of patients with symptomatic hemorrhage in the placebo group. Despite this increased risk of symptomatic hemorrhage, there was no increase in overall mortality in the treated group. It is important to note that several similar trials (none exactly comparable) failed to duplicate the benefits of the NINDS trial and have emphasized the risks of intracerebral bleeding, especially in patients treated more than 3 hours after symptom onset.[11–13]

Clinical experience with thrombolytic therapy has been quite variable, depending in part on the clinical setting. A recent large study of 3,948 acute stroke patients conducted in a group of 29 community hospitals resulted in only 1.8% of the patients actually being treated with tPA. Protocol violations occurred in 50% of treated patients. Symptomatic intracerebral hemorrhage occurred in 15.7% of treated patients, and in-hospital mortality was significantly higher in treated patients.[14]

By contrast, in a recent smaller study of 269 patients treated in a single institution, an experienced and dedicated stroke team was able to treat 9% of their stroke patients (nearly 15% near the end of the study), with a symptomatic hemorrhage rate of only 4.5%. Even with this highly experienced team, protocol violations occurred in 13% of patients; the hemorrhage rate in those patients was 15%.[15]

At this time, the usefulness of thrombolytic therapy in many clinical settings remains uncertain. Clinical experience continues to accumulate rapidly, and several recent reviews have attempted to summarize these extensive and sometimes conflicting data and to propose specific recommendations for the appropriate use of tPA in patients with acute stroke.[16–19] Based on these reviews, the following recommendations seem reasonable:

1. Safe and effective use of tPA requires that it be used only in patients with acute stroke and only in those patients in whom intracerebral hemorrhage has been excluded. Reference has already been made to the potentially high rates of clinical and radiographic diagnostic errors in patients with stroke. Accordingly, all such patients should be evaluated by physicians with adequate expertise in neurologic diagnosis and CT interpretation. The Canadian Association of Emergency Physicians additionally recommends that all such patients be evaluated by a neurologist prior to treatment.[17]

2. It is essential that the current inclusion and exclusion criteria, and the treatment protocol recommended by the NINDS, be followed scrupulously (Table 4-6). Based on the available data, there is no reason to "push the envelope" by giving tPA to patients who do not meet strict eligibility criteria or in whom the diagnosis or the time of symptom onset is uncertain.

3. tPA should be given only in settings where there are adequate staff and facilities for the close observation and immediate management of patients with bleeding complications (intracranial or elsewhere) from tPA. Neurosurgical consultation and treatment should be available within 2 hours.

4. At this time, the safety and efficacy of thrombolytic therapy remain controversial; it should be given with with the fully informed consent of the patient or other appropriate decision makers.

TABLE 4-6

INCLUSION/EXCLUSION CRITERIA FOR
THROMBOLYTIC THERAPY

Inclusion Criteria
 1. Ischemic stroke with a measurable defect on NIHSS[a]
 2. Clearly defined time of onset within 3 hours of start of treatment[b]
 3. Age >18 years

Exclusion Criteria
 1. Evidence of ICH on pretreatment CT scan[c]
 2. Clinical presentation consistent with subarachnoid hemorrhage, even if
    CT scan is negative
 3. Known arteriovenous malformation or aneurysm
 4. Prior intracranial hemorrhage
 5. Active internal bleeding
 6. Known bleeding diathesis including, but not limited to:
    platelet count <100,000/mm³
    prothrombin time >15 sec; international normalized ratio >1.7, or current
       use of oral anticoagulants
    use of heparin within 48 hr and prolonged partial thromboplastin time
 7. Systolic blood pressure >185 mmHg, or diastolic blood pressure
    >110 mmHg (repeated measurements at the time treatment is to begin);
    aggressive measures should not be used to reduce blood pressure to
    these limits
 8. Intracranial surgery, serious head trauma, stroke within past 3 months
 9. Major surgery with past 14 days
 10. Pregnancy
 11. Post myocardial infarction myocarditis

Warnings
 1. Rapid improvement of neurologic signs
 2. Mild stroke or isolated neurologic deficits[d]
 3. Gastrointestinal or genitourinary bleeding within past 21 days
 4. Recent lumbar puncture
 5. Recent arterial puncture at noncompressible site
 6. Blood glucose <50 or >400 mg/dL
 7. Seizure at stroke onset

---

[a] NIHSS, National Institutes of Health Stroke Scale—see Table 4-4 and text.

[b] Note that time interval is from symptom onset to time of treatment (not time of presentation). Time of
onset is the last time at which the patient was known to be normal. For patients in whom stroke onset
was not observed or in whom stroke occurs during sleep, this will often preclude treatment.

[c] The scan must be interpreted by a physician with demonstrated expertise in the interpretation of
brain CT. See text for discussion.

[d] Some isolated deficits (e.g., aphasia) may be devastating even without a high NIHSS score, and treatment
may well be appropriate.

At this time, thrombolytic therapy should not be considered standard or routine treatment for patients with acute stroke. Safe and effective use of such treatment requires a highly organized and experienced team to provide immediate evaluation and treatment of appropriate patients. Even in the best circumstances, intracranial bleeding will occur in some patients. Patients should be monitored closely during and after tPA infusion: sudden deterioration in the patient's condition may signal bleeding. The tPA infusion should be stopped and an immediate CT scan obtained. If bleeding is confirmed, neurosurgical consultation should be obtained. Cryo-precipitate (6 to 8 U) may be beneficial but is of unproven effectiveness.

Anticoagulant Therapy

Anticoagulation with heparin, and more recently with low molecular weight heparins, has been widely used in the management of patients with acute ischemic stroke for many years. Despite this extensive clinical experience, and multiple clinical trials, there are as yet no data to suggest that acute anticoagulation with heparin or similar agents offers any benefit in the management of acute stroke. Even in patients with progressing strokes or with presumed cardioembolic stroke, groups in whom anticoagulation is most commonly advocated and used, there is little evidence of any benefit. It is generally agreed (based on several studies) that anticoagulation does reduce the long-term risk of recurrent stroke in patients with cardiogenic embolism; it is treatment in the acute setting that remains controversial. The use of anticoagulation for the treatment of acute stroke remains a matter of preference of the treating physician.[9,19–22] A recent review by a joint committee of the American Academy of Neurology and the American Stroke Association concluded that there was no evidence that either heparin or low molecular weight heparin were beneficial in the treatment of patients with acute stroke, regardless of the presumed mechanism of the stroke, and that use of these agents was not recommended.[23]

Antiplatelet Therapy

Several recent clinical trials indicate that aspirin produces a small but definite net reduction in the risk of early recurrent stroke in patients with acute stroke.[23–25] The optimum dose of aspirin remains unclear; either 81 or 325 mg/day can be used based on the preference of the treating physician.

Supportive Care

Hypertension is common in patients with acute stroke. In most cases, immediate treatment is unnecessary and may be contraindicated. The normal autoregulation of cerebral blood flow is thought to fail in the region of the ischemic penumbra; blood flow in this zone of relative ischemia is therefore pressure-dependent, and any reduction in systemic blood pressure will worsen the ischemia, potentially enlarging the zone of infarction.[26] Current American Heart Association guidelines suggest cautious treatment if the systolic pressure exceeds 220 mmHg or if the mean arterial pressure exceeds 130 mmHg.[9] If patients have evidence of acute end-organ damage or other risk from acute hypertension (acute myocardial infarction, congestive heart failure, aortic dissection, etc.), they should be treated as necessary for these conditions.

If thrombolytic therapy is being considered, current guidelines suggest that the blood pressure not exceed 185/110 at the time of treatment (Table 4-6). The guidelines are based on those utilized in the NINDS trial and are not supported by experimental evidence. If blood pressure exceeds the recommended level, nitroglycerin paste or one or two small doses of IV labetolol (10 to 20 mg) may be given to reduce blood pressure to this level. If these measures are ineffective, the patient should not be treated with tPA. If there is a marked increase in blood pressure following tPA administration, more aggressive measures should be used as needed to maintain blood pressure no higher than 185/110. For any emergency department using thrombolytic therapy, a specific written protocol for blood pressure management should be immediately available.[10,17]

Hypotension is much less common following acute ischemic stroke. Because of the risk that diminished perfusion will lead to infarct extension, aggressive measures to manage hypotension (volume expansion, inotropic agents, vasopressors) should be used to maintain blood pressure in the normal range.[16]

Hyperglycemia has been associated with worsened outcome in acute stroke. It is not clear whether the hyperglycemia actually causes worsening, possibly by facilitating continued anaerobic metabolism in areas of relative brain ischemia, or whether the elevated blood sugar is a stress reaction in patients with more severe stroke.[27,28] Treatment with insulin may be appropriate to achieve normal glucose levels, but no clinical trials are available that bear directly on this point.[29]

Hyperthermia is also associated with worse outcome in patients with stroke. Even mild elevations in temperature may have a measurable deleterious effect. Accordingly, antipyretics should be used when temperature is elevated; of course, the cause of the elevated temperature should be sought and treated.[30]

Seizures occur in approximately 5% of patients with stroke. When present, seizures should be treated in the usual fashion; there is general agreement that prophylactic treatment with anticonvulsants is not indicated.

Increased intracranial pressure resulting from brain edema is not usually a problem in early stages of acute stroke; when present, it is usually maximum 3 to 5 days after the stroke. In patients with large cerebellar strokes, early swelling may cause progressive brainstem compression during the acute phase; in occasional patients, obstruction of normal cerebrospinal fluid (CSF) drainage may lead to acute hydrocephalus. Management is difficult. Corticosteroids are not helpful; hyperventilation, mannitol, or CSF drainage via ventriculostomy may be beneficial. Neurosurgical consultation should be sought; especially in patients with cerebellar infarcts or hemorrhages; early neurosurgical treatment may be life-saving and may be associated with a good outcome.[9]

General Medical Care

Common secondary medical problems in stroke patients include aspiration pneumonia, urinary tract infection, and deep venous thrombosis (DVT) with pulmonary embolism. Although the continuing care of stroke patients is often not the responsibility of the acute care physician, appropriate care should be initiated in the acute care setting. Patients should be kept NPO until there is no doubt about their swallowing function; in case of any doubt, a formal swallowing study should be obtained, if available. Indwelling bladder catheters are usually unnecessary and should be used only when clearly required, not for the convenience of physicians and nursing staff. Appropriate prophylaxis for DVT should be initiated, but all anticoagulants should be withheld for 24 hours in patients treated with thrombolytic agents.

Intracerebral Hemorrhage

Approximately 15% of acute strokes are due to intracerebral hemorrhage (ICH) rather than to ischemia. In many cases, ICH cannot be reliably distinguished from ischemic infarction on clinical grounds. Clinical symptoms suggesting ICH include severe headache or vomiting at the onset of the stroke, sudden loss of consciousness at the onset of the stroke, or rapid decline in consciousness soon after onset. Continuing progression of a neurologic deficit over several hours, especially with a decline in mental status, also suggests ICH. The deterioration in mental status may be due to mass effect, increased intracranial pressure, or intraventricular or subarachnoid extension of the hemorrhage.

The most common cause of ICH is degenerative disease of small blood vessels associated with chronic hypertension, diabetes, or advanced age. ICH can occur as a complication of anticoagulant therapy. Other potential causes include primary vascular disorders such as amyloid angiopathy, vascular malformations, aneurysms (congenital or mycotic), hemorrhage into tumors (primary or metastatic), and trauma. Rare causes include vasculitis, moya-moya disease, and others. Small vessel disease most commonly results in bleeding in the basal ganglia, the pons, and the cerebellum; more peripheral hemorrhages suggest one of the other etiologies.

The diagnosis of ICH is usually confirmed by CT scanning; in experienced hands, CT is virtually 100% sensitive for ICH. As noted above, smaller or more subtle hemorrhages can be overlooked by less experienced physicians. Lumbar puncture is not indicated. It is important to stress that these guidelines apply only to *intracerebral* hemorrhage, not to *subarachnoid* hemorrhage.

Treatment of patients with ICH is largely supportive, as outlined for patients with acute ischemic stroke. Management of hypertension in patients with acute ICH remains controversial; these patients often have chronic hypertension and frequently develop severe reactive hypertension. Although it seems intuitively obvious that lowering the blood pressure would reduce the risk of further bleeding, patients with ICH often have raised intracranial pressure, and reducing the systemic pressure may lower the cerebral perfusion pressure, compromising cerebral blood flow and worsening the neurologic injury. Although no controlled trials data are available, current guidelines suggest that the mean arterial pressure (MAP) be kept below 130 mmHg. For patients with marked elevations in blood pressure (systolic pressure >230 mmHg or diastolic pressure >140 mmHg), intravenous nitroprusside should be used. For patients with systolic pressures between 180 and 230 mmHg or diastolic pressures between 105 and 140 mmHg, labetalol or similar agents can be used. As in patients with ischemic stroke, hypotension should be avoided and treated if necessary.[29]

Neurosurgical intervention may be beneficial in selected patients with cerebral hemorrhage, especially those with initially less severe deficits who show signs of progressive deterioration. There is little reason to expect any benefit from surgery in patients with massive hemorrhages or in those who are moribund at presentation. In patients with *cerebellar* hemorrhage, neurosurgical intervention may be life-saving and may result in surprisingly good outcome. The clinical picture of cerebellar hemorrhage is characterized by the abrupt onset of headache, dizziness, and ataxia, as well as vomiting. Brainstem signs are often present. The diagnosis is confirmed by CT scanning.

Transient Ischemic Attack

A TIA may be defined as ". . . a temporary and focal episode of neurologic dysfunction of presumed vascular origin, typically lasting from 2 to 15 minutes, but occasionally as long as 24 hours, which clears without residua."[31] It is important to stress that most TIAs are very brief and that many will have resolved by the time the patient comes to medical attention. The diagnosis must therefore be based entirely on the history. The onset of the attack is usually abrupt, with symptoms developing over only a few seconds or minutes. A detailed account of the attack should be obtained to establish that the symptoms were consistent with a focal lesion of the brain or brainstem. An especially subtle form of TIA, often ignored by patients, is *amaurosis fugax*, an episode of transient monocular blindness cause by acute retinal ischemia. Patients typically describe a "shade" coming down over the eye with temporary loss of vision; the other eye is unaffected. Normal vision is restored after a few minutes. As with virtually all TIAs, the episode is painless and its significance often unrecognized. In general, nonfocal symptoms such as syncope or lightheadedness are not due to TIA. Similarly, symptoms such as vertigo, dysarthria, double vision, etc., occurring in isolation are not usually due to TIA.

A TIA should be regarded as a stroke with complete resolution. It is well established that patients with TIA are at substantially increased risk for subsequent strokes; their evaluation and treatment are directed toward preventing subsequent attacks. In general, the causes of TIA are the same as the causes of stroke, except that cardiogenic embolism is thought to be an unusual cause of TIA. Accordingly, the initial diagnostic evaluation (imaging, laboratory, and other studies) are the same as for patients with stroke. Since the highest risk of stroke is within the first few days after TIA, the workup should be carried out expeditiously.

Treatment depends on the presumed cause of the TIA. For patients with high-grade (>70%) stenosis in an accessible neck vessel, surgical endarterectomy is often the procedure of choice; percutaneous endovascular surgery is under study and may be an effective alternative in some patients. For patients with atrial fibrillation or presumed cardiogenic emboli, anticoagulation is beneficial. For patients with non-critical vascular stenosis (<70%), or in whom no cause for TIA can be discovered, antiplatelet therapy is usually recommended. Available agents include aspirin, ticlopidine (Ticlid), clopidogrel (Plavix), and aspirin combined with sustained-release dipyridamole (Aggrenox). Despite the claims of aggressive marketers, convincing data on the relative merits of these agents are lacking. Aspirin at 81 or 325 mg/day is usually appropriate for initial treatment; management of persons who cannot take aspirin or whose symptoms occur while they are on aspirin remains highly controversial. Consultation with a neurologist is probably the best course.

Migraine

The diagnosis and management of migraine are discussed in Chapter 7. Focal neurologic symptoms are common in patients with migraine. Most common are the familiar visual auras, which may include central or peripheral scotomas, visual field loss, or even complete blindness. Although both eyes are usually involved, unilateral visual loss (amaurosis fugax) may occur and be mistaken for TIA.[32] Other focal neurologic symptoms may include aphasia or speech arrest, motor weakness, or paralysis (even hemiplegia) or sensory symptoms. The attacks may or may not be associated with headaches.

Recognition of this syndrome, and distinction from TIA, requires a careful history. A history of previous similar attacks, some associated with typical migraine headaches, may be diagnostic. In general, migraine symptoms evolve gradually over a period of 5 to 10 minutes or more; patients may describe numbness or weakness beginning in one hand, gradually spreading up the arm, and then spreading to the face, the trunk, or elsewhere. When present, this history is virtually diagnostic and is quite different from the abrupt onset characteristic of TIA and stroke. In some cases, of course, the story will not be so clear. There is no laboratory or imaging study that will permit a clear distinction between migraines and TIA; when in doubt, it is reasonable to pursue the workup for TIA.

Cerebral Vein Thrombosis

Thrombosis of the cortical veins and venous sinuses is much less common than arterial occlusive disease. The diagnosis is often difficult but is suggested by somewhat slower evolution of clinical symptoms and frequently by the presence of bilateral signs. Signs of raised intracranial pressure (especially depressed level of consciousness, vomiting, and papilledema) are often present, and seizures are often prominent. The CT scan may reveal extensive bilateral cortical and subcortical hemorrhagic infarction, but the diagnosis is often difficult to confirm. MR or contrast angiography may be needed.

Cerebral vein thrombosis occurs most often in the setting of an underlying coagulopathy such as pregnancy (or recent delivery), systemic cancer, sickle cell disease, or primary coagulopathy. Mutations in the factor V Leiden gene have been highly associated with cerebral vein thrombosis in several recent studies.[33] Because of the frequent association with primary coagulopathy, extensive medical evaluation may be needed in these patients.

Treatment remains controversial. A recent retrospective review of 42 patients concluded that heparin anticoagulation was safe, but benefit could not be confirmed.[34]

Direct local infusion of thrombolytic agents at the site of the venous occlusion is under investigation but requires the availability of an interventional neuroradiologist.

Other Disorders

The clinical picture in patients with *brain abscess* is nonspecific, with headache, seizures, and focal signs; signs of increased intracranial pressure may be present as well. As in patients with tumors, the onset of clinical symptoms is usually subacute rather than abrupt. The diagnosis is often suggested by CT or MRI evidence of a mass lesion, often enhancing following contrast administration. These lesions may be difficult to distinguish from neoplasms, although the correct diagnosis may be suggested by the clinical context. Brain abscess should be considered in patients with evidence of systemic infection, patients with sinus or mastoid infections, patients with suspected endocarditis, congenital or valvular heart disease, patients using IV drugs, and patients with a history of recent head trauma or neurosurgery. Biopsy may be needed to confirm a diagnosis and to identify the causative organism. Brain abscesses can be caused by a wide variety of bacterial infections, both aerobic or anaerobic, and polymicrobial infections are common. In immunocompromised hosts (especially patients with AIDS), fungal infections, or protozoan infections (e.g., toxoplasmosis), should also be considered. Although many brain abscesses are caused by hematogenous spread of infection, fever and signs of systemic infection may be absent.

Definitive treatment ultimately depends on the size and location of the lesion(s), the stage of development of the lesion (early "cerebritis" or a well-developed mature abscess with a thick capsule), and identification of the causative organism. Neurosurgery may be needed both for diagnosis and treatment, and early consultation is appropriate. Depending on the clinical urgency of the situation, treatment may be delayed until a definitive diagnosis is established, or empiric antibiotic treatment can be started, based on the most likely clinical diagnoses. For patients with probable bacterial infection from sinus infection or cardiac sources, a third-generation cephalosporin (e.g., ceftriaxone 2 g IV q12h) and metronidazole 30 mg/kg/day (divided into four doses) is appropriate. For patients with head trauma or neurosurgery, coverage for staphylococci should be given. For patients with AIDS, coverage for toxoplasmosis should be considered. Early consultation with a specialist in infectious diseases should be sought.[35,36]

The clinical syndrome of acute *encephalitis* is characterized by fever, headache, altered mental status, and sometimes focal neurologic signs. The most common cause of acute encephalitis is *Herpes simplex virus* (HSV), but a wide variety of other viruses, as well as bacterial and other infections, can cause a similar picture. Treatment with acyclovir or other antiviral agents may be beneficial in HSV encephalitis (see Chap. 3 for further discussion).

Intracranial tumors occasionally present with the apparent onset of acute focal neurologic deficits; in many of these cases, a careful history will reveal a more subacute or chronic course. However, symptoms are occasionally abrupt in onset. Potential mechanisms include sudden hemorrhage into a previously "silent" tumor, the onset of seizure activity, or disruption of local blood supply by the tumor. Either primary or metastatic tumors may present in this way.

Brain metastases may be suspected in patients with a prior history of systemic cancer, but either primary or metastatic tumors may present with no antecedent history. The diagnosis is often first suggested by the appearance of a mass lesion on CT scanning, although low-grade primary brain tumors may easily be overlooked on nonenhanced CT scans. MRI with enhancement is usually the imaging procedure of choice but is rarely needed in the acute setting. Emergency treatment is usually not required unless there is substantial mass effect or impending herniation, in which case intravenous corticosteroids (e.g., dexamethasone 10 mg initially, then 4 mg q6h) may be beneficial. Patients with marked decrease in their level of consciousness should be managed as outlined in Chapter 3. Prophylactic anticonvulsants are not necessary.

Epidural hematomas are generally due to arterial bleeding secondary to head trauma with a skull fracture. The classic clinical picture is that of a patient with a head injury who acutely loses consciousness and then recovers, at least in part, before beginning progressive deterioration. Focal signs are common, as are signs of progressive herniation. The diagnosis is usually evident on CT scanning. The treatment is neurosurgical intervention. *Subdural hematomas* may be much more subtle. They result from venous bleeding and may evolve over a prolonged period as a result of small recurrent hemorrhages. There is often, but not always, a history of head trauma, sometimes seemingly trivial. Diagnosis is by CT scan. As with epidural hematomas, neurosurgical consultation should be obtained.

Hypoglycemia and hyperglycemia typically present with altered mental status, as discussed in Chapter 3. However, either condition may cause focal signs; these usually resolve promptly with treatment. If focal signs persist following normalization of blood glucose, alternative causes should be sought.

Focal motor seizures ordinarily cause no diagnostic difficulty. However, sensory seizures, unaccompanied by any abnormal movements, may occur as well and may be very difficult to recognize. Simple focal seizures (either motor or sensory) are not associated with any alteration of consciousness. Focal seizures imply the presence of an underlying focal brain lesion; focal seizures of new onset should prompt a thorough evaluation. This can usually be done on a nonurgent or elective basis. Focal seizures (with or without secondary generalization) may result in focal weakness (Todd's paralysis) that persists after the seizure has resolved. This can cause diagnostic confusion in a patient who comes to medical attention after an unwitnessed seizure; the clinical picture is of altered mental status with focal weakness, with a large differential diagnosis. Usually the correct diagnosis will be suggested by rapid improvement. It is important to recall that the presence of a Todd's paralysis implies a focal onset to the seizure, even if the seizure was apparently generalized at onset (see Chap. 11).

Multiple sclerosis (MS) may present with acute focal neurologic deficits. In one classic study, nearly 20% of patients presented with acute deficits of abrupt onset.[37] In such cases, the clinical picture may be difficult to distinguish from acute stroke. CT scans may be normal or may reveal one or more low-density lesions. MRI scanning is far more sensitive and specific for MS lesions but may also be nondiagnostic in new-onset cases. The subsequent workup of patients with suspected MS may include evoked potential studies and lumbar puncture, none of which need to be accomplished in the acute care setting.

In patients with established MS, acute focal deficits may result either from new lesions or from acute exacerbation of previous lesions because of fever, infection, or other causes. Of course, a history of MS does not exclude other causes of acute focal weakness. Patients with MS can therefore present a major diagnostic and therapeutic challenge to the acute care physician.

ACUTE FOCAL LESIONS OF THE SPINAL CORD

The clinical anatomy of the spinal cord is reviewed in Chapter 9; only a few brief points will be discussed here. The spinal cord extends from the foramen magnum to approximately the level of the L1 vertebral body. It should be noted that there is no spinal cord in the lumbar spinal canal; imaging studies of the lumbosacral spine are not indicated in patients with suspected spinal cord lesions! There are 31 pairs of spinal nerves, numbered according to the vertebral levels at which they exit the spinal canal via the neural foramina. These numbers are also used to designate the spinal cord levels at which each pair of nerves originates. Since the spinal cord is shorter than the vertebral column, the spinal levels and the vertebral levels do not match. It is important to remember this fact when planning and interpreting clinical findings and imaging studies of the spine and spinal cord in patients with suspected spinal cord lesions (Table 4-7 and Figure 4-1).

Several anatomic features make the spinal cord highly susceptible to injury from compression by mass lesions within the spinal canal. The cord is tightly confined within the spinal canal, with little room for displacement by a mass lesion. In addition, the major blood supply to the spinal cord (the anterior spinal artery) depends on a small number of feeding vessels derived from segmental branches from the aorta, with the result that much of the cord depends on a somewhat tenuous blood supply. Compression of these vessels can result in irreversible infarction of the spinal cord. The spinal cord may also be injured by intrinsic processes. Table 4-8 lists some

TABLE 4-7

SPINAL CORD LEVELS AND VERTEBRAL LEVELS

Spinal Cord Level	Vertebral Level
C1	C1
T1	C7–C8
T6	T4
T12	T9–T10
L1–L5	T10–T12
S1–S5	T12–L1

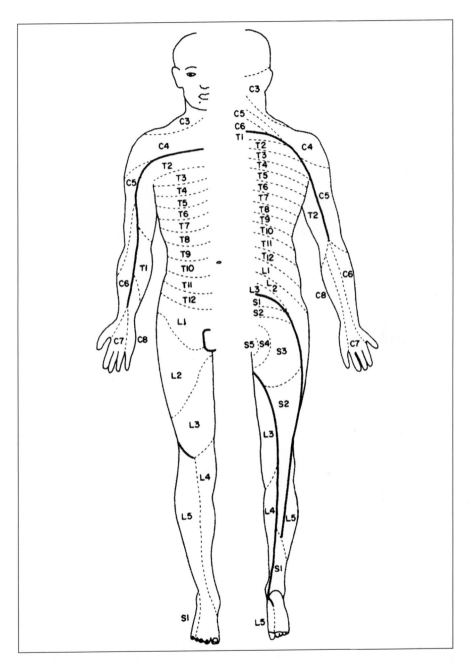

FIGURE 4-1   The sensory dermatomes.   (From Victor M, Ropper AH. *Adams and Victor's Principles of Neurology,* 7th ed. New York: McGraw-Hill, 2000, with permission.)

TABLE 4-8 ————————————————————————
ETIOLOGIES OF SPINAL CORD LESIONS

Extrinsic (Compressive) Lesions
Spondyloarthropathy
Disc protrusion/herniation[a]
Neoplasms (primary/metastatic)[a]
Epidural abscess[a]/hematoma[a]
Trauma[a]

Intrinsic Lesions
Vascular (spinal cord infarction)[a]
Neoplasms (primary/metastatic)
Inflammatory/granulomatous
    Multiple sclerosis[a]
    Transverse myelitis[a] (idiopathic or postinfectious)
    Vasculitis

[a] Lesions most likely to present with acute spinal cord dysfunction. See text for details.

of the more common lesions that may affect the spinal cord. It is imperative that extrinsic compression of the spinal cord be recognized as quickly as possible, since emergency treatment may lead to dramatic improvement. Conversely, delay in treatment can lead to irreversible injury to the spinal cord.

Clinical Assessment

The most common cause of acute lesions of the spinal cord is trauma; the possibility of spinal cord injury should be considered in all injured patients and appropriate steps taken to evaluate and treat such injuries (see Chap. 9). Nontraumatic injuries to the spinal cord are less common and are more easily overlooked; recognition of a spinal cord lesion may require a high index of suspicion and a high degree of skill in the performance and interpretation of the neurologic examination. The neurologic examination is reviewed in Chapter 2; clinical findings that indicate a spinal cord lesion are summarized in Table 4-1 and are discussed below. It is important to remember that symptoms involving the face and head (e.g., facial weakness or numbness) are not caused by spinal cord lesions.

A *sensory level*, with impairment of sensation below a specific spinal level on the trunk or neck, is diagnostic for a spinal cord lesion; the anatomic organization of the nervous system is such that a true sensory level will not result from lesions elsewhere in the nervous system. It is important to recall that the patient may be completely unaware of the sensory impairment, which can therefore be overlooked unless specifically sought by the examiner. Sensory levels may be very difficult to recognize in the extremities and may be difficult to distinguish from the distal sensory impairment seen in patients with peripheral nerve lesions.

A *motor level* is usually characterized by weakness in the lower extremities more than in the upper extremities. This finding is less clearly diagnostic than a true sensory level, but a spinal cord lesion should be suspected especially if there is severe weakness in the lower extremities with normal strength in the upper extremities. Careful examination can sometimes reveal weakness in the lower abdominal or trunk muscles more than the upper muscles, suggesting a lesion in the lower thoracic spinal cord, but this is frequently very subtle and difficult to detect.

Sensory dissociation means impairment of pain and temperature sensation on one side of the body and impairment of position and vibration sense on the opposite side; this finding can *only* result from a spinal cord lesion and implies a lesion affecting one side of the spinal cord but sparing the other side.

Sensory-motor dissociation means impairment of motor function on one side of the body and impairment of pain and temperature sensation of the opposite side; as with sensory dissociation, this can only result from a spinal cord lesion.

Additional symptoms that should suggest a spinal cord lesion include early involvement of bladder function, bowel function, or sexual function. The presence of neck pain or back pain in association with weakness of the lower extremities or impaired bowel, bladder, or sexual function should strongly suggest a spinal cord lesion. Finally, the presence of both "lower motor neuron" and "upper motor neuron" signs should suggest a spinal cord disorder.

If a spinal cord lesion is suspected, additional clinical history may suggest the etiology. The patient should be asked about recent trauma. A history of localized pain in the neck or back, especially in association with percussion tenderness, suggests a lesion of the spine or meninges. A history of prior cancer, even if remote, should suggest metastatic disease. A history of systemic infection, or of unexplained fever, especially if associated with back pain, should suggest a spinal or epidural abscess. A history of HIV infection suggests opportunistic infection or abscess, or HIV myelopathy. Chest pain or abdominal pain in association with signs of spinal cord injury may be due to thoracic or abdominal aortic aneurysm.

Once a spinal cord lesion is suspected, it is essential to try to determine whether the lesion is extrinsic or intrinsic to the spinal cord. Although various clinical clues have been used to make this distinction (e.g., the presence or absence of "sacral sparing"), none is sufficiently reliable to preclude the need for an adequate imaging study.

Spinal Cord Imaging

MRI with contrast enhancement is the study of choice for patients with suspected lesions of the spinal cord. MRI provides detailed images of the spinal cord, the subarachnoid space, and surrounding structures. The images distinguish extrinsic from intrinsic lesions and often indicate the specific diagnosis. Even in patients with x-ray evidence of an acute spine lesion (e.g., collapse of a vertebral body), MRI will indicate the extent of injury to the spinal cord. Accordingly, emergency MRI, if available, should be obtained in virtually all patients with acute spinal cord syndromes. If emergency MRI is not immediately available, contrast myelography, preferably with

CT imaging, should be obtained. Plain radiographs, or CT without intrathecal contrast, are rarely, if ever, adequate. If neither MRI or myelography is immediately available, arrangements should be made for emergency transfer of the patient with a suspected acute spinal cord lesion to an appropriate facility. Diagnostic imaging should not be delayed any more than is absolutely necessary.

As noted above, careful clinical assessment is needed to ensure that the appropriate region of the spine is scanned; even exquisitely detailed images of the thoracic spinal cord are of no diagnostic value in a patient with a cervical spinal cord lesion. Consultation with a radiologist may help to ensure that the appropriate regions are scanned and the appropriate imaging sequences are obtained.

Extrinsic Compression of the Spinal Cord

Epidural metastasis from systemic cancer is a common cause of extrinsic compression of the spinal cord. The most common mechanism is metastasis to the vertebral bodies with direct extension of tumor into the epidural space. Less common mechanisms include extension of extraspinal tumors through the intravertebral foramina or (rarely) direct metastasis to epidural fat. Especially in the case of vertebral metastasis, neurologic symptoms are usually preceded by several weeks or more of steadily increasing localized back pain. Unlike most mechanical back pain, the pain is not relieved by rest or changes in position and may actually become worse when the patient lies down. The diagnosis of vertebral metastasis should be suspected in any patient with systemic cancer and worsening back pain, but it should be considered as well in patients with a similar pattern of steadily progressive pain even without known cancer. Epidural metastasis with cord compression is not rare as the initial manifestation of systemic cancer. The initial neurologic symptoms may be mild and subtle, with vague numbness or tingling or mild weakness of heaviness of the legs. Bladder, bowel, or sexual dysfunction may occur early, and the patient should be questioned carefully about these symptoms. Once neurologic symptoms develop, progression may be very rapid, and diagnosis and treatment are urgent. It is a rule of thumb that patients who lose their ability to walk will never regain it. As noted above, once the diagnosis is suspected, emergency MRI scanning is mandatory.

Treatment usually consists of high-dose corticosteroids (e.g., dexamethasone 100 mg IV immediately, then 25 mg IV q6h), followed by emergent radiation therapy.[38] Surgery is generally reserved for those patients in whom the diagnosis is unclear, in whom there is evidence of spinal instability, or who have undergone prior radiation of the affected area.

Epidural abscess is an unusual but important potential cause of spinal cord compression. The abscess may develop as a result of direct extension from osteomyelitis of a vertebral body or from direct seeding of the epidural space from the blood. Important predisposing causes include diabetes mellitus, immunodeficiency syndromes (including AIDS), and systemic sepsis. The clinical symptoms generally include severe and progressive pain, similar to that seen in patients with metastatic disease. Fever and malaise are common. Neurologic symptoms, once present, may evolve rapidly; as with metastatic disease, treatment should begin as soon as possible after diagnosis. The diagnosis is most often made by MRI. Treatment is with antibiotics and surgical drainage; surgery serves to decompress the spinal cord and to obtain positive identification of the causative organism (most often *Staphylococcus aureus*).

Herniation of an intervertebral disc is an occasional cause of acute spinal cord compression, most often as a result of trauma (see Chap. 9). Degenerative disease of the spine can also cause spinal cord compression, as a result of either disc disease or spondylosis, or both. This is most often a chronic process, and a good history will usually indicate the presence of chronic, slowly evolving symptoms. If the process is long-standing, emergency treatment is not usually required, and an appropriate referral should be made. Unusual causes of spinal cord compression include epidural hematomas (most often the result of trauma) and intraspinal tumors (often benign). Diagnosis usually depends on imaging studies obtained in a patient with a clinically suspected spinal cord lesion.

Intrinsic Lesions of the Spinal Cord

Infarction of the spinal cord (spinal cord stroke) can occur as a result of occlusion of the anterior spinal artery or of one of the segmental arteries that supply blood to the cord. The most common cause is occlusion of segmental arteries by aortic dissection or as a result of surgery on the aorta. Other potential causes include systemic lupus, polyarteritis nodosa, decompression sickness (the bends), and cocaine use; occasional cases are seen with no evident cause. The clinical syndrome is characterized by the abrupt onset of paralysis (including sphincter paralysis) below the level of the lesion. There is commonly a sensory level to pain and temperature sensation below the level of the lesion; there is often relative sparing of posterior column sensory functions such as vibration sense, light touch sensation, and joint position sense. The clinical findings are typically bilateral and symmetric. The infarction is usually seen on MRI scanning of the spine. Unfortunately, there is no effective treatment.

Multiple sclerosis is the most common cause of acute intrinsic lesions of the spinal cord in adults. Usually the onset of symptoms is subacute, over a period of several days or longer, but abrupt onset is not rare. The diagnosis is usually straightforward in patients with previously diagnosed MS, but acute myelopathy may be the presenting symptom of MS. The clinical signs are frequently asymmetric. The diagnosis is often suggested by the finding of an acute inflammatory focal lesion on MRI scanning (often enhancing with contrast); confirmation of the diagnosis requires demonstrating other lesions within the central nervous system. Acute treatment usually consists of intravenous corticosteroids (e.g., methylprednisolone 1,000 mg IV q day × 3 to 5 days).

Patients with MS may also experience acute deterioration in their clinical symptoms as a result of fever or other systemic illness (e.g., urinary tract or respiratory infections). These symptoms need not indicate any activity of their underlying MS and will improve rapidly when the secondary disease is treated. Therefore, in patients with known MS who present with sudden worsening of their symptoms, a careful evaluation is needed to exclude some other disorder. Treatment is directed toward the secondary disorder, and steroids are not required.

Acute intrinsic lesions of the spinal cord may result as well from a variety of infectious agents (viruses, mycoplasma, Lyme disease), granulomatous disorders (e.g., sarcoidosis), and postinfectious and postimmunization immune-mediated disorders. Other remote considerations (usually with a subacute or chronic course) include primary or metastatic spinal cord tumors, syringomyelia, and arteriovenous malformations. Diagnosis in most of these cases depends on imaging studies and an extensive diagnostic workup. No emergency treatment is available.

ACUTE FOCAL LESIONS OF THE PERIPHERAL NERVES

Although acute focal lesions of peripheral nerves are fairly common, they often cause diagnostic difficulty in the acute care setting. Of course, many peripheral nerve lesions are due to obvious trauma such as lacerations, penetrating injuries, and fractures, and they ordinarily present no diagnostic difficulty. Acute nontraumatic lesions of peripheral nerves, also fairly common, may be less easily recognized for several reasons. First, it is probably fair to say that acute care physicians, presented with a patient with an acute focal neurologic deficit, are "predisposed" to consider potentially life-threatening or serious "central" lesions and may overlook clinical clues suggesting a peripheral lesion. Second, nontraumatic lesions are often incomplete and result in clinical syndromes that are partial or incomplete rather than "classical." Finally, some symptoms of peripheral nerve lesions, such as pain, paresthesias, or sensory loss, are entirely subjective and difficult to define accurately.

In the following discussion, the term *peripheral nerve* will include cranial nerves III through XII, the motor and sensory spinal roots, the brachial and lumbosacral plexuses, and the peripheral nerves. Potential causes of focal lesions of peripheral nerves are listed in Table 4-9.

TABLE 4-9

ETIOLOGIES OF ACUTE FOCAL LESIONS
OF PERIPHERAL NERVES

Extrinsic Lesions
Direct trauma (blunt trauma, lacerations, avulsions, etc.)
Mass lesions (neoplasms, spondyloarthropathy, disc protrusion/herniation)
Pressure palsies

Intrinsic Lesions
Vascular (diabetes, vasculitis, etc.)
Inflammatory
Idiopathic

Clinical Assessment

As in the case of spinal cord lesions, recognition of peripheral nerve disorders depends on the clinical acumen of the examining physician. The task for the physician is to recognize that a patient's clinical symptoms indicate a lesion of a specific peripheral root or nerve rather than a more "central" lesion. This requires detailed knowledge of the clinical anatomy of the peripheral nervous system. There are hundreds of peripheral nerves, and it is virtually impossible for the physician to recall all of the relevant anatomic and clinical details (Table 4-10 and Figure 4-2). Fortunately, there are several excellent references available that summarize the anatomy and the necessary techniques for an effective clinical examination.[39,40] A copy of one of these or similar references should be part of the basic armamentarium of every physician who confronts neurologic disorders. With such a reference, and with the willingness to consider the possibility of peripheral nerve disorders, accurate diagnosis is usually straightforward. For example, the syndrome of severe pain in the postero-lateral aspect of the lower extremity, weakness of plantar flexion of the foot, and loss of the ankle reflex suggests a lesion of the S1 nerve root; if weakness of dorsiflexion of the foot were also present, the lesion would more likely affect the sciatic nerve, since the clinical findings are not compatible with a single root lesion (S1 does not innervate the anterior tibial muscle) but would be consistent with a sciatic nerve lesion. Similarly, weakness of the wrist and finger extensor muscles in the forearm, without weakness of other muscles, suggests a radial nerve lesion; a brain or spinal cord lesion would not cause symptoms limited to the distribution of a single peripheral nerve.

Laboratory and Imaging Studies

Laboratory studies are usually of little value, especially in the acute care setting. Electromyography (EMG) and nerve conduction velocity (NCV) studies are often crucial in characterizing and confirming the localization of peripheral nerve lesions but are usually not done in the acute care setting. In addition, EMG and NCV abnormalities may not become detectable until 2 to 3 weeks or more after an acute injury, making such studies unhelpful even if performed.

MRI has revolutionized the diagnostic evaluation of peripheral nerve injuries due to structural lesions, but it is usually of little help in other cases. Effective use of MRI requires that an accurate "anatomic" diagnosis be made (so that the appropriate body region can be imaged). As a practical matter, MRI is rarely needed in the acute care setting.

Cranial Nerve Lesions

Trigeminal neuralgia is characterized by severe pain in the distribution of one or more divisions of the trigeminal nerve (most often the mandibular and maxillary divisions). The pain is typically very intense and occurs in brief paroxysms, each lasting only a few seconds; the pain usually has a burning, stabbing, or searing quality. The

TABLE 4-10 PRINCIPAL MUSCLES AND THEIR NERVE SUPPLY

Action tested	Roots	Nerves	Muscles
CRANIAL			
Closure of eyes, pursing of lips, exposure of teeth	Cranial 7	Facial	Orbicularis oculi Orbicularis oris
Elevation of eyelids, movement of eyes	Cranial 3, 4, 6	Oculomotor, trochlear, abducens	Levator palpebrae, extraocular
Closing and opening of jaw	Cranial 5	Motor trigeminal	Masseters Pterygoids
Protrusion of tongue	Cranial 12	Hypoglossal	Lingual
Phonation and swallowing	Cranial 9, 10	Glossopharyngeal, vagus	Palatal, laryngeal, and pharyngeal
Elevation of shoulders, anteroflexion and turning of head	Cranial 11 and upper cervical	Spinal accesory	Trapezius, steromastoid
BRACHIAL			
Adduction of extended arm	**C5**, C6	Brachial plexus	Pectoralis major
Fixation of scapula	C5, C6, C7	Brachial plexus	Serratus anterior
Initiation of abduction of arm	**C5**, C6	Brachial plexus	Supraspinatus
External rotation of flexed arm	**C5**, C6	Brachial plexus	Infraspinatus
Abduction and elevation of arm up to 90°	**C5**, C6	Axillary nerve	Deltoid
Flexion of supinated forearm	C5, C6	Musculocutaneous	Biceps, brachialis
Extension of forearm	C6, **C7**, C8	Radial	Triceps
Extension (radial) of wrist	C6	Radial	Extensor carpi radialis longus
Flexion of semipronated arm	C5, **C6**	Radial	Brachioradialis
Adduction of flexed arm	C6, **C7**, C8	Brachial plexus	Latissimus dorsi

Action	Root	Nerve	Muscle
Supination of forearm	C6, C7	Posterior interosseous	Supinator
Extension of proximal phalanges	*C7*, C8	Posterior interosseous	Extensor digitorum
Extension of wrist (ulnar side)	**C7**, C8	Posterior interosseous	Extensor carpi ulnaris
Extension of proximal phalanx of index finger	**C7**, C8	Posterior interosseous	Extensor indicis
Abduction of thumb	*C7*, C8	Posterior interosseous	Abductor pollicis longus and brevis
Extension of thumb	**C7**, C8	Posterior interosseous	Extensor pollicis longus and brevis
Pronation of forearm	C6, C7	Median nerve	Pronator teres
Radial flexion of wrist	C6, C7	Median nerve	Flexor carpi radialis
Flexion of middle phalanges	C7, **C8**, T1	Median nerve	Flexor digitorum superficials
Flexion of proximal phalanx of thumb	**C8**, *T1*	Median nerve	Flexor pollicis brevis
Opposition of thumb against fifth finger	C8, *T1*	Median nerve	Opponens pollicis
Extension of middle phalanges of index and middle fingers	C8, *T1*	Median nerve	First, second lumbricals
Flexion of terminal phalanx of thumb	**C8**, T1	Anterior interosseous nerve	Flexor pollicis longus
Flexion of terminal phalanx of second and third fingers	C8, T1	Anterior interosseous nerve	Flexor digitorum profundus
Flexion of distal phalanges of ring and little fingers	C7, **C8**	Ulnar	Flexor digitorum profundus
Adduction and opposition and fifth finger	C8, *T1*	Ulnar	Hypothenar

(continued)

TABLE 4-10   PRINCIPAL MUSCLES AND THEIR NERVE SUPPLY (*continued*)

Action	Root	Nerve	Muscle
Extension of middle phalanges of ring and little fingers	C8, *T1*	Ulnar	Third, fourth lumbrical
Adduction of thumb against second finger	C8, *T1*	Ulnar	Adductor pollicis
Flexion of proximal phalanx of thumb	**C8**, T1	Ulnar	Flexor pollicis brevis
Abduction and adduction of fingers	C8, *T1*	Ulnar	Interossei
CRURAL			
Hip flexion from semiflexed position	*L1, L2*, L3	Femoral	Iliopsoas
Hip flexion from externally rotated position	L2, L3	Femoral	Sartorius
Extension of knee	L2, *L3, L4*	Femoral	Quadriceps femoris
Adduction of thigh	*L2, L3*, L4	Obturator	Adductor longus, magnus, brevis
Abduction and int. rotation of thigh	*L4, L5*, S1	Superior gluteal	Gluteus medius
Extension of thigh	*L5, S1*, S2	Inferior gluteal	Gluteus maximus

Flexion of knee	L5, **S1**, S2	Sciatic	Biceps femoris Semitendinosus Semimembranosus
Dorsiflexion of foot (medial)	**L4**, L5	Peroneal (deep)	Anterior tibial
Dorsiflexion of toes (proximal and distal phalanges)	**L5**, S1	Peroneal (deep)	Extensor digitorum longus and brevis
Dorsiflexion of great toe	**L5**, S1	Peroneal (deep)	Extensor hallucis longus
Eversion of foot	L5, S1	Peroneal (superficial)	Peroneus longus and brevis
Plantar flexion of foot	**S1**, S2	Tibial	Gastrocnemius, soleus
Inversion of foot	L4, **L5**	Tibial	Tibialis posterior
Flexion of toes (distal phalanges)	L5, **S1**, **S2**	Tibial	Flexor digitorum longus
Flexion of toes (middle phalanges)	**S1**, **S2**	Tibial	Flexor digitorum brevis
Flexion of great toe (proximal phalanx)	S1, S2	Tibial	Flexor hallucis brevis
Flexion of great toe (distal phalanx)	L5, **S1**, **S2**	Tibial	Flexor hallucis longus
Contraction of anal sphincter	S2, S3, S4	Pudendal	Perineal muscles

SOURCE: from Victor M, Ropper AH. *Adams and Victor's Principles of Neurology*, 7th ed. New York: McGraw-Hill, 2001, pp 1468–1469. (with permission)

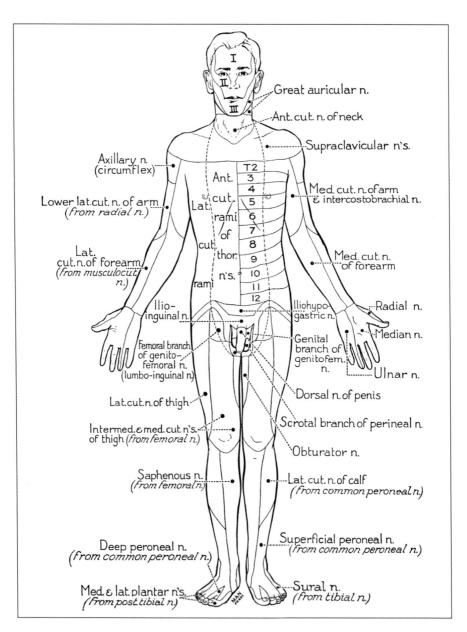

FIGURE 4-2   Cutaneous fields of the peripheral nerves.   (From Victor M, Ropper AH. *Adams and Victor's Principles of Neurology*, 7th ed. New York: McGraw-Hill, 2000, with permission.)

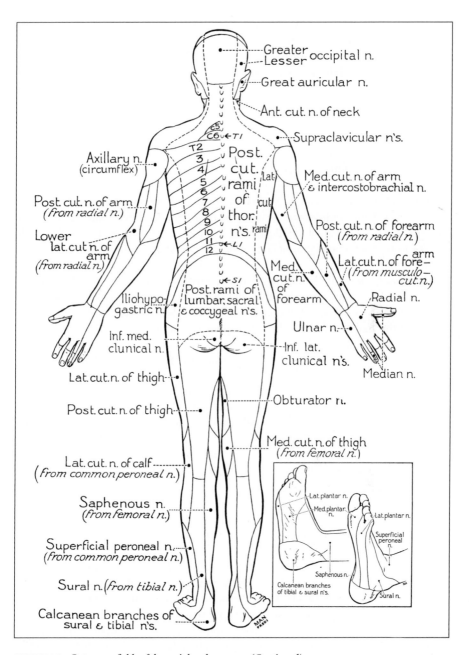

FIGURE 4-2   Cutaneous fields of the peripheral nerves.   *(Continued)*

stabs of pain may be isolated or occur in bursts. Bursts of pain may be associated with involuntary twitches or jerks of the face, hence the synonym *tic douloureux*. Attacks are often stimulated by touching trigger zones on the face or in the mouth, by chewing or eating, or even by a breath of wind; patients will often walk about with a hand held over the face (not touching the face) to ward off any contact. The physical examination is normal, and there are no associated neurologic signs. The syndrome may occur without warning in a previously healthy patient and thus provoke a visit to the emergency department. It is important to distinguish this condition from more slowly evolving pain or sensory loss in the face, which suggest infiltration or compression of the trigeminal nerve by tumor, infection, connective tissue disease, dental disease, or other causes. This syndrome is usually called *trigeminal neuropathy*, and diagnosis may require a very detailed workup that would not be undertaken on an emergency basis.

For patients with classic trigeminal neuralgia, emergency imaging studies are not required. Pain medication is usually of little benefit. Many patients respond promptly to anticonvulsant medications; carbamazepine is commonly used with success. Long-term management is complicated, and patients should be referred to a neurologist.

Facial nerve palsy is characterized by acute weakness or paralysis of the muscles on one side of the face. Typically, in lesions of the facial nerve, the upper and lower portions of the face are affected equally; in "central" lesions (e.g., stroke), the lower portion of the face is affected while the upper portion is spared. This well-known "clinical pearl" is not entirely reliable; some patients with acute hemispheric strokes will have weakness affecting both the upper and the lower face, and some patients with more distal lesions of the facial nerve, for example in the parotid gland, may have selective weakness of the lower face. A more reliable approach is to examine the patient carefully for evidence of any other neurologic deficit; if the only deficit is weakness of the face, a peripheral lesion is likely. Weakness of an arm or leg on the ipsilateral side suggests a contralateral hemisphere lesion; an ipsilateral abducens palsy or gaze palsy or a contralateral hemiparesis indicates an ipsilateral brainstem (pons) lesion. Since weakness of the facial muscles makes it difficult or impossible to close the eye on the affected side, many patients complain of "blurred vision" on the affected side, but careful examination shows no actual visual impairment. Some patients with facial nerve palsy may experience hyperacusis on the affected side; some will complain of an abnormal sense of taste, but actual loss of taste sensation is difficult to demonstrate.

The most common cause of facial nerve palsy is *Bell's palsy*; by definition this is idiopathic, although recent data suggest that a significant proportion of these cases may be due to infection by HSV. A similar clinical picture with the added features of pain in the ear and a vesicular eruption in the external ear canal is caused by *herpes zoster* (the Ramsay-Hunt syndrome). In typical Bell's palsy, the onset is acute, and weakness develops over a few hours to a day or two, occasionally longer. The onset of weakness may be preceded by a few days or hours of temporal headache or pain behind the ear. If the weakness develops more slowly, over a period of weeks or longer, infiltration or compression of the nerve should be suspected. In general, in cases of isolated facial weakness, diagnostic study is not an emergency and can be undertaken on an elective basis.

Treatment of Bell's palsy remains somewhat controversial. Fortunately, most patients (70% to 80%) make a full recovery over several weeks to months. Corticosteroids (prednisone 40 to 60 mg/day for 5 to 10 days), if started early, may shorten the course and improve outcome; they may be used if there are no contraindications. As a result of the possible role of HSV, some physicians advocate a course of oral acyclovir. Regardless of any specific treatment, it is important to remember to protect the patient's eye on the affected side; because they are unable to close the eye, patients are at risk for excessive drying of the eye, foreign bodies, and infection. Depending on the severity of the weakness, treatment may range from liberal use of eye drops to patching or taping the eye shut, or even to tarsorrhaphy. Patients should be instructed to seek medical attention without delay if they develop pain or other problems in the eye.

Isolated lesions of other cranial nerves may occur as well. Lesions of the oculomotor (III), trochlear (IV), and abducens (VI) nerves cause diplopia; oculomotor lesions may also cause ptosis and pupillary abnormalities. Careful physical examination is needed to decide which nerve is affected and to look for any evidence of brainstem involvement. These are discussed in Chapter 8. Isolated mononeuropathies of the lower cranial nerves are much less common.

Spinal Root Lesions

The most common symptom of lesions affecting single spinal roots is pain in the dermatome of the affected root. Sensory loss is highly variable or may be absent entirely. Reflexes are typically reduced or absent in the affected root distribution. Weakness, if present, is confined to muscles innervated by the affected root; complete paralysis does not occur because individual muscles are innervated by nerve fibers from several roots (Table 4-10). The most common cause of an *acute* root lesion is herniation of an intervertebral disc; the cervical and lumbosacral roots are most often affected. The patient can often recall some specific activity, trauma, or other cause that provoked the symptoms. Other structural lesions such as osteophytes, tumors, and others can also cause root lesions, more often with a subacute or chronic course.

The clinical diagnosis of an acute root lesion ordinarily presents no difficulty. A careful examination is necessary to look for any evidence of spinal cord involvement. In the usual case of an isolated single root lesion, urgent imaging studies are not required. Initial treatment usually consists of aspirin, NSAIDs, and sometimes muscle relaxants. In patients with severe pain, a short course of steroid therapy may be beneficial (e.g., prednisone 1 mg/kg/day for 5 to 7 days followed by a tapering dose over the next 5 to 7 days). Narcotic analgesics may be needed if the pain is very severe.

There are three situations in which urgent imaging (MRI) and neurosurgical referral may be needed. First is the patient with marked weakness in the affected muscles. Second is the patient with signs and symptoms suggesting spinal cord compression. Third is the patient with pain in the perineum or pain and sensory loss in a "saddle" distribution involving the perineum and medial thighs. These findings suggest compression of the cauda equina; bladder and bowel function may be compromised as well. Urgent surgical treatment may be needed to minimize the extent of permanent injury.

Brachial and Lumbosacral Plexus Lesions

Plexus lesions should be suspected when symptoms are not confined to the distribution of a single nerve or nerve root, but instead indicate injury to several anatomically related nerves. The anatomy of the brachial and lumbosacral plexuses is quite complex,[38,39] and detailed analysis of these lesions requires careful examination and often EMG and NCV studies. Fortunately, detailed assessment is not required in the acute care setting, and these patients can be referred for elective evaluation.

Acute lesions of the brachial plexus are often due to trauma. Violent stretching or twisting of the neck, shoulder, or upper arm are obvious potential causes. Less immediately obvious are compression injuries from shoulder straps. An idiopathic (possibly inflammatory or immune-mediated) brachial plexopathy (Parsonage-Turner syndrome) is also well described. It is usually characterized by severe pain in the shoulder and upper arm; weakness of arm muscles, sensory loss, and impaired reflexes involving several different nerve distributions are also seen. Acute treatment consists of pain management and rest; steroids are often prescribed but are of unknown benefit.

Acute lesions of the lumbosacral plexus can result from pelvic fractures. Other potential causes of particular interest in the acute care setting include leaking abdominal aortic aneurysm or retroperitoneal hemorrhage (in patients on anticoagulant therapy). Infiltration of the plexus by cancer or compression from retroperitoneal or psoas muscle abscess also occur but generally have a subacute or chronic course.

Peripheral Mononeuropathy

Isolated acute lesions can affect virtually every peripheral nerve, each resulting in a characteristic clinical syndrome. As noted previously, recognition of these syndromes depends on the skill of the examining physician; because of the bewildering variety of these syndromes, liberal use should be made of appropriate tables and references. Many of these syndromes are sufficiently common that they should be easily recognized by acute care physicians. In the upper extremity, common syndromes include those of the median, ulnar, and radial nerves. In the lower extremity, the common syndromes are those of the lateral femoral cutaneous, femoral, sciatic, and peroneal nerves. It is important to recall that the clinical syndromes are frequently incomplete; it is generally best to base the diagnosis on those findings that *are* present rather than on those that are absent. For example, weakness of the extensor muscles of the wrist and fingers should suggest a radial nerve palsy even in the absence of the typical sensory findings.

As noted above, many peripheral nerve injuries are caused by obvious trauma. However, the peripheral nerve injury itself may *not* be obvious, especially in the face of pain, or limited motion, caused by the primary injury. The acute care physician should always consider the possibility of peripheral nerve injury in trauma patients and should carry out any needed examination. A less obvious cause of peripheral nerve injury is *pressure palsy,* resulting from sustained compression of a nerve, often against a bony surface. There is usually no obvious trauma, and the patient may be unaware of the cause of the injury. There are several quite common pressure palsies in the acute care setting.

Radial nerve palsy results from compression of the radial nerve against the medial surface of the humerus in the upper arm. This can result when an arm is allowed to hang over the back of a chair or over the side of a bed for an extended period (Saturday night palsy), or when a heavy object (such as a companion's head) is allowed to rest on the inside of the upper arm (honeymooner's palsy). The nerve is occasionally injured in the axilla in patients using crutches. A more restricted radial palsy, characterized by pain and numbness on the back of the hand, but without weakness, can result from compression of the superficial sensory branches of the nerve from handcuffs.

Median and *ulnar* nerve palsies can also result from compression of the nerves in the axilla, at the elbow, and at the wrist. The median nerve can be injured at the wrist (carpal tunnel syndrome) by a variety of mechanisms. Although usually chronic, these are occasionally seen as an acute problem in pregnant women or following forceful hyperextension of the wrist (as in motor vehicle accidents).

Sciatic nerve palsies can result from local pressure on the sciatic nerve from prolonged sitting in a fixed position, particularly in patients who drive long distances; a large billfold in a hip pocket may be the culprit. The sciatic nerve may also be injured when a leg is allowed to hang over the edge of the bed for a prolonged period, as when a patient falls asleep while intoxicated.

Peroneal nerve palsy results from compression of the peroneal nerve where it passes under the head of the fibula. This occurs when patients sit for long periods with one leg crossed over the other, or in bedridden patients who are unable to move their legs. The nerve is sometimes injured when the legs are placed in stirrups to maintain the lithotomy position during obstetrical delivery, gynecologic examinations, and so on.

Femoral nerve palsy can result from compression of the femoral nerve at the inguinal ligament; this can result from hematomas following arterial puncture or from forceful flexion of the hips during childbirth or gynecologic procedures. Compression of the femoral nerve within the abdomen by an enlarged uterus is an occasional complication of pregnancy. The femoral nerve can also be injured with retroperitoneal bleeding.

Lateral femoral cutaneous nerve injury causes pain and paresthesias in the anterolateral thigh (meralgia paresthetica). This is a pure sensory nerve and there are no motor symptoms. The cause is usually obscure, but the nerve is occasionally injured by pressure from the enlarged abdomen in pregnant patients or grossly obese patients, or occasionally by tight undergarments.

Finally, isolated peripheral nerve palsies may occur for an number of other reasons. Some of these, especially in patients with diabetes or other microangiopathic diseases, are thought to result from nerve infarction; others are probably immune-mediated. In some cases, no explanation can be found.

In most cases, no urgent treatment is necessary or available. Fortunately, the prognosis is usually good unless the nerve is transected. It is important to be able to reassure the patient that he or she has not had a stroke or other neurologic catastrophe.

Mononeuritis multiplex is a rare clinical syndrome in which two or more isolated peripheral nerves are affected nearly simultaneously. This is most often the result of microvascular infarction of nerves and may be seen in polyarteritis nodosa or other vasculitides, or in diabetes. Other potential causes include multifocal motor neuropathy (an autoimmune-mediated disorder), sarcoidosis, and others.

Summary

Patients with acute focal weakness are frequently seen in the acute care setting. The crucial step in the evaluation of these patients is localization of the anatomic lesion causing the clinical symptoms. A useful technique is for the physician to consider, in each case, whether the symptoms could be caused by a lesion in the brain, the brainstem, the spinal cord, the peripheral nerves, or the muscles. The clinical history and neurologic examination are the sources of the necessary information. Accurate localization of the lesion and the clinical course should suggest a differential diagnosis; the differential diagnosis should then suggest the appropriate laboratory and imaging studies. There are relatively few causes of acute focal weakness that require emergency management; often the task of the acute care physician is to determine that the patient does *not* require emergency intervention.

The most common emergency condition is acute stroke. At this time, the best management of acute stroke is highly controversial, and physicians can expect a continuing flood of new data and conflicting opinions; the matter is likely to remain unsettled for some time. Regardless, the cornerstone of management is meticulous attention to suppportive measures ensuring oxygenation and perfusion. Whatever approaches ultimately prove to be superior, the pathophysiology of stroke implies that effectiveness of any treatment will depend in large measure on rapid identification of appropriate patients. It seems likely that the choice of therapy will vary depending on the probable mechanism of the stroke, placing a high premium on rapid clinical assessment.

A second category of patients who may benefit from urgent intervention are those with acute brainstem lesions. Although such conditions are less likely to respond to specific treatment, these patients are at substantial risk from respiratory failure and aspiration, and protection of the airway and support of ventilation should be considered.

The final category of patients who require emergency treatment are those with spinal cord syndromes, especially spinal cord compression from mass lesions. Urgent decompression may reduce or prevent permanent damage to the spinal cord.

REFERENCES

1. Hakim AM. Ischemic penumbra: the therapeutic window. *Neurology* 1998;51:544–546.
2. Kothari RU, et al. Emergency physicians: accuracy in diagnosis of stroke. *Stroke* 1995;26:2238–2241.
3. Libman RB, et al. Conditions that mimic stroke in the emergency department. *Arch Neurol* 1995;52:1119–1122.
4. Culebras A, et al. Practice guidelines for the use of imaging in transient ischemic attacks and acute stroke: a report of the Stroke Council, American Heart Association. *Stroke* 1997;28:1480–1497.
5. Schriger DL, et al. Physician accuracy in determining eligibility for thrombolytic therapy. *JAMA* 1998;279:1293–1297.
6. Parsons MW, et al. Diffusion- and perfusion-weighted MRI response to thrombolysis in stroke. *Ann Neurol* 2002;51:28–37.
7. Warach S. Thrombolysis in stroke beyond three hours: targeting patients with diffusion and perfusion MRI. *Ann Neurol* 2002;51:11–13.
8. Schellinger PD, et al. Stroke: magnetic resonance imaging within 6 hours after onset of hyperacute cerebral ischemia. *Ann Neurol* 2001;49:460–469.
9. Adams HP, et al. Guidelines for the management of patients with acute ischemic stroke. A statement for healthcare professionals from a special writing group of the Stroke Council, American Heart Association. *Stroke* 1994;25:1901–1914.
10. The National Institute of Neurological Disorders and Stroke rt-PA Stroke Study Group. Tissue plasminogen activator for acute ischemic stroke. *N Engl J Med* 1995;333:1581–1587.
11. Hacke W, et al. Intravenous thrombolysis with recombinant tissue plasminogen activator for acute hemispheric stroke. The European Cooperative Acute Stroke Study. *JAMA* 1995;274:1017–1025.
12. Hacke W, et al. Randomised double-blind placebo-controlled trial of thrombolytic therapy with intravenous alteplase in acute ischaemic stroke (ECASS II). Second European-Australasian Stroke Study Investigators. *Lancet* 1998;352:1245–1251.
13. Clark WM, et al. Recombinant tissue-type plasminogen activator (Alteplase) for ischemic stroke 3 to 5 hours after symptom onset. The ATLANTIS Study: a randomized controlled trial. Alteplase Thrombolysis for Acute Noninterventional Therapy in Ischemic Stroke. *JAMA* 1999;282:2019–2026.
14. Katzan IL, et al. Use of tissue-type plasminogen activator for acute ischemic stroke: the Cleveland area experience. *JAMA* 2000;283:1151–1158.
15. Grotta JC, et al. Intravenous tissue-type plasminogen activator therapy for ischemic stroke. Houston experience 1996–2000. *Arch Neurol* 2001;58:2009–2013.
16. Lewandowski C, Barsan W. Treatment of acute ischemic stroke. *Ann Emerg Med* 2001;37:202–216.
17. Adams HP, et al. Guidelines for thrombolytic therapy for acute stroke: a supplement to the guidelines for the management of patients with acute ischemic stroke. A statement for healthcare professionals from a special writing group of the Stroke Council, American Heart Association. *Circulation* 1996;94:1167–1174.
18. Canadian Association of Emergency Physicians Committee on Thrombolytic Therapy for Acute Ischemic Stroke. Thrombolytic therapy for acute ischemic stroke. *Canadian Journal of Emergency Medical Care* 2001;3.
19. Albers GW, et al. Antithrombotic and thrombolytic therapy for ischemic stroke. *Chest* 1998;114:683S–698S.

20. Berge E, et al. ASA or low-molecular-weight heparin in the initial management of acute ischemic stroke complicating atrial fibrillation? *Lancet* 2000;355:1205–1210.

21. Counsell C, Sandercock P. Low-molecular weight-heparins or heparinoids versus standard unfractionated heparin for acute ischaemic stroke (Cochrane Review) In: *The Cochrane Library,* Issue 3, 2001.

22. Gubitz G, et al. Anticoagulants for acute ischaemic stroke (Cochrane Review). In: *The Cochrane Library,* Issue 3, 2001.

23. Joint Stroke Guideline Committee of the American Academy of Neurology and the American Stroke Association. Anticoagulants and antiplatelet agents in acute ischemic stroke. *Neurology* 2002;59:13–22.

24. International Stroke Trial Collaborative Group. The International Stroke Trial (IST): a randomized trial of aspirin, subcutaneous heparin, both, or neither among 19,435 patients with acute ischaemic stroke. *Lancet* 1997;349:1569–1581.

25. Chinese Acute Stroke Trial (CAST) Collaborative Group. CAST: a randomized placebo-controlled trial of early aspirin use in 20,000 patients with acute ischemic stroke. *Lancet* 1997;349:1641–1649.

26. Powers WJ. Acute hypertension after stroke: the scientific basis for treatment decisions. *Neurology* 1993;43:461–467.

27. Bruno A, et al. Acute blood glucose level and outcome from ischemic stroke. *Neurology* 1999;52:280–284.

28. Tracy D, et al Hyperglycemia and mortality from acute stroke. *Q J Med* 1993;86:439.

29. Kagansky N, Levy S, Knobler H. The role of hyperglycemia in acute stroke. *Arch Neurol* 2001;58:1209–1212.

30. Broderick JP, et al. Guidelines for the management of spontaneous intracerebral hemorrhage: a statement for healthcare professionals from a special writing group of the Stroke Council, American Heart Association. *Stroke* 1999;30:905–915.

31. Committee on Cerebrovascular Diseases. Classification and outline of cerebrovascular diseases II. *Stroke* 1975;6:564–616.

32. Harbison J, Palmer K, Ochs A. Migraine amaurosis fugax? Investigate. (abstract). *Stroke* 1987;18:225.

33. Victor M, Ropper AH. *Adams and Victor's Principles of Neurology,* 7th ed. New York: McGraw-Hill, 2001, pp 821–924.

34. Bruckner AB, et al. Heparin treatment in acute cerebral sinus venous thrombosis: a retrospective clinical and MRI analysis of 42 cases. *Cerebrovasc Dis* 1998;8:331–337.

35. Sagar SM, McGuire D. Infectious diseases. In: Samuels MA, ed. *Manual of Neurologic Therapeutics,* 6th ed. Philadelphia: Lippincott Williams & Wilkins, 1999.

36. Pruitt AA. Infections of the nervous system. *Neurol Clin North Am* 1998;16:419–447.

37. McAlpine D, Lumsden CE, Acheson ED. *Multiple Sclerosis: A Reappraisal,* 2nd ed. Edinburgh: Churchill Livingstone, 1972.

38. Weiss HD. Neoplasms. In: Samuels MA, ed. *Manual of Neurologic Therapeutics,* 6th ed. Philadelphia: Lippincott Williams & Wilkins, 1999.

39. Guarantors of Brain. *Aids to the Examination of the Peripheral Nervous System,* 2nd ed. London: Baillière-Tindall, 1986.

40. Devinsky O, Feldmann E. *Examination of the Cranial and Peripheral Nerves.* New York: Churchill Livingstone, 1988.

5

ACUTE GENERALIZED WEAKNESS

A large portion of the central and peripheral nervous system is dedicated to the initiation and control of voluntary movement. As a result, abnormal function in virtually any part of the nervous system may result in weakness of voluntary muscles. Chapter 4 discusses focal lesions of the nervous system that may result in localized weakness; this chapter reviews the evaluation and management of patients with more diffuse or generalized weakness. Many of the disorders causing generalized weakness are chronic or even lifelong; this discussion focuses on those disorders that develop over a few hours or days rather than over periods of weeks or longer.

Strictly speaking, the term *weakness* means loss of muscle power or strength. However, the term is often used by patients to denote a variety of different symptoms in addition to actual loss of strength. The term weakness is sometimes used to describe such symptoms as malaise, fatigue, or lassitude, conditions characterized more by a disinclination to move than by actual weakness. Patients with movement disorders, such as Parkinson's disease, often describe themselves as weak even though their actual muscle power is normal. (Even the classic term *paralysis agitans* implies weakness, although this is not a typical symptom of Parkinson's disease.) Patients with pain may also describe themselves as weak, due to their inability to move around as they wish. A careful history is often necessary to distinguish patients with actual weakness from those with other symptoms. If true weakness is present, the next step is to localize the likely cause within the nervous system. As with focal lesions, the location of the lesion should then suggest the likely diagnostic possibilities.

Clinical Assessment

History

The first and most important step in clinical diagnosis is to be as clear as possible about exactly what symptom is to be diagnosed. The differential diagnosis of true generalized weakness of acute onset is fairly limited, whereas the differential diagnosis of the multiple symptoms that may masquerade as weakness is enormous. The single best clinical clue to the presence of true muscle weakness is loss or impairment of function. It is often helpful to ask patients to describe their symptoms without using the term "weakness" or to ask them to describe any specific activities that are limited or prohibited by their supposed weakness. A patient who is unable to climb stairs is more likely to have true weakness than the patient who feels tired or exhausted after climbing stairs. A patient who cannot get up from a chair is more likely to have true weakness than one who gets up slowly and with difficulty. A patient unable to lift his arms over his head is more likely to have true weakness than one who feels exhausted after carrying out her usual daily activities. If true weakness seems likely, the physician should try to determine which muscles are affected and to what extent.

Once the basic nature of the patient's complaints is clear, the usual questions should be asked regarding the onset, progression, and severity of the symptoms. Patients commonly date the onset of their symptoms from the time they first became aware of them; what seems to the patient to be acute weakness may actually have been slowly evolving for months or even years. Careful questioning may reveal subtle changes in function that began well before the patient became aware the weakness. It is crucial to determine whether the weakness is constant or variable, provoked by activity, or relieved by rest. The patient should be questioned carefully about any recent or chronic illnesses and recent or chronic use of drugs, whether prescribed or otherwise, including alcohol. Other drugs of particular importance include diuretics, thyroid replacement, steroids, and lipid-lowering agents such as the statins. A prior history of similar symptoms should be sought. The presence or absence of bladder or bowel dysfunction, sexual dysfunction, pain, paresthesias, sensory loss, or muscle cramps and spasms should be determined. A family history of similar symptoms should be sought.

Physical Examination

A general physical examination should be performed. Special attention should be directed to any signs of chronic systemic illness, occult neoplasms, chronic infection, or endocrine dysfunction such as hyper- or hypothyroidism or Cushing's disease or syndrome. A fairly comprehensive neurologic examination is usually necessary. Especially for less experienced physicians, a "focused" neurologic examination carries a risk of missing essential information. When in doubt, it is usually better to be over- rather than underinclusive. The neurologic examination is discussed in Chapter 2; only a few points will be reviewed here.

The goals of the neurologic examination, as always, are to

1. Clarify the exact nature of the clinical symptoms. Does the patient have true loss of strength?
2. Identify clinical symptoms not recognized by the patient. For example, is weakness of the legs accompanied by mild but less evident weakness in the arms? Is the weakness accompanied by sensory loss not recognized by the patient?
3. Clarify the anatomic basis for the symptom. For example, is the weakness accompanied by altered reflexes or an upgoing toe, or by muscle atrophy and fasciculations?

The evaluation of muscle strength is commonly regarded as a fairly "objective" matter, a misconception reinforced by the common practice of rating muscle strength on a numerical scale. In fact, assessment of muscle strength is quite subjective and is highly dependent, as is most of the physical examination, on the skill and insight of the physician. It is important to recall that assessment of strength requires that the patient exert a maximum effort; patients' apparent strength can thus be affected by their willingness and ability to cooperate with the examiner. It may be difficult or impossible to assess strength reliably in an individual with severe pain or who is unwilling to make a maximum effort. Patients with severe anxiety or depression may not be motivated to make a full effort. Although true malingering is uncommon, patients with subjective weakness may try to "help" the examiner by exaggerating the extent of their weakness.

A substantial disparity between the strength of the examiner and the patient may also cause confusion. It is not uncommon for elderly patients to have their strength graded as "4/5," indicating a degree of weakness, when in fact their only problem is that they were examined by younger (and presumably stronger) house officers! Similarly, a small or slight examiner may be unable to detect even significant weakness in a much stronger patient. Accordingly, assessment of strength is ultimately a subjective judgement by the physician that an individual is as strong or less strong than expected. When in doubt, it is better simply to admit that strength cannot be adequately assessed than to "guess" that the patient is or is not weak.

The best way to assess strength is usually to observe the patient attempting to perform the specific activities that are affected by the reported weakness. Watching the patient get up from a chair and walk may be much more revealing than direct manual muscle testing. Careful observation of the patient's spontaneous activity during the interview and when his or her attention is distracted can yield important information.

If weakness is present, the distribution of the weakness should be determined. Are all four limbs affected? Are axial muscles (especially the neck and back) affected? Is there any involvement of the cranial nerve muscles such as extraocular muscles, the eyelids, or the face? Is there any involvement of speech or swallowing? A careful search should be made for any sign of an underlying focal disorder. Weakness affecting only the legs and sparing the arms may indicate a spinal cord lesion; weakness affecting all four extremities but completely sparing the face may indicate a lesion of the upper cervical spinal cord. Involvement of cranial muscles, especially if asymmetric, may indicate a brainstem lesion. A sensory "level" indicates a spinal cord lesion. The presence of hyperactive reflexes or a Babinski sign indicates a central (brain or spinal cord) lesion, but recall that complete arreflexia may be seen in patients with acute lesions of the spinal cord (see Chaps. 4 and 9 for further discussion).

Laboratory Studies

Routine blood studies (electrolytes, complete blood count [CBC], and others) are unlikely to be of much value in the initial assessment of patients with acute generalized weakness. Specific laboratory studies should be obtained as indicated by the clinical context. For example, in patients taking diuretics or laxatives, severe *hypokalemia* may be the cause of marked weakness; patients with periodic paralysis may develop severe weakness from either *hypokalemia* or *hyperkalemia*. Patients with cancer may develop severe weakness as a result of *hypercalcemia*. Necrosis of muscle cells (rhabdomyolysis) may result in marked elevation of serum *creatine kinase* (CK) levels and urine *myoglobin* levels. The *erythrocyte sedimentation rate* (ESR) may be elevated in patients with inflammatory muscle disease but is nonspecific and therefore often of little help. In general, appropriate laboratory studies will be suggested by the differential diagnosis; screening studies are usually not indicated.

In contrast to patients with acute focal weakness, imaging studies (such as computed tomography [CT] and magnetic resonance imaging [MRI]) are rarely necessary or helpful in evaluation of patients with generalized weakness. Electrodiagnostic studies (electromyography [EMG] and nerve conduction velocity [NCV]) are often helpful to confirm a clinical diagnosis but are rarely needed or available on an urgent basis. In patients with severe generalized weakness, bedside tests of pulmonary function (negative inspiratory pressure and forced vital capacity) can estimate respiratory reserve and indicate the need for ventilator support. In selected patients, an *edrophonium (Tensilon) test* can confirm the diagnosis of myasthenia gravis (see below). Lumbar puncture may reveal elevated protein and relatively normal cells in patients with Guillain-Barré syndrome but is frequently normal (and therefore not helpful) early in the course of the disease (see below).

DIFFERENTIAL DIAGNOSIS

Acute generalized weakness can result from disorders affecting virtually any part of the nervous system; as noted earlier, the differential diagnosis and diagnostic strategy depend on the likely location of the lesion. In the case of brain disorders, for example, generalized weakness is the result of diffuse brain dysfunction and is likely to be associated with abnormalities of consciousness and mentation; the primary focus of the evaluation will be the altered mental status, which is discussed in Chapter 3. Similarly, focal disorders of the brainstem and spinal cord may cause generalized weakness; their evaluation is discussed in Chapter 4. As noted in Chapter 4, any clinical suspicion of an acute spinal cord lesion should prompt an urgent imaging study.

In the acute care setting, the most important causes of acute generalized weakness *without localizing signs* are disorders affecting the peripheral nerves, the neuromuscular junction, and the muscles themselves. Clinical features that help to distinguish among these are listed in Table 5-1. Inspection of the table reveals that the clinical features of these disorders are often highly variable; as a result, a reliable diagnosis cannot often be based on one or two features but rather depends on the entire clinical picture.

Peripheral nerve disorders may involve isolated nerves, as discussed in Chapter 4; disorders that affect the peripheral nerves in a more diffuse or generalized fashion, such as the Guillain-Barré syndrome, are termed *polyneuropathies.* These conditions may affect either primarily myelin (*demyelinating polyneuropathies*) or the axons themselves (*axonal polyneuropathies*) or both. Depending on the particular population of nerve fibers affected, symptoms may be primarily motor weakness, primarily sensory (pain, paresthesias, sensory loss), or any combination of these. Because longer nerve fibers are commonly affected first, symptoms often begin distally and spread proximally. There may be atrophy of distal muscles, and fasciculations are occasionally seen. Reflexes are often markedly diminished or absent, even in muscles not obviously weak or otherwise affected. Muscle enzymes (e.g., creatine kinase [CK]) are normal.

Neuromuscular junction disorders, such as myasthenia gravis, are characterized by highly variable weakness that may be relieved by rest. The weakness is fre-

TABLE 5-1

GENERALIZED WEAKNESS: PERIPHERAL LOCALIZATION

Clinical Sign	Neuropathy	N-M Junction	Myopathy
Weakness (pattern)	Distal > proximal	Variable	Proximal > distal
Weakness (severity)	Constant, progressive	Variable	Constant, progressive
Sensory loss	Distal > proximal	Absent	Absent
Pain	Variable, distal	Absent	Usually absent
Muscle atrophy	Variable, often early	Absent	Variable, usually late
Reflexes	Decreased or absent	Normal	Normal or slightly decreased
Fasciculations	Sometimes	Absent	Absent
CSF protein	Normal or increased	Normal	Normal
CK level (serum)	Normal	Normal	Increased
Edrophonium test	No response	May respond	No response

quently asymmetric and often does not respect anatomic boundaries. Cranial nerve muscles and spinal nerve muscles are often affected together. Sensory symptoms and pain are absent. Reflexes are generally preserved unless the weakness is severe. Muscle enzymes are usually normal.

Muscle disorders are characterized by fairly symmetric weakness affecting proximal more than distal muscles; axial muscles are often affected as well. Although muscle pain and tenderness are sometimes present, sensory symptoms are absent. Reflexes are generally preserved unless weakness is severe. Muscle enzymes may be normal or markedly elevated.

By the time a patient's illness has progressed to the point of severe generalized weakness, these clinical patterns may be obscured. However, a careful history can often reveal how the symptoms began and progressed and thus suggest the likely location of the disorder.

Peripheral Nerve Disorders

Many of the disorders that affect the peripheral nervous system are chronic. The chronic polyneuropathies due to diabetes and other metabolic disorders, chemotherapeutic drugs, genetic disorders, and other causes may sometimes cause patients to present to the acute care setting seeking treatment for pain, weakness, gait disorders, or other symptoms. A brief history will reveal that the neuropathy is long-standing, and the focus of care will be relief of the acute symptoms rather than diagnosis and management of the underlying disorder. There are, however, a few conditions in which peripheral nerve disorders cause acute or subacute weakness and that therefore require urgent evaluation and treatment (Table 5-2).

TABLE 5-2
ACUTE PERIPHERAL NERVE DISORDERS

I. Acute Motor Paralysis[a]
  A. Guillain-Barré syndrome
  B. Diphtheritic polyneuropathy
  C. Porphyric polyneuropathy
  D. Tick paralysis
  E. Critical illness polyneuropathy

II. Acute or Subacute Sensorimotor Neuropathy[b]
  A. Deficiency states (alcoholism, beriberi, pellagra, vitamin B_{12})
  B. Toxic polyneuropathy

[a] Although acute motor weakness is the most prominent symptom in these conditions, sensory symptoms such as pain, paresthesias, or sensory loss commonly occur as well. See text for details.
[b] Either motor or sensory symptoms may predominate; the clinical picture varies from one syndrome to another and may vary among patients with the same condition. See text.

Guillain-Barré syndrome (GBS) is known by a variety of eponyms, most derived by stringing together the various names of the many authors who have described components of the clinical syndrome during the past century. In an effort to avoid such eponymic confusion, the term *acute idiopathic demyelinating polyradiculoneuritis (AIDP)* has been widely adopted. The cause of AIDP remains unclear; about 50% to 60% of cases appear to develop a few weeks after apparent viral illness (often mild), but many cases develop without any evident prodrome. Recently, infection with *Campylobacter jejuni* has been identified as a cause in some cases. The syndrome has been associated with multiple other infectious agents including HIV. The mechanism of the disorder involves an autoimmune-mediated attack on peripheral nerves.

The major clinical symptom of AIDP is progressive weakness. This usually begins in the lower extremities and may spread to involve the upper extremities, the trunk, the cranial muscles. and sometimes even the eye muscles. Bilateral facial weakness develops in about 50% of cases. The weakness may be mild or may progress to total motor paralysis. Approximately 30% of patients develop marked weakness of respiratory muscles and thus require ventilator support. Reflexes are markedly reduced and frequently absent, even relatively early in the clinical course when weakness may be mild. Aching pain, especially in the thighs and back, is common. Some sensory loss is also quite common but is often overlooked since position and vibration sensation are more likely affected than pain sensation. The symptoms usually evolve over a few days to a week or so; in some cases maximal weakness may not be evident for several weeks, and, in rare instances, severe weakness may develop within less than a day. Autonomic symptoms, such as tachycardia, bradycardia, labile hypertension and hypotension, and hyperthermia, are common and potentially life-threatening.

The key to the diagnosis is recognition by an alert physician. In patients with the typical clinical syndrome, the diagnosis is usually straightforward. The differential diagnosis includes the other entities listed in Table 5-2. Variant forms of AIDP also occur and may pose a diagnostic challenge. In some cases, the initial symptoms may be pain in the back and legs with only mild or minimal weakness; these patients may be erroneously diagnosed with muscle strain, acute viral illnesses, and other conditions. Rarely, the muscles of the face, neck, and upper trunk are affected first. In the so-called *Fisher variant*, the initial symptoms are complete ophthalmoplegia, limb ataxia, and arreflexia. In these cases such conditions as brainstem strokes, myasthenia gravis, or botulism may be suspected; these are discussed below.

Laboratory studies are of little help. The cerebrospinal fluid (CSF) formula is classically characterized by elevated protein with only minimal or no pleocytosis, but this finding is often absent early in the course of the disease and may not develop until several days or more after onset. Accordingly, normal CSF studies do not exclude the diagnosis. Even when present, the elevation of CSF protein is too nonspecific to be considered diagnostic. Respiratory function should be assessed as soon as the diagnosis is suspected and should be followed closely. Inspiratory pressure and vital capacity are useful measures that can be easily assessed at the bedside. A downward trend in vital capacity is an ominous sign; intubation is performed if vital capacity falls to 12 to 15 mL/kg (25% to 35% of normal).

Virtually all patients with known or suspected AIDP should be admitted to the hospital, usually to an ICU or other setting where close observation of vital signs and respiratory function can be provided. The only exceptions are those patients with normal respiratory function and very mild weakness that has been present for a week or more and that is clearly stable, and who can be closely watched by a responsible person who can immediately return them to the hospital if there is any deterioration. Severe hypotension should be managed with volume expansion and with pressors if necessary; severe hypertension should be managed with short-acting agents that can easily be titrated, such as esmolol or nitroprusside since blood pressure may be very labile, and elevated pressures may suddenly fall. Specific treatment either with plasma exchange (200 to 250 mL/kg over four to six treatments) or intravenous immune globulin (0.4 g/kg each day for 5 days) has been shown to shorten the duration of ventilator support and hospitalization and to hasten recovery. Steroids are of no benefit. Otherwise, care is largely supportive. Long-term prognosis is generally good, with 85% to 90% of patients eventually making a good functional recovery.[1–3]

Diphtheria and *acute intermittent porphyria* can cause acute generalized weakness essentially identical to that caused by AIDP; both are quite rare. In diphtheria, mild weakness of cranial muscles may be present during the acute phase of the illness, but the polyneuropathy may not develop until some 6 to 8 weeks later. Treatment is supportive. Acute intermittent porphyria is characterized by recurrent attacks of colicky abdominal pain and vomiting, sometimes associated with confusion and delirium; attacks may be precipitated by a wide variety of drugs and other causes. The polyneuropathy is very similar to that of AIDP, although the facial and cranial muscles are less likely to be affected. Treatment is directed at the porphyria; treatment of the neurologic disorder is supportive.

Tick paralysis is a relatively rare syndrome of acute ascending weakness caused by a toxin secreted by the bite of a female tick (most often *Dermacentor* or *Ixodes*). The identity of the toxin and its mode of action remain obscure; the clinical syndrome is virtually indistinguishable from AIDP except that there are no sensory symptoms and the CSF protein remains normal. The weakness can be profound and can cause respiratory failure and death. The disease is more common in children (perhaps due to their relatively smaller body mass) and occurs when ticks are active. Diagnosis depends on finding the tick; there is no other diagnostic test. A careful search for ticks should be made in all patients with suspected AIDP during appropriate seasons. Treatment consists of removal of the tick; improvement is rapid and complete recovery is expected. Treatments used for AIDP are ineffective in tick paralysis.

Critical illness polyneuropathy is an important cause of acute weakness, admittedly unlikely to present in the usual acute care setting. However, it is important for primary care physicians to be aware of this syndrome. The disorder typically occurs in critically ill patients in ICUs, especially patients with sepsis and multiple organ failure. It is characterized by an acute axonal neuropathy, primarily affecting motor function; it may cause profound and prolonged weakness, delaying weaning from ventilator support. There is no specific treatment, and recovery is very prolonged. This syndrome is distinct from the critical illness myopathy discussed below.[4]

Toxic polyneuropathies may be caused by a bewildering variety of environmental and occupational toxins, plant and animal poisons, and drugs.[5-7] A partial list of potential neurotoxins is given in Table 5-3; the list is by no means complete and is intended to give the physician some indication of the variety of possible offending substances. The keys to the correct diagnosis are a high index of suspicion and a history of exposure to an appropriate toxin. Obtaining an adequate history may involve considerable detective work since patients may be unaware of their exposure or, in the case of some toxins, unwilling to admit their exposure.

Toxic neuropathies are often subacute or chronic in onset but can present acutely. In fact, the clinical picture of an acute, rapidly progressive mixed sensory and motor neuropathy should suggest the diagnosis. The clinical picture is highly variable; a given neurotoxin may cause quite different clinical syndromes in different patients.

TABLE 5-3
NEUROTOXIC SUBSTANCES

Heavy Metals
Arsenic
Lead
Thallium
Mercury

Chemical Compounds
Acrylamide
Allyl chloride
Carbon disulfide
Chlorinated phenoxy herbicides
Ethylene oxide
Hexacarbons
Methyl bromide
Organophosphate esters
Polychlorinated biphenyls
Trichloroethylene
Vacor

Plant and Animal Toxins
Tick paralysis
Snake and sea snake venoms
Ciguatera
Paralytic shellfish poisoning
Neurotoxic shellfish poisoning
Puffer fish (*Fugu*) poisoning
Buckthorn poisoning

(continued)

TABLE 5-3

NEUROTOXIC SUBSTANCES *(continued)*

Drugs
Antibiotics
  Isoniazid
  Ethambutol
  Nitrofurantoin
  Metronidazole
  Chloramphenicol
  Dapsone
Antineoplastic agents
  Vinca alkaloids
  Cisplatin
  Thalidomide
  Doxorubicin
Others
  Phenytoin
  Pyridoxine
  Nitrous oxide
  Tacrolimus
  Colchicine
  Disulfiram
  Procainamide
  Amiodarone
  Gold
  Antiretroviral agents

Toxic neuropathies are usually characterized by both motor and sensory symptoms, although either may predominate. Pain is common. The symptoms most often begin in the distal parts of the extremities and spread proximally. In their more chronic forms, toxic neuropathies may be difficult to distinguish from chronic congenital or metabolic disorders (such as diabetes), but this is unlikely to be an issue in the acute care setting. A few representative toxic neuropathies are reviewed here.

Arsenic is an occasional cause of acute polyneuropathy. Arsenic may be encountered in industrial settings and in some insecticides and is occasionally used with suicidal or homicidal intent. Acute ingestion of arsenic causes severe abdominal pain, vomiting, and diarrhea and may be rapidly fatal. If the patient survives the acute exposure, the acute symptoms resolve, to be followed within a few days or weeks by the neuropathy. This commonly takes the form of a acute, rapidly progressive, often very painful motor and sensory neuropathy that begins in the feet and spreads proximally. It can easily be mistaken for AIDP, especially early in the course. Diagnosis depends on a high index of suspicion; high levels of arsenic in the urine, hair, and fingernails confirm the diagnosis. The classic findings of arsenic intoxication (Mees' lines in the nails, pigmented dermatitis, and others) may not occur for several weeks. Poisoning with *thallium, lead,* and *mercury* may cause a similar syndrome.

Chemical neuropathies may result from exposure to a wide variety of industrial and domestic chemicals; some seemingly exotic chemicals can be easily encountered in the everyday environment. *Ethyl alcohol* may cause polyneuropathy either directly or as a consequence of prolonged nutritional deficiency. *Trichloroethylene* is used in the dry cleaning industry, and *ethylene oxide* is used in gas sterilization systems. *Hexacarbon* solvents are the cause of the neuropathy and encephalopathy encountered in glue sniffers. *Organophosphate* compounds, employed as insecticides, cause acute neuromuscular blockade (see below) but may also be associated with a delayed peripheral neuropathy. The list of potential chemical toxins is large and constantly growing; appropriate references,[5-7] Material Safety Data Sheets, and poison control centers should be consulted as needed.

Animal and plant venoms and toxins can cause a variety of neuropathic syndromes. *Tick paralysis* has already been discussed above. Some *snake venoms,* such as that of the Eastern coral snake, are highly neurotoxic and can quickly cause paralysis and death. Treatment consists of supportive care and administration of the appropriate antivenin; a poison control center should be consulted. Many species of *marine fish and shellfish* produce neurotoxins; clinically these cause a combination of gastrointestinal, autonomic, and neurologic symptoms. Treatment is mostly supportive.

Drug-induced neuropathies are fairly common and may be due to a wide variety of agents. Most often these conditions follow a subacute or chronic course and are unlikely to require emergency diagnosis or management. When more rapid in onset, they may present in the acute care setting and may be confused with AIDP or other acute neuropathy; unfortunately, there are no reliable clinical findings specific to these syndromes. Usually, a careful history will reveal that the clinical symptoms began well before and evolved slowly; the patients present when their symptoms become noticeable or intolerable. Treatment is largely supportive; the offending substance should be withdrawn if possible. Agents such as amitriptyline or gabapentin may help to relieve the discomfort.

Neuromuscular Junction Disorders

The neuromuscular junction is a highly specialized structure at which acetylcholine (ACh), released from a nerve terminal in response to a nerve action potential, diffuses across a narrow synaptic cleft to interact with receptors on a specialized area of muscle membrane (the motor end plate). In response to this chemical stimulus, a muscle action potential is generated that results in contraction of the muscle fibers. Clinical disorders that impair or prevent the release of ACh, or that interfere with its effective binding to the muscle receptors, thus prevent normal muscle contraction and result in weakness of the affected muscles. As noted earlier, there are no sensory symptoms, and reflexes are generally preserved. Disorders of neuromuscular transmission that may be seen in the acute care setting are listed in Table 5-4.

Myasthenia gravis (MG) is the most important primary disorder of neuromuscular transmission. MG is an autoimmune disorder in which antibodies are

TABLE 5-4
NEUROMUSCULAR JUNCTION DISORDERS

Myasthenia gravis
Lambert-Eaton myasthenic syndrome
Drugs and toxins
    Botulism
    Tetanus
    Black widow spider bite
    Strychnine poisoning
    Organophosphate poisoning
    Drug-induced neuromuscular blockade

produced that bind with ACh receptors on the motor end plate. Those receptors occupied by antibody are unable to bind ACh; although normal amounts of ACh are released into the synaptic cleft, the lack of adequate receptor sites results in failure of neuromuscular transmission and muscle weakness. Over time, permanent structural changes occur in the motor end plate leading to chronic weakness.

The cause of MG remains unknown. It may appear in isolation or in association with other autoimmune disorders such as Graves' disease or systemic lupus erythematosus. The peak age of onset is between 20 and 30 years in women and between 50 and 60 years in men. In most cases the onset is insidious, and patients may have consulted several physicians before a diagnosis is made; in a few cases the onset is quite abrupt, and such patients may well present to acute care settings. Some patients with well-established and treated MG may experience periodic crises of markedly increased weakness and require treatment in the acute care setting.

The cardinal symptom of MG is fluctuating weakness; repeated use of an affected muscle results in progressive weakness and exhaustion, whereas rest often results in at least partial recovery. Weakness of the extraocular muscles and levator palpebrae (causing ptosis) is a common presenting symptom and eventually occurs in more than 90% of patients. Other bulbar muscles (facial expression, mastication, speech, and swallowing) are affected in 80%. Skeletal muscles may be affected as well; although proximal muscles are more often and more severely affected than distal muscles, virtually any pattern of muscle weakness can be seen. The degree of weakness can be severe, with compromise of respiration, inability to swallow or speak, and other symptoms.

MG should be considered in any patient who presents with weakness of sudden onset, especially if the weakness is variable. The presence of weakness affecting the face, the levator palpebrae, and extraocular movements with sparing of the pupils is virtually diagnostic. If the patient can cooperate, repeat testing of an affected muscle may result in worsening weakness, and rest results in improvement; when present, this finding is diagnostic. A common maneuver is to ask the patient to count backward from 100 until her speech is slurred and indistinct; a short period of rest will restore normal speech. In patients with diplopia, sustained gaze in one direction will result in worsening diplopia; allowing the patient to rest for several minutes with the eyes closed will temporarily restore normal vision. The diagnosis can be confirmed with the *edrophonium test* (Table 5-5); a positive test confirms the diagnosis, but a negative test does not exclude MG.

Treatment of MG is complex and should usually be managed by a neurologist. Severely affected patients should be admitted to the hospital, and a neurologist should be consulted. Patients with significant impairment of respiration or at risk for aspiration may require intubation and ventilator support until their condition can be improved. For patients with less severe symptoms, treatment with pyridostigmine 30 to 90 mg PO q6h may provide symptomatic relief until they can be seen by a neurologist. A common starting dose is 60 mg PO q6h. If desired, the response to pyridostigmine can be assessed by giving the first dose IM or IV using 1/30 of the PO dose (i.e., 1 to 2 mg).

A special problem in the acute care setting concerns those patients with established myasthenia who present with abrupt worsening of their symptoms (myasthenic crisis). This is most often due to worsening of their disease and may result from intercurrent illness (often a respiratory or other infection), from treatment with certain drugs (Table 5-6), or from no evident cause. If these patients are not

TABLE 5-5 ────────────────────────────────

THE EDROPHONIUM TEST[a]

1. The strength of several affected muscles should be assessed as objectively as possible, e.g.:
   Measure the palpebral fissures in patients with ptosis.
   Observe the severity of ocular misalignment in patients with diplopia.
   Have the patient count out loud until unable to continue.
   Measure grip strength with a dynamometer; clinical assessment is less reliable.
   Assess respiratory function—maximum inspiratory force and vital capacity.
2. Administer 10 mg (1 mL) edrophonium chloride intravenously:
   Give 1 mg (0.1 mL) initially; observe for improvement or side effects.
   Give 3 to 6 mg (0.3 to 0.6 mL); observe for 45 seconds for improvement or side effects.
   If no effect, give the remainder; observe for improvement or side effects.
3. A *positive* result is objective improvement in the strength of one or more of the muscles assessed. There should be complete resolution of diplopia or ptosis and a measurable increase in muscle strength or respiratory function. Subjective improvement or equivocal results are not reliable.

[a] Side effects of edrophonium include nausea, vomiting, sweating, salivation, and occasionally bradycardia and hypotension. These can be prevented by pretreatment with atropine 0.4 to 0.8 mg SC. There is a very small risk of cardiac standstill, especially in older patients; facilities for resuscitation should be available.

TABLE 5-6

DRUGS THAT MAY WORSEN MYASTHENIA GRAVIS[a]

Neuromuscular blocking agents
Aminoglycoside antibiotics
Tetracyclines[b]
β-blockers[b]
Antiarrythmics
Calcium channel blockers
Magnesium
Procaine, lidocaine
Iodinated contrast agents
Corticosteroids[c]

[a] This is not an exhaustive list. Drugs are listed by class to give the reader a sense of the wide variety of agents that may exacerbate myasthenia gravis. Any new drug should be used with caution in patients with myasthenia.

[b] These agents may exacerbate myasthenia even when used as topical agents (eyedrops).

[c] Although corticosteroids are used in the treatment of myasthenia, they may cause temporary worsening, especially if introduced at full doses. A common strategy is to introduce corticosteroids at very low doses and to titrate the dose upward as tolerated.

taking anticholinesterase drugs, a trial of pyridostigmine (see above) may be helpful. Patients with myasthenic crisis may progress rapidly to severe weakness and respiratory collapse and should be hospitalized, preferably in the ICU, until their condition has been stabilized. Endotracheal intubation should be carried out as needed.

In myasthenic patients treated with anticholinesterase drugs, a similar clinical syndrome of progressive weakness can result from drug toxicity (cholinergic crisis). A common clinical scenario is that of the patient who experiences apparent worsening of her myasthenic weakness and attempts self-treatment by increasing the dose of anticholinesterase medication. Excess cholinergic effect causes further weakness, leading to a vicious circle. Weakness due to excess cholinergic effect may be difficult to distinguish from myasthenic weakness, although the presence of miosis and increased secretions suggests excessive cholinergic effect. Unfortunately, both myasthenic and cholinergic weakness can coexist in the same patient, further complicating both diagnosis and treatment. Although small doses of edrophonium can be used to distinguish the two syndromes (cholinergic weakness will get worse and myasthenic weakness may improve), this approach may be quite hazardous, leading to increased pharyngeal secretions and respiratory collapse simultaneously. The safer course in such cases is to be certain that the airway is secure, by intubation if needed, stop all cholinergic (anticholinesterase) medications until the patient is stable (as the effects of the drugs wear off), and then cautiously restart therapy. Hospital admission to an acute care unit is necessary.

In summary, MG is an important cause of acute weakness in the acute care setting. The acute care physician should remember the following points:

1. Myasthenia gravis should be considered in all patients who present with acute weakness. A positive edrophonium test confirms the diagnosis; a negative or equivocal test does not exclude the diagnosis.
2. Severe myasthenic weakness, especially when the muscles of the pharynx or respiratory muscles are involved, is a medical emergency. The focus of initial management is to protect the airway and ensure adequate respiration.
3. Myasthenic patients with abrupt worsening may have either myasthenic or cholinergic crises; these are difficult to distinguish on clinical grounds. The safest approach is to withhold medication, protect the airway and respiration, and wait for the situation to stabilize.

Lambert-Eaton myasthenic syndrome (LEMS) is another cause of muscle weakness that worsens with progressive exercise. The onset is usually subacute; in contrast to MG, the weakness in LEMS most commonly initially affects the proximal muscles of the legs, trunk, and shoulders rather than the bulbar muscles. Strength may actually increase with the first few contractions of an affected muscle, but this is often difficult to detect on clinical examination. Autonomic symptoms (impotence, dry mouth, difficult urination) are common. There is little or no response to anticholinesterase drugs (edrophonium, neostigmine, or pyridostigmine). LEMS occurs most commonly in association with small cell carcinoma of the lung; it may appear before the underlying tumor is detectable and may also occur in the absence of cancer. No emergency treatment is available.

Botulism is a rare cause of acute muscle weakness. It is caused by an exotoxin of *Clostridium botulinum,* an anaerobic bacterium that may contaminate improperly canned foods. There are at least seven serotypes of the toxin; types A, B, and E cause disease in humans. The toxin is heat-labile and is inactivated by adequate cooking. The toxin acts at the neuromuscular junction to prevent the release of acetylcholine, thus blocking neuromuscular transmission.

Clinical symptoms typically begin within 12 to 36 hours after ingestion of the contaminated food. The first symptoms usually involve the extraocular, facial, and pharyngeal muscles; ptosis, blurred vision, diplopia, facial weakness, dysarthria, dysphagia, and hoarseness may all occur. These early symptoms are similar to those of MG except that in botulism the pupillary reflexes are affected early; the pupils are rarely affected in MG. The weakness spreads rapidly to the muscles of the trunk and extremities and may progress to complete paralysis. As the weakness advances, it can be mistaken for AIDP; however, in botulism there are no sensory symptoms, and reflexes are preserved. There is no response to edrophonium.

Treatment is largely supportive; trivalent botulism antitoxin (obtained from the Centers for Disease Control and Prevention in Atlanta, Georgia) may shorten the course of the clinical illness. Recovery is very prolonged. Botulism is a reportable disease, and local health authorities should be notified.

Tetanus, although technically not a disorder of peripheral neuromuscular transmission, is included here because, like botulism, it is caused by a bacterial exotoxin (tetanospasmin), produced by the anaerobic bacterium *Clostridium tetani.* The spores of *C. tetani* are widespread in the environment, especially in soil; introduced into a wound, the spores become vegetative and elaborate the toxin. The primary action of the toxin is to block inhibitory neurotransmitters (especially γ-aminobutyric acid) at spinal cord and brainstem levels.

The clinical illness begins with a sensation of stiffness and cramping in the muscles of the jaws and face. Weakness is not prominent, but the stiffness may be initially described as weakness by the patient. As the disease advances, severe, prolonged, and very painful muscle spasms develop and spread to involve the neck, the trunk, and the extremities; these symptoms can progress to a state of generalized rigidity. The differential diagnosis includes poisoning from strychnine or black widow spider bite, neuroleptic malignant syndrome (see Chap. 6), and malignant hyperthermia (see below); the correct diagnosis is usually clear from the clinical context.

Treatment for tetanus includes administration of tetanus antitoxin. Subsequent care is largely supportive; sedation, muscle relaxants (such as benzodiazepines), and neuromuscular blockade may be used; ventilator support is almost always required. Local wound care (debridement, antibiotics, and other measures) can prevent further toxin production. Of course, tetanus is a preventable disease, hence the emphasis on the regular use of tetanus toxoid. An attack of tetanus does not confer immunity, and regular immunization is required.[8]

Black widow spider venom acts at the nerve terminals to provoke rapid release of acetylcholine, initially causing severe painful cramps, spasms, and muscle rigidity. As the supply of ACh becomes depleted, muscle weakness and paralysis develop and may be severe. The disorder can be fatal, especially in children (presumably because of their smaller body mass). Treatment is usually supportive; an antivenin is available. Complete recovery is expected with proper supportive care.

Organophosphate compounds are widely used as insecticides; they can be used as well as chemical warfare agents and by terrorists. These agents act by inhibiting acetylcholinesterase; in effect, they act as cholinergic agents. Symptoms of acute organophosphate poisoning develop immediately after exposure and include nausea and vomiting, abdominal cramps and diarrhea, increased salivation and lacrimation, bronchospasm, and muscle weakness. The pupils are usually miotic. In severe cases, death results from respiratory paralysis. The clinical picture is similar to that resulting from overdose of antimyasthenic drugs such as edrophonium, neostigmine, and pyridostigmine.

Treatment with pralidoxime (2-PAM) can reverse the effect of the toxin if administered within 24 to 48 hours of exposure. After that time, binding between the toxin and the acetylcholinesterase becomes irreversible, and recovery depends on the synthesis of new enzyme, a process that may take weeks or months. Treatment with anticholinergic drugs such as atropine will reverse the effects of excessive cholinergic stimulation of *muscarinic* receptors (salivation, lacrimation, GI symptoms, and others) but will not reverse the skeletal muscle weakness (resulting from overstimulation of *nicotinic* receptors. With appropriate support and treatment, full recovery is expected.[9]

Drug-induced neuromuscular blockade is sometimes seen in the acute care setting. Neuromuscular blocking agents are widely used in the acute care and intensive care settings and are not ordinarily a cause of diagnostic confusion. However, these drugs may occasionally be given in error, or with homicidal intent; possible intoxication with these agents should be suspected in a patient who abruptly develops generalized flaccid weakness. The clinical picture is similar to that of MG except for the abrupt onset of the symptoms. Use of these drugs in patients with MG (even in very mild or unsuspected cases) can result in prolonged paralysis and very delayed recovery.

A wide variety of other drugs can induce some degree of neuromuscular blockade (Table 5-6). These drugs do not cause clinically significant weakness in most patients but can potentially cause significant weakness in patients with MG. Treatment in these cases consists in withdrawal of the offending agent and supportive care as outlined for MG.

Disorders of Muscle

As with peripheral nerve diseases, most of the disorders of skeletal muscle are chronic and slowly progressive. Although not rare, chronic diseases such as the muscular dystrophies and most metabolic myopathies are unlikely to present in the acute care setting, except perhaps as the underlying cause of an acute disorder such as pneumonia. In general, no specific therapy for these conditions is available. There are, however, a few muscle disorders that can present with acute weakness (Table 5-7).

The hallmark of muscle disease is symmetric weakness, usually affecting proximal more than distal muscles. Although pain and muscle tenderness may be present, sensory symptoms are absent, and reflexes are usually preserved unless the weakness is very severe. Elevation of muscle enzyme levels (CK, aldolase, SGOT) in the serum confirms the clinical diagnosis of a myopathy. In severe myopathies, necrosis of muscle cells (*rhabdomyolysis*) liberates myoglobin; high concentrations of myoglobin in the serum can result in acute renal failure, and aggressive treatment to maintain high urine volumes is necessary. The presence of myoglobin in the urine results in dark discoloration that can be mistaken for blood; laboratory tests can confirm the presence of myoglobinuria even if blood is present.

Polymyositis is characterized by muscle weakness that usually develops over several weeks or longer. As is typical for muscle disease, the weakness affects the proximal muscles more than distal muscles; the face is often spared. The weakness is usually painless but some aching, especially in the thighs and hips may occur. The ESR is usually (but not always) elevated, and the serum CK is elevated. EMG examination and muscle biopsy may be needed to confirm the diagnosis. Unless the weakness is very severe, urgent treatment is not necessary, and the patient may be referred to a neurologist or rheumatologist for further evaluation and management. *Dermatomyositis* is clinically similar to polymyositis, with the addition of a skin rash on the extensor surface of the joints and a purple or "lilac" (heliotrope) rash over the face. Dermatomyositis has been variably associated with an increased risk of systemic cancer, and an extensive workup may be appropriate.

Trichinosis is rare in the United States; it occurs occasionally as a result of eating improperly cooked pork or wild game. The encysted larvae of the parasitic nematode *Trichina spiralis* mature in the gut after ingestion by the host; the mature

TABLE 5-7

MUSCLE DISORDERS CAUSING ACUTE WEAKNESS

Inflammatory Disorders
Polymyositis/dermatomyositis
Trichinosis

Toxic Myopathies
Alcohol
Drugs
   Statins
   Amiodarone
   Colchicine
   Vincristine
   Zidovudine
   Labetolol
   Rifampin
Mushroom poisoning
Venoms
Malignant hyperthermia
Critical illness myopathy

Metabolic Disorders
Electrolyte disorders
   Hyper/hypokalemia
   Hypercalcemia
   Hypermagnesemia
Periodic paralysis

nematodes lay eggs and the resulting larvae then spread throughout the body where they induce an intense inflammatory reaction. Clinical symptoms begin a week or so after ingestion and consist of fever, muscle pain and swelling, weakness, and malaise. Laboratory studies reveal an elevated ESR and marked eosinophilia. Thiobendazole, given early in the course of the disease, or even before symptoms occur in cases of known exposure, may prevent production of larvae and reduce the severity of the disease. Prednisone at 40 to 60 mg/day may give symptomatic relief. The symptoms may last for many weeks, but complete recovery can be expected.

Toxic myopathy may be due to a wide variety of drugs and poisons. These may be indolent or subacute, as in the case of *steroid-induced myopathy.* These patients present with slowly evolving weakness; muscle enzyme levels are normal, and myoglobinuria is not present. Diagnosis depends greatly on clinical suspicion; a careful drug history and a careful search through drug information resources may yield the diagnosis. Treatment consists in withdrawal of the offending substance. Other toxic myopathies present with an acute or fulminating course with severe weakness and rhabdomyolysis, with dramatic elevation of muscle enzyme levels, hyperkalemia, myoglobinuria, and renal failure. Potential causes include alcohol, many drugs including statins and other lipid-lowering agents, and toxins from snake bites, mushroom poisoning, and others.[10–12] A similar clinical picture with acute weakness and rhabdomyolysis can be caused by strenuous exercise, especially in patients with preexisting congenital muscle diseases. Rhabdomyolysis may result from pressure necrosis in patients with prolonged immobility or crush injuries, in cases of the neuroleptic malignant syndrome (see Chap. 6) malignant hyperthermia (see below). In all these cases, diagnosis depends on recognition of the general clinical syndrome and a careful search for potential causes. Treatment is largely supportive and includes withdrawal of the offending substance, aggressive hydration to maintain urine output, and other care as indicated.

Malignant hyperthermia is a rare and potentially catastrophic disorder associated with the use of certain anesthetics and neuromuscular blocking agents used in the acute care setting. Symptoms usually develop shortly after exposure to the causative agent but may begin several hours later. Initial symptoms are tachycardia and tachypnea, followed by dramatic muscle rigidity and severe hyperpyrexia. The syndrome is due to the sudden release of calcium from the sarcoplasmic reticulum, resulting in sustained muscle contraction. Treatment is aggressive management of the hyperpyrexia and administration of dantrolene 1 mg/kg IV initially, with additional doses as needed to maintain muscle relaxation. The syndrome is nearly always fatal if not recognized and treated immediately. Susceptibility to this disorder is inherited as an autosomal dominant trait, so a family history may be available. In potentially susceptible individuals, a muscle-biopsy-based laboratory test may be used to estimate risk prior to elective procedures.

Critical illness myopathy is not likely to present in the usual acute care settings, but it is an important cause of acute weakness that may be encountered by primary care physicians. As with critical illness polyneuropathy, with which it may coexist, critical illness neuropathy occurs in severely ill patients, especially those treated with corticosteroids and neuromuscular blocking agents. It becomes clinically evident as the patient begins to recover from the acute illness, is found to have severe weakness, and cannot be weaned from ventilator support. There is no treatment other than continuing supportive care. Recovery may take many months.[4]

Electrolyte disorders are an infrequent but important cause of acute muscle weakness. Either hyper- or hypokalemia from any cause can cause muscle weakness; serum potassium levels below 2 mEq/L or above 7 mEq/L can cause flaccid arreflexic paralysis similar to that seen in the Guillain-Barré syndrome. This is distinct from the genetic syndromes of periodic paralysis described below. Severe hypercalcemia, hypophosphatemia, and hypermagnesemia can cause a similar picture. Abnormalities in serum potassium are likely to be detected in "routine" blood work often obtained in the acute care setting, but their significance as a cause of severe generalized weakness may be overlooked. Other electrolyte abnormalities may be found only if specifically sought. Treatment consists of correction of both the acute electrolyte abnormality and the underlying cause.

The unusual disorders termed *periodic paralysis syndromes* are examples of a much larger group of muscle diseases collectively referred to a *channelopathies*.

They are caused by mutations in the genes that control the structure of various ion channels (chloride, sodium, and calcium) in skeletal muscle. The periodic paralysis syndromes, as the name implies, are characterized by acute attacks of muscle weakness; between attacks the patients are clinically normal. Because these disorders are inherited as autosomal dominant traits, a family history is often present.

Hypokalemic periodic paralysis, the most common and best known of these disorders, is caused by a genetic defect in the calcium channel. The first attacks usually occur before age 20. Attacks often develop during sleep, especially after strenuous exercise or a meal rich in carbohydrates. Patients awaken with generalized muscle weakness that may be severe enough to prevent the patient's getting out of bed or even calling for help. The muscles of the face and trunk are usually spared so that respiration is not compromised. Reflexes may be diminished or lost, but sensation is preserved. Diagnosis depends first on a high index of suspicion and a positive family history. Laboratory studies usually reveal low levels of potassium, but the reductions need not be profound. Untreated, attacks may last from hours to days; administration of supplemental potassium (orally or IV) leads to rapid improvement. Regular administration of supplemental potassium may prevent subsequent attacks.

Hyperkalemic and normokalemic periodic paralysis are less common than hypokalemic periodic paralysis. The genetic defect is in the sodium channel. The clinical attacks are relatively brief (less than 1 hour) and typically occur after exercise.

The cranial muscles and trunk muscles are usually spared. In mild attacks, no treatment is required, and the clinical symptoms may have resolved by the time the patient is evaluated. In patients with severe weakness, intravenous calcium gluconate (1 to 2 g) or intravenous glucose may be helpful.

Summary

Acute generalized weakness can result from disorders involving any level of the nervous system. Accurate diagnosis and appropriate treatment depend first and foremost on accurate localization of the likely lesion within the nervous system; accurate localization, in turn, depends on the results of the history and physical examinations. A careful search should be made for any alteration of consciousness, behavior, or mentation that suggests brain disease, or for any localizing signs, no matter how subtle, suggesting lesions of the brainstem or spinal cord (see Chaps. 3 and 4). If there are no signs of a central nervous system disorder, then a disorder of peripheral nerves, the neuromuscular junction, or the muscles should be considered.

The initial assessment of a patient with acute generalized weakness has several goals:

1. To ensure that the patient's airway is secure and that respiratory function is adequate. Remember that early mortality in these patients is most often the result of ventilatory failure. Other vital functions should be assessed and stabilized as needed.

2. To determine whether the likely cause affects the peripheral nerves, the neuro-muscular junction, or the muscles, determine the likely diagnosis, and obtain the necessary laboratory studies to secure the diagnosis.
3. To decide whether emergency treatment is required, either for the primary disorder (e.g., myasthenia gravis or Guillain-Barré syndrome) or for secondary effects (e.g., myoglobinuria in patients with rhabdomyolysis).
4. To initiate appropriate management and referral.

It is important to recall that many of the disorders causing acute weakness, such as the Guillain-Barré syndrome, can progress rapidly to severe weakness and respiratory failure even though the initial symptoms are quite mild. Accordingly, hospital admission and close observation should be considered even for patients with relatively mild symptoms, until the diagnosis is secure and until it is clear that the patient's condition has been stabilized.

REFERENCES

1. Walsh TM. Diseases of nerve and muscle. In: Samuels MA, ed. *Manual of Neurologic Therapeutics*, 6th ed. Philadelphia: Lippincott Williams & Wilkins, 1999, pp 403–442.
2. van der Meche FGA, van Doorn PA. Guillain-Barré syndrome. *Curr Treat Options Neurol* 2000;2:507–516.
3. Bella I, Chad DA. Neuromuscular disorders and acute respiratory failure. *Neurol Clin* 1998;16:391–417.
4. Hund E. Neurological complications of sepsis: critical illness polyneuropathy and myopathy. *J Neurol* 2001;248:929–934.
5. Spencer PS, Schaumberg HH, eds. *Experimental and Clinical Neurotoxicology*, 2nd ed. New York: Oxford University Press, 2000.
6. Goldfrank LR, ed. *Goldfrank's Toxicologic Emergencies*, 6th ed. Stamford, CT: Appleton & Lange, 1998.
7. Aminoff MJ. Effects of occupational toxins on the nervous system. In: Bradley WG, et al., eds. *Neurology in Clinical Practice*, 3rd ed. Boston: Butterworth-Heinemann, 2000, pp 1511–1599.
8. Farrar JJ, et al. Tetanus. *J Neurol Neurosurg Psychiatry* 2000;69:292.
9. Robey WC, Meggs WJ. Insecticides, herbicides, rodenticides. In: Tintinalli JE, Kelen GD, Stapczynski JS, eds. *Emergency Medicine: A Comprehensive Study Guide*, 5th ed. New York: McGraw-Hill, 2000, pp 1174–1182.
10. Curry SC, Chang D, Connor D. Drug and toxin-induced rhabdomyolysis. *Ann Emerg Med* 1989;18:1068.
11. Visweswaran P, Guntupalli J. Rhabdomyolysis. *Crit Care Clin* 1999;15:415–428.
12. Hodel C. Myopathy and rhabdomyolysis with lipid lowering drugs. *Toxicol Lett* 2002;128:159–168.

6
MOVEMENT DISORDERS

The term *movement disorders* refers to a large group of heterogeneous disorders characterized primarily by decomposition and disorganization of motor control rather than by weakness or paralysis. These disorders are usually due to abnormal function in the so-called extrapyramidal motor system, including the frontal cortex, the basal ganglia, the cerebellum, and related structures.

The symptoms of these disorders include the following:

1. Abnormalities of muscle tone (rigidity or hypotonia).
2. Slowing down or paucity of spontaneous movement (bradykinesia or akinesia).
3. Involuntary movements.
4. Inhibition of normal postural reflexes.

Movement disorders are quite common but are usually insidious in onset and only slowly progressive, so they do not commonly present in the acute care setting. However, these disorders may confound the evaluation of other diseases, and their symptoms may worsen abruptly in the face of medical illness or on exposure to some drugs; it is important therefore to have a working knowledge of the more common of these disorders. In addition, a few of these disorders may present as true medical emergencies. For virtually all these conditions, laboratory and imaging studies are of little help; diagnosis depends largely on the time-honored skills of clinical medicine.

CLINICAL ASSESSMENT

History

The clinical history should seek to obtain as accurate a description as possible of the patient's symptoms. It is important to recall that many of the symptoms of the movement disorders are more apparent to family members than to the patients themselves; it is not uncommon to encounter patients who are unaware of, or even flatly deny, involuntary movements that are obvious to everyone around them. When did the symptoms begin; was the onset abrupt or insidious? Have the symptoms progressed over time; have new symptoms developed? How have the symptoms interfered with the patient's regular function? How have the symptoms been affected by sleep, fatigue, anxiety? How have the symptoms been affected by any drugs (alcohol, caffeine, prescribed or over-the counter medications)? Can the patient exert any control over the movements, even for a short time? Have any family members had the same or a similar disorder?

Physical Examination

In addition to the usual general physical and neurologic examinations, there are several observations of special importance. The patient should be carefully watched for any involuntary movements or abnormal or bizarre postures of the trunk or extremities, both with the patient at rest and when engaged in some activity such as walking or talking. Note should be made as well of any evident decrease or absence of normal spontaneous movements. In patients with Parkinson's disease, for example, there is often a striking lack of spontaneous movement; such patients rarely blink, and there is often little or no movement of the face when they are speaking. Special attention should be paid to the patient's gait and to control of fine movements (finger-nose-finger, heel-knee-shin, finger tapping, and others). Muscle tone should be assessed. Relevant findings are often quite subtle, and their recognition requires considerable skill and experience on the part of the examining physician. The physician should try to characterize the findings in detail, as this will usually be the key to differential diagnosis.

Symptom Definitions

Abnormalities of Muscle Tone

Rigidity is an increase in the resistance of resting muscle to passive movement. The increased tone is not dependent on the rate at which the muscles are moved (in contrast to *spasticity*). The increased tone may be constant (sometimes called "lead-pipe" rigidity) or may have a curious racheting quality (so-called "cogwheel" rigidity).

Spasticity is an increase in resting muscle tone that depends on the rate at which the muscle is moved—if the affected muscles are moved slowly, the increase in tone may not be evident. It is generally associated with increased muscle stretch reflexes and is more characteristic of disorders of the voluntary (pyramidal) motor system.

Hypotonia is a reduction in resting muscle tone. It occurs in some disorders of the cerebellum and is associated with some kinds of involuntary movements such as chorea. It is usually quite subtle and likely to be detected only by an experienced clinician.

Slowing or Absence of Spontaneous Movement

Bradykinesia is a slowing down of spontaneous or voluntary movement. Patients seem to move slowly and deliberately. Such spontaneous movements as blinking, swallowing saliva, gesticulating with the hands while speaking, etc. are reduced both in their frequency and in their speed. The virtual absence of such spontaneous movements is termed *akinesia*. This can be very dramatic in patients with Parkinson's disease and related disorders, who may sit virtually immobile, with a fixed, unblinking "reptilian" stare.

Involuntary Movements

The most familiar, obvious, and characteristic symptoms of the movement disorders are involuntary movements. These involuntary movements are referred to by the collective term *dyskinesias* and are identified by classical terminology that may create the impression that the various movements are separate and distinct. In fact, there is considerable overlap among the various varieties of involuntary movements. The dyskinesias share some features in common; they are generally worsened by anxiety and stress and generally disappear with sleep. They can often be temporarily suppressed by the patient but will eventually recur despite the patient's efforts to prevent them. In past times, these movements were often considered to be psychogenic in origin, but it is now clear that they are definitely "organic."

Although certain kinds of movements have been classically associated with specific diseases, there is considerable overlap here as well. This section will briefly define the various symptoms of the movement disorders; the following section will consider some of the more important clinical conditions associated with these symptoms.

Tremor is defined as a rhythmic, regular, purposeless, oscillating movement that may involve the extremities, the trunk, and the head and neck. Most individuals have experienced tremor at some time, usually when anxious or fatigued, or in association with alcohol, caffeine, or medications; such tremors are usually self-limited, and such persons do not seek medical attention. In other individuals, tremor may be much more persistent and severe and may cause considerable personal distress and functional impairment.

Tics are irregular, shock-like, or twitching or jerking movements that may involve the head and face, the trunk, or the extremities. Tics may involve the coordinated movement of multiple muscles and may resemble voluntary movements. A given patient may have one or more different tics, each of which will be quite stereotyped from one occurrence to the next. The tics can often be temporarily suppressed by the patient, who will then develop an irresistible urge to perform the tic.

Akathisia is a state of motor restlessness; patients have a constant urge to move some part of the body and find it impossible to relax. Patients constantly shift position; they may constantly move their legs or bodies or get up and walk about. They find the sensation difficult to describe but extremely distressing. Akathisia is a common side effect of many drugs (see below); it is often unrecognized.

Choreiform movements (*chorea*) are irregular, purposeless, brief movements that move randomly from one part of the body to another. They often involve the distal extremities but may also involve the tongue and face, the head, or the trunk; they are not stereotyped and are more prolonged than tics. They may be modified by patients into apparently purposeful movements. The movements frequently disrupt normal activity such as speaking, writing, walking, and so on. Slower, more sinuous movements are described by the term *athetosis;* there is considerable clinical overlap, and the term *choreoathetosis* is used to refer to the whole complex of abnormal movements.

Ballism refers to wild flinging or flailing movements, usually of the extremities. The movements can be very violent and may result in serious injury. Ballism is considered by many authors to be a variant of chorea[1] This condition, fortunately quite rare, is one of the most dramatic of involuntary movements.

Dystonic movements are slower and more prolonged than choreoathetoid movements, with which they often coexist. *Dystonia* may result in prolonged abnormal or even bizarre postures of individual muscles, groups of related muscles, or even the entire body.

Myoclonus is a very brief lightning-like contraction. Twitching movements may involve individual muscles, groups of related muscles, or even major portions of the body. The twitches may be isolated or recurrent and may be confined to small groups of muscles or may flit randomly from one body region to another. Unlike *tics,* which they may superficially resemble, myoclonic movements are not stereotyped.

Asterixis, in contrast to the involuntary movements described thus far, is characterized by sudden brief *lapses* in muscle tone. Thus, when a muscle is held in a fixed position, there will be sudden movements as the muscles suddenly lose their tone. This is best seen when the hands are held outstretched with the wrists extended; the sudden loss of tone results in an irregular peculiar "flapping" movement of the hands. Asterixis is considered by some authors to be a variant of tremor or of myoclonus and by others to represent an entirely distinct phenomenon.[1,2] Asterixis may be seen in a variety of toxic-metabolic encephalopathies and is characteristic of hepatic encephalopathy.

Fasciculations are brief spontaneous contractions of groups of muscle fibers; they may produce visible twitching in the skin overlying the muscle but are not strong enough to actually move joints. They may occur in normal individuals, especially after vigorous exercise, and are characteristic in diseases affecting anterior horn cells. As a rule, fasciculations that occur in the absence of weakness, muscle atrophy, or other abnormalities on neurologic examination may be regarded as benign.

Spasm is a nonspecific term that refers to any sustained contraction of muscle. Painful spasms are referred to as *cramps.*

CLINICAL SYNDROMES

Tremor

Tremor is an extremely common symptom; most persons have experienced tremor at one time or another, usually in association with anxiety or fatigue, use of caffeine or other stimulant drugs, or following excessive alcohol use. Most of these tremors are benign and self-limited, cause no significant functional impairment, and rarely lead to medical attention. In some patients, tremors become severe and persistent; by themselves they may cause significant embarrassment or even substantial functional impairment, and they may be a sign of severe underlying disease.

Tremors are classified as either resting tremors or action tremors, depending on when they are most evident. Resting tremor, as the name implies, occurs when the involved extremity is at rest and is commonly suppressed by voluntary movement. Action tremors, conversely, are most evident when the involved extremity is active in some way, and they commonly improve with rest. The distinction is not absolute; also, more than one variety of tremor may be present in a given patient.

Physiologic tremor can be detected in virtually everyone. It is a low-amplitude, very rapid (8 to 12 Hz) tremor most evident in the hands and fingers when they are held in a fixed position. Physiologic tremor can be embarrassing but rarely causes functional impairment. It is exacerbated by a wide variety of drugs and other influences (Table 6-1). A similar tremor may be present in patients with thyrotoxicosis and other metabolic disorders, and an appropriate history should be sought. Treat-

TABLE 6-1 ———————————————————————
FACTORS ACCENTUATING PHYSIOLOGIC TREMOR

Anxiety
Fatigue
Weakness
Hypercapnia
Drug withdrawal
Hypocalcemia
Hypoglycemia
Hypomagnesemia
Uremia
Severe liver disease
Heavy metal intoxication
Drugs (catecholamines, theophylline, caffeine, lithium, tricyclic antidepressants, steroids, antipsychotic drugs, sodium valproate, antihistamines, amphetamines)
Thyrotoxicosis
Hysteria

ment of simple physiologic tremor consists of reassurance, elimination of offending substances, and, rarely, mild (temporary) sedation.

Essential tremor is a low- or medium-amplitude tremor that may occur in the hands, the legs, or the head and trunk. It is generally lower in frequency than physiologic tremor (5 to 10 Hz). It is worsened by sustained contraction of muscles and often interferes with fine movements such as writing, eating, and so on. Essential tremor can develop at any age and, once present, tends to slowly worsen as the patient ages. Essential tremor can be worsened by the same factors that worsen physiologic tremor; the two tremors can often not be easily distinguished. Essential tremor is typically relieved by even small amounts of alcohol; this does not mean that the tremor is the result of excess drinking. Because of their concern about this implication, patients will often not mention the fact that their tremors improve after drinking. Depending on the clinical circumstances, essential tremor has also been called senile tremor and familial tremor.

Other than the tremor, the neurologic examination of patients with essential tremor should be normal. A careful search should be made for signs of Parkinson's disease (see below), both to avoid missing the diagnosis and to reassure those patients who do not have that condition. Note that essential tremor and Parkinson's disease can coexist. One important clinical clue is that essential tremor often involves the head, whereas parkinsonian tremor rarely does so.

Acute treatment for essential tremor is rarely needed. Occasional use of small amounts of alcohol or anxiolytics can be helpful, but neither should be encouraged for chronic regular use. For many patients, propranolol may be helpful. Primidone is occasionally helpful, but sedation is often limiting. For patients with severe tremor, referral to a neurologist is appropriate.

Intention tremor is the least common form of tremor but frequently the most disabling. It is typically higher in amplitude and lower in frequency (3 to 5 Hz) than other action tremors. As the name implies, it is usually most evident during controlled movements, particularly near the end of the movement. On examination it is often best demonstrated by the classic tests of coordination such as the finger-nose-finger or heel-knee-shin maneuvers. Intention tremor is classically associated with cerebellar disorders; in young patients it is a common finding with multiple sclerosis. However, intention tremor may also result from drug intoxication (especially anticonvulsant drugs and alcohol), or from lesions affecting the motor and sensory pathways as diverse as stroke or peripheral neuropathy. Accordingly, the presence of intention tremor indicates the need for a comprehensive neurologic evaluation.

Treatment depends on the underlying disorder; the results are frequently disappointing.

Resting tremor, as the name implies, is most evident when the involved extremity is in repose; it is suppressed and may disappear entirely with movement. It is not unusual to see patients with quite severe resting tremor who can perform the finger-nose-finger maneuver or drink a cup of coffee without difficulty. Resting tremor is characteristic of Parkinson's disease (see below). These patients typically exhibit a pronation-supination movement of the hands and fingers (the so called pill-rolling tremor). It is usually asymmetric and may be entirely confined to one side or the other.

The head is rarely involved. Careful examination of these patients will usually reveal other signs of parkinsonism, as discussed below. Recall that resting tremor and physiologic or essential tremor can coexist in the same patient. Treatment is discussed below under parkinsonism.

Tics

Tics can range from very simple movements such as eye blinking, shoulder shrugging, or head jerking through much more complex movements involving multiple muscles or large portions of the body. Vocal tics are common as well and may range from simple grunts or barks through words or short phrases. The movements are apparently purposeless and inappropriate to the situation, but sometimes they can be modified by the patient into an apparently purposeful movement. As noted above, the tics can often be suppressed by the patient, who will then experience a steadily mounting, and eventually irresistible, urge to perform the movement. A given patient may exhibit only one or a few simple motor tics or may have multiple motor tics and vocal tics (Gilles de la Tourette syndrome). Tics often occur in association with other conditions such as obsessive-compulsive disorder or the attention deficit-hyperactivity disorder.[3]

Like the other movement disorders, tics are frequently increased with stress and anxiety; they are absent during sleep. Management is difficult and frequently requires the use of neuroleptic drugs; treatment is not required in the acute care setting.

Akathisia

The term *akathisia* refers to a sense of motor restlessness; patients feel an irresistable urge to move. These patients are in constant motion—standing up and sitting down, rubbing various parts of their bodies, picking at their clothing, fidgeting, and so on. The sensations are very distressing to patients (and others) and sometimes painful. Akathisia occurs most often as a complication of neuroleptic drug use and may occur in 30% to 40% of patients on these agents. It is common as well in patients taking selective serotonin reuptake inhibitors (SSRIs). The syndrome is thought to be quite common but very often unrecognized.[4,5]

Akathisia is a common side effect of neuroleptics (such as prochlorperazine) used in the acute care setting to manage nausea and vomiting; if recognized, it can be effectively treated with diphenhydramine.[6]

Choreoathetosis

Choreiform movements may occur in a wide variety of neurologic disorders (Table 6-2). Most of these are chronic disorders, with the abnormal movements developing gradually. Accordingly, these patients will rarely present to the acute care setting for their initial evaluation. There are a few situations in which choreiform movements may develop acutely, and these will be discussed briefly.

TABLE 6-2
CAUSES OF CHOREA

Drugs (levodopa, other dopaminergic agents, neuroleptics, amphetamines, tricyclic antidepressants, and others)

Pregnancy (chorea gravidarum) and oral contraceptives

Toxic/metabolic disorders (carbon monoxide, anoxia, hypomagnesemia, electrolyte derangements, hypo- and hyperglycemia, and others)

Huntington's disease, Wilson's disease, other hereditary and degenerative disorders

Rheumatic fever

Lupus erythematosus

Vascular disease (particularly lacunar infarction)

Senile chorea

Levodopa and other dopaminergic drugs used in the management of Parkinson's disease are common causes of choreoathetoid movements. The movements can develop quite abruptly, especially after dose adjustment or after an accidental overdose. The abnormal movements are usually more distressing to family members or other observers than to the patient, who may be unaware of even quite dramatic involuntary movements. The movements may affect the extremities, the head and trunk, the face and voice, or any combination of these. A similar clinical picture may result from drugs such as neuroleptics (tardive dyskinesia) or from other drugs such as amphetamines and tricyclics. Treatment is withdrawal of the offending substance (when possible).

Rarely, acute chorea may be seen in pregnancy or with oral contraceptives (chorea gravidarum). This syndrome has become exceedingly rare with the virtual disappearance of Syndenham's chorea. The abrupt onset of chorea in children should suggest Syndenham's chorea, one of the major manifestations of rheumatic fever (fortunately rare).[1,7]

Dystonia

Like other involuntary movements, dystonia may occur in a wide variety of primary and secondary neurologic disorders, many of which are quite rare and few of which are likely to be encountered in the acute care setting. Acute dystonias do occur, most often as a consequence of neuroleptic drug treatment. Since these agents are often used in the management of nausea and vomiting, the acute care physician should be familiar with these unusual but dramatic events. Patients may present any of a wide variety of bizarre movements such as forced deviation of the eyes and head, twisting of the face and slurred speech, torticollis, hyperextension of the head and trunk (opisthotonus), and choreoathetoid movements. Despite their often bizarre (and frequently painful) postures, patients remain awake and alert with normal mental function. The diagnosis can be confirmed (and the symptoms relieved) by giving diphenhydramine 25 to 50 mg IV or IM or benztropine 1 to 2 mg IM. This will result in rapid, often spectacular, resolution of the abnormal posture and movements. Since the duration of action of the offending drug may be quite long, repeat treatment may be needed.

A much more rare, but dangerous and potentially fatal complication of neuroleptic drug use is the *neuroleptic malignant syndrome*. It may occur acutely, following a single dose of the inciting agent, or as a late complication of the chronic use of these drugs, most often in psychiatric patients. The syndrome may also develop rarely following sudden withdrawal of agents such as levodopa. The clinical picture is characterized by generalized muscle rigidity, dramatic elevation of temperature, obtundation, and elevated serum creatinine kinase, often to spectacular levels. The clinical syndrome may develop over several days and should be suspected in patients taking neuroleptic drugs who develop increasing agitation, muscle stiffness, and fever. Treatment remains controversial but generally includes aggressive use of benzodiazepines to manage muscle rigidity. Neuromuscular blockade (with nondepolarizing agents) may be required. Dopaminergic drugs such as bromocriptine 5 to 20 mg via NG tube q8h may be beneficial and are widely used. These patients require intensive management in a critical care unit.[8]

Myoclonus

As noted above, myoclonus may involve single muscles, groups of related or adjacent muscles (termed segmental myoclonus), or even the entire body. The movements may be isolated or recurrent; they are usually irregular but may occur in rhythmic bursts. They may occur spontaneously or in response to tactile stimulation or attempts to move the affected body part. As with other involuntary movements, myoclonus is nonspecific and may occur in a wide variety of neurologic conditions, including many chronic disorders. (Table 6-3). Several causes of myoclonus are more likely to be seen in the acute setting and these are discussed briefly.

Benign myoclonus is common. The most familiar form is "sleep starts," the sudden jerks that occur just as one is falling asleep. These are occasionally mistaken for seizures and can be a source of anxiety. Exercise-related myoclonus is

TABLE 6-3
CAUSES OF MYOCLONUS

Benign myoclonus—sleep starts, hiccoughs, exercise-induced
Drug-induced—tricyclics, penicillins, meperidine, tacrolimus, many others
Toxic-metabolic encephalopathies—especially hypoxia/ischemia, heat stroke, electric shock, hepatic and renal failure, dialysis, heavy metal poisoning
Encephalitis—herpes simplex, other viral encephalites, Creutzfeld-Jakob disease, and others causes
Epileptic myoclonus
Degenerative diseases of the central nervous system (multiple)

another benign phenomenon; as with exercise-related fasciculations, this can safely be ignored if the neurologic examination and history are otherwise unremarkable. Finally, myoclonus occasionally occurs in association with syncope, especially if the patient is held upright and cannot fall to a supine position. Myoclonus in this setting can easily be mistaken for seizure activity.

Myoclonus can occur in a wide variety of toxic and metabolic encephalopathies, including drug intoxication, hypoxia, hyponatremia, and others. Multifocal myoclonus is common following hypoxic-ischemic injury (as in cardiac arrest) and may be difficult to distinguish from seizure activity. Multifocal myoclonus is also prominent in intoxication with tricyclic antidepressants and SSRIs. In patients receiving repeated doses of meperidine, especially in the face of renal insufficiency, accumulation of normeperidine, a toxic metabolite, may cause encephalopathy and dramatic myoclonus. A similar picture has been seen in patients treated with tacrolimus (Prograf and others) following organ transplantation.

Myoclonus per se does not cause any alteration of consciousness. Patients and witnesses should be questioned carefully in the case of episodic myoclonus—if there is any alteration of consciousness, seizure activity should be suspected.

Spasms and Cramps

Most muscle spasms result from local irritation or injury of muscle. Pain from any cause may create reflex spasm in local muscles, as is commonly seen near sites of injury such as fracture. Muscle spasm may also occur spontaneously or as a result of some activity; when prolonged and painful, these spasms are called cramps. During the cramp, the muscle will be very hard on palpation. The cramp can usually be overcome by massage and passive forceful stretching; it will often recur if the muscle is allowed to relax too soon. Most of these spasms and cramps are benign. Treatment consists of treatment of the underlying injury, if any. Analgesics and antiinflammatory agents may be helpful. Muscle relaxants may be helpful. In elderly patients with recurrent nocturnal cramps, quinine sulfate 300 mg PO may be useful.

Irritation or injury to peripheral nerves may cause spasm of isolated muscles or groups of muscles. Hemifacial spasm is characterized by repetitive twitching of the muscles on one side of the face and may occur as a primary process or following Bell's palsy. Injury to other peripheral nerves may result in similar spasms in affected muscles, especially during recovery.

Spasm may result from a variety of electrolyte abnormalities. Hypocalcemia, hypomagnesemia, and other electrolyte abnormalities can result in muscle cramps. Hyperventilation, by causing an abrupt fall in ionized calcium, can cause muscle spasm and cramp. The classic clinical sign of hypocalcemia is Chvostek's sign, in which tapping the facial nerve at the angle of the jaw induces reflex spasms of the facial muscles.

More ominous acute causes of muscle spasm include tetanus and strychnine poisoning. The diagnosis of tetanus must be based on clinical suspicion. Common early symptoms of tetanus include jaw tightness, irritability, and headache. Later, more pronounced spasm of the masseter muscles (trismus) prevents jaw opening (lockjaw), and tonic contraction of facial muscles cause a fixed facial grimace (risus sardonicus). The painful spasms spread progressively, eventually leading to complete rigidity and immobility. The spasms are intensified with any external stimulation. Treatment is complex and requires intensive nursing and medical care.

Strychnine is found as a common adulterant in many street drugs and in products used to kill animal pests; it is occasionally taken intentionally. It can produce symptoms within 15 to 30 minutes of ingestion. Initial restlessness and agitation may be followed by heightened auditory and visual acuity. Usually spasms and convulsions lasting up to 2 minutes occur, followed by periods of relaxation. Extensor muscle spasm may produce opisthotonus, and risus sardonicus may occur. Convulsions, hyperthermia, lactic acidosis, and rhabdomyolysis can occur. Whereas initially the differential diagnosis centers around that of spasms, the presentation is more that of repetitive seizures (but consciousness is preserved during paroxysm).

Parkinsonism

The most common clinical syndrome associated with disease of the basal ganglia and extrapyramidal motor system is parkinsonism. Although not usually a medical emergency, the syndrome is common, especially in older patients, and all physicians should be familiar with its major features. The clinical syndrome is usually characterized by slowing or paucity of movement (bradykinesia/akinesia), increased muscle tone (rigidity), tremor or other involuntary movements, and impaired posture and gait. The most common cause of the syndrome is Parkinson's disease, but a similar clinical picture can result from a wide variety of other conditions.

For the acute care physician, perhaps the single most important aspect of the disorder is that it be recognized, particularly in its early stages. The early symptoms are gradual in onset, mild, and nonspecific. Patients and their families report that patients seem dull and lifeless, with decreased interest in their daily activities. Their gait is slow, shuffling, and unsteady, with frequent falls. They often have trouble sleeping. Not surprisingly, they are often misdiagnosed as depressed or "senile," or given a meaningless diagnosis such as "mini-strokes." Once it is familiar to the physician, the syndrome of bradykinesia and increased muscle tone, often with "cogwheeling," is virtually unmistakable. Parkinson's disease should always be considered in an older patient with abnormal gait and frequent falls. Note that resting tremor, although common, is not always present. Patients with Parkinson's disease frequently have a dramatic response to treatment. Emergency treatment is not necessary, and the effective management of Parkinson's disease requires a long-term commitment from both physician and patient. Referral to a neurologist is usually appropriate.

The acute care physician should also be aware of the common side effects of anti-Parkinson's drugs. These symptoms may develop quite abruptly and may well provoke a visit to the acute care setting. As noted above, dyskinesias, especially choreiform and dystonic movements, are common side effects of dopaminergic drugs. Confusion and hallucinations may occur, especially with some of the newer agents such as ropinirole (Requip) and pramipexole (Mirapex). Episodes of syncope should suggest autonomic insufficiency or postural hypotension, possibly exacerbated by medications. Later in the course of Parkinson's disease, patients may experience sudden and dramatic fluctuations in motor function, including episodes of sudden immobility ("freezing"). All these complications are difficult to manage and require referral to the patient's treating physician.

It is important to remember that not all "parkinsonism" is due to Parkinson's disease. A similar clinical syndrome may be seen in many other degenerative disorders of the central nervous system (Table 6-4). It is often difficult to distinguish among these conditions, especially early in their courses, and a convincing diagnosis can sometimes be made only after prolonged observation. Much more important in the acute care setting is parkinsonism caused by specific, sometimes treatable causes, primarily drugs and toxins. Parkinsonism is common and well known in patients treated with neuroleptics. Less obvious are agents such as lithium and metoclopramide (Reglan). Possible toxins include manganese, mercury, carbon disulfide, and alcohols, among others. A complete list is obviously impossible; a physician confronted by a patient with recent onset of parkinsonian symptoms should obtain a detailed history of drug use and toxic exposure. Treatment is withdrawal, if possible, of the offending agent.

SUMMARY

It is common to think of involuntary movements as manifestations of rare, mostly untreatable diseases of interest only to neurologists. However, involuntary movements are commonly caused by systemic disorders, drugs, and toxins, and effective treatment may well be possible. Confronted by a patient with an apparent movement disorder, the acute care physician should first try to classify the involuntary

TABLE 6-4

CAUSES OF PARKINSONISM

Parkinson's Disease

Secondary Parkinsonism
Drugs and toxins
    Phenothiazines, butyrophenones, other neuroleptics
    Lithium, metoclopramide, and so on.
    Manganese, mercury, ethanol, methanol, and so on.
Vascular disease—small vessel vasculopathies, multiinfarct state
Structural lesions—head injury, neoplasms, hydrocephalus
Anoxic/ischemic—cardiac arrest, carbon monoxide
Degenerative diseases—multisystem atrophies, Lewy body disease, cortical-basal ganglionic degeneration, progressive supranuclear palsy, and so on.

TABLE 6-5 ———————————————————————————————————
MOVEMENT DISORDERS—EMERGENCIES

Acute dystonic reactions to neuroleptics and other drugs
Neuroleptic malignant syndrome
Muscle cramps and spasms due to tetanus, strychnine poisoning[a]
Myoclonus due to electrolyte abnormalities, drug intoxication, hypoxemia

[a] These conditions are also discussed in Chapter 5.

movements; a correct classification will often suggest the likely diagnoses. Second, it is important to obtain a detailed history of drug use and toxin exposure. Except in the case of obvious "repeat offenders," it is often necessary to look up each drug or toxin in an appropriate reference source, since even common agents, familiar to the physician, may produce uncommon side effects.

Only a few movement disorders require emergency management (Table 6-5). Although admittedly rare, these disorders may well be seen from time to time in the acute care setting, and urgent intervention may be life-saving.

Finally, the physician must remember that the presence of bizarre and incomprehensible movements or behaviors need not imply a psychiatric disorder. A careful assessment may be needed to establish a convincing and correct diagnosis.

REFERENCES

1. Lang AE. Movement disorder symptomatology. In: Bradley WG, et al., eds. *Neurology in Clinical Practice*, 3rd ed. Boston: Butterworth-Heinemann, 2000.
2. Victor M, Ropper AH. *Adams and Victor's Principles of Neurology*, 7th ed. New York: McGraw-Hill, 2001.
3. Weiner WJ, Lang AE. *Movement Disorders: A Comprehensive Survey*. Mt. Kisco, NY: Futura, 1989.
4. Bakheit A. The syndrome of motor restlessness—a treatable but unrecognized disorder. *Postgrad Med J* 1997;73:529.
5. Weiden PJ, et al. Clinical nonrecognition of neuroleptic induced movement disorders; a cautionary study. *Am J Psychiatry* 1987;144:1148–1153.
6. Vinson DR, Drotts DL. Diphenhydramine for the prevention of akathisia induced by prochlorperazine: a randomized, controlled trial. *Ann Emerg Med* 2001;37:125–131.
7. Shoulson I. On chorea. *Clin Neuropharmacol* 1986;9:585.
8. Lavonas EJ, Ford MD. Antipsychotics. In: Marx JA, et al., eds. *Rosen's Emergency Medicine: Concepts and Clinical Practice*, 5th ed. St. Louis: Mosby, 2001, pp 2174–2179.

7
HEADACHE

The evaluation of headache is a common task for any physician working in the acute care setting. Sorting the benign from the serious causes of headache represents a challenge because of the wide variety of systemic and intracranial abnormalities that can cause headache. Generally, headaches do not represent serious disease; however, rarely they may be the manifestation of a severe systemic or intracranial process.[1,2] Patients often regard pain in the head as potentially more significant than pain elsewhere, with brain tumor being a common but frequently unexpressed fear.

Headache is a common problem and frequent complaint to physicians.[1] It is the ninth most common cause of physician visits and one of the most common causes for emergency department visits.[2] Whereas muscle contraction and migraine are the most common causes of headache, the potential list of causes is extensive. This chapter will discuss an approach to the headache patient. Because physicians practicing acute care medicine will see headache problems that encompass the entire spectrum from acute to chronic, many etiologies will be covered. Some will simply be listed to serve as a reference starting point and to keep some uncommon etiologies under consideration. Some etiologies will be dealt with in more detail because of their frequency or seriousness.

History

The history may serve as the sole basis for a diagnosis, because physical signs are frequently lacking or nonspecific. A focused workup proceeds from a careful history. Table 7-1 lists important historical facts to elicit. Of those listed, the temporal relationships and pattern profile are most important. A headache that begins and becomes maximal in an instant suggests etiologies that are vastly different from those with a vague, poorly defined onset. The significance of these historical clues will be

TABLE 7-1

HEADACHE HISTORY

1. Temporal relations: time of day, time to maximum intensity, frequency, duration
2. Pattern profile: prodrome, correlation with medications, menstruation
3. Site of pain: unilateral, bilateral, frontal, occipital, facial, head, neck
4. Quality of pain: pulsatile, steady, shock-like, tightness
5. Intensity
6. Associated symptoms: nausea, vomiting, loss of consciousness, flushing, lacrimation, drop attack, neck stiffness, photophobia, dizziness, phonophobia
7. Precipitating or aggravating factors: exertion, position, foods, drugs, weather, anxiety
8. Relieving factors: dark room, position, pressing on scalp, medication
9. Medical history: past headache history, past headache evaluations, medications, hypertension, cancer, travel, trauma, HIV history/risk
10. Family history
11. Occupational history: solvents, vapors, chemicals, fumes

covered in the individual discussions of headache etiologies. Some of these historical aspects warrant brief discussion.

The intensity of the pain does not necessarily correlate with the severity of the causative illness. Sudden excruciating pain, however, points to subarchnoid hemorrage (SAH).

Of the associated symptoms listed, many, such as lacrimation, can point specifically to a given entity, e.g., cluster headache. Loss of consciousness should always be considered serious and the result of important entities such as SAH or third ventricular tumor.

When questioning concerning the effect of position, one should be careful to note whether it is the exertion of getting to any position that worsens the pain, as with vascular headache, or the actual position itself that is important, as with a colloid cyst.

A travel history may cause one to suspect etiologies not common in North America, such as parasitic infection. Likewise, an occupational history should expand beyond the stress that virtually everyone believes accompanies their work and consider exposure to chemicals, solvents, carbon monoxide, and other substances.

When taking a family history, one should beware of patients labeling chronic-recurrent headaches as sinus and try to seek details of the headaches themselves. Frequently lay people mislabel any commonly occurring headache as sinus and any intense headache as migraine.

Many patients in the general population with significant headaches have migraines, despite the lack of a formal diagnosis by a physician.[3]

Examination

In addition to the routine vital signs, general physical, and neurologic exam, one should pay particular attention to palpation of the head and neurophthalmic exam.[4] Tender scalp arteries may occur with migraine or cranial arteritis. Conversely, many patients with migraine experience relief of pain with arterial compression. Scalp tenderness may accompany unrecognized trauma, cranial neuralgias, or underlying infection. Stiffness of the neck or other meningeal signs should be elicited. Examination of the fundus should be done with the patient seated, because venous pulsations can be lost in the supine positions. Abnormalities on mental status testing, or on evaluation of extraocular movements or pupils, should prompt consideration of serious underlying pathology.

Procedures and Laboratory Evaluation

An unsuspected diagnosis in the headache patient is uncommonly made by laboratory evaluation alone. Several exceptions occur and should be kept in mind. An elevated sedimentation rate virtually always occurs in temporal arteritis and should be considered in patients over the age of 55 unless an alternative diagnosis is certain. Carbon monoxide levels may be useful in the appropriate setting. Although anemia and anoxia can cause headache, it is unlikely that they would pass unsuspected clinically.

Of the studies that will provide the basis for or against a given diagnosis, lumbar puncture and computed tomography (CT) scan are the most useful. The indications for emergent spinal tap are clinical suspicion of intracranial infection or subarachnoid blood. It should be noted that elevated pressure alone is not worrisome for herniation, but unilateral mass or posterior fossa mass can precipitate herniation syndromes. It is uncommon for these to present with the clinical picture of meningitis. A special discussion of this potential problem will be given at the end of this chapter. When high pressure alone is found, one should still obtain cerebrospinal fluid (CSF) for analysis. One may need to begin an osmotic diuretic such as mannitol to reduce the pressure, plan for an emergency CT scan to rule out mass, or call for neurosurgical evaluation emergently in this setting.

Lumbar puncture is used to detect blood from SAH hemorrhage if the CT scan fails to, or if a scan is not obtainable and no signs to suggest an intracranial mass exist. When the suspicion of bleed is low but must be excluded, lumbar puncture can be done as the primary procedure in certain clinical settings.

CT scan is by far the most useful tool in evaluating intracranial disease in the headache patient. It should be used, however, on a selected basis when the history and/or exam suggest an intracranial lesion and not as a screening tool.[5] A plain, unenhanced CT is the test of choice. It will not, however, reliably diagnose cerebral venous sinus thrombosis or carotid or vertebral artery dissection, which are rare but important causes for headache. These are discussed later.

Some CT scans will be falsely negative for SAH. Small amounts of subarachnoid blood may not be seen because of obscuring artifact, proximity to bone, poor resolution of the scan, low iron content of the blood[6] (from anemia or old bleed with partial resorption), or resolution of the scanner. Small amounts of subarachnoid blood, which carry a similar prognostic significance to larger amounts, are frequently a very subtle finding on CT. More chronic, or "isodense," collections of blood near bone, especially bilaterally without shift, may be difficult to detect. If one has not directed specific attention to the base of the brain, such as the pituitary fossa, routine cuts may not visualize lesions there. Bony abnormalities such as basilar fractures likewise must be clinically suspected in order to direct specific techniques to reveal them. Small aneurysms and arteriovenous anomalies may not be seen by CT and may require angiography in patients with SAH.

Plain skull x-rays now play an extremely small role in the definitive evaluation of headache.[7] The most they can do is lead one to do a CT.[8] Sinus films, however, may help confirm or exclude a diagnosis of sinusitis, but are frequently over- and under-read. CT may find slight sinus inflammation in many patients without clinical suspicion of sinusitis.

PAIN MECHANISMS IN HEADACHE

It is not the intent of this chapter to deal specifically with the pathophysiology of pain in headache, but it may be of interest to refer to Table 7-2 for structures that are pain-sensitive and -insensitive and to Table 7-3 for some general mechanisms of pain genesis.

INITIAL APPROACH TO THE HEADACHE PATIENT

Because of the wide diversity of etiologies of headache, one must develop an approach to narrow the possibilities yet not overlook potential etiologies. For a variety of reasons, patients will present to emergency facilities with chronic and possibly acutely exacerbated problems. Although it is not necessarily the goal to achieve a final diagnosis on each patient on initial presentation, certain etiologies require more acute diagnosis and treatment than do others.

One of the more important etiologies to consider in a patient with a sudden-onset severe headache is SAH. This entity is not necessarily a common cause of headache, but its detection is important because morbidity and mortality dramatically increase with rebleeding.[9] Details on SAH are discussed below in the section covering specific etiologies.

Because of its potential for rapid progression and morbidity, meningitis should also be constantly considered in the headache patient. Although most cases will occur in the young age group and most have meningeal signs, there are strong exceptions to these generalities. If the suspicion persists in one's mind after examination, spinal tap should be considered.

TABLE 7-2
PAIN SENSITIVITY OF CRANIAL STRUCTURES

Structure	Pain-Sensitive	Pain-Insensitive
Intracranial	Cranial venous sinuses with afferent veins	Brain parenchyma
	Arteries of the dura	Ependyma
	Arteries at base of brain and their major branches	Choroid
	Dura near base of brain and large arteries	Pia
		Arachnoid
		Dura over the convexity
		Skull
Extracranial	Skin	
	Scalp appendages	
	Periosteum	
	Muscles	
	Mucosa	
	Arteries	
Nerves	Trigeminal	
	Facial	
	Vagal	
	Glossopharyngeal	
	Second and third cranial nerves	

TABLE 7-3
GENERAL MECHANISMS OF HEADACHE

1. Traction on major intracranial vessels
2. Distention, dilation of intracranial arteries
3. Inflammation near pain-sensitive structures
4. Direct pressure on cranial or cervical nerves
5. Sustained contraction of scalp or neck muscles
6. Stimulation from disease affecting the eye, ear, nose, and sinuses

SUBARACHNOID HEMORRHAGE

Although SAH is an uncommon cause for headache in the acute care setting (less than 1%), it is a particularly important etiology to consider. Spontaneous hemorrhage into the subarachnoid space usually results in sudden cataclysmic headache, maximizing quickly (usually over seconds), commonly in the occipital region but occasionally in the frontal region. It is typically very severe, different from past headaches, and of sudden onset. Spontaneous SAH is graded using the system proposed by Hunt and Hess (Table 7-4). Those patients with grades I and II have the best prognosis. These patients have a normal neurologic exam and represent about one-half of all SAH patients. The pain of SAH goes away over time, particularly with small hemorrhages. The typically severe headache of SAH may improve with both narcotic and nonnarcotic analgesics. Such improvement should not serve as the sole basis for excluding the diagnosis. Undiagnosed small hemorrhages that resolve spontaneously or with treatment, followed by subsequent diagnosed SAH, have been termed "warning leaks." This diagnosis can only be applied, by definition, in retrospect. The concept, however, that the pain of small leaks improves spontaneously or with treatment, is important to bear in mind

Nausea and vomiting, photophobia, and stiff neck commonly occur with typical SAH. Obtundation is common within 15 minutes in one-fourth of patients, and one-half will lose consciousness, with 10 to 30% experiencing unconsciousness at the outset.[10,11] Unless the hemorrhage has entered the brain substance, there are usually no focal neurologic signs.[4] Posterior communicating artery aneurysms can compress the third nerve locally and cause a dilated pupil and/or other features of third nerve palsy. Later vasospasm can produce focal cerebral ischemia. The pain may radiate into the neck and at times low back, rarely causing sciatica. Fever may develop. Hypertension is common at the time of presentation either as a result of hemorrhage or as a predisposing factor. Seizures may occur at the time of hemorrhage and recur with rebleeding. Subhyaloid hemorrhage may occasionally be seen on examination of the fundus and is more common on the side of the hemorrhage.[12] Electrocardiographic (ECG) changes, usually diffuse nonspecific T-wave changes, may occur.[13] These and other concomitants are listed in Table 7-5. Of

TABLE 7-4

HUNT AND HESS CLASSIFICATION OF SAH

Grade 1. Asymptomatic, or minimal headache and slight nuchal rigidity

Grade 2. Moderate to severe headache, nuchal rigidity; no neurologic deficit other than cranial nerve palsy

Grade 3. Drowsiness, confusion, or mild focal deficit

Grade 4. Stupor, moderate to severe hemiparesis, possible early decerebrate rigidity and vegetative disturbances

Grade 5. Deep coma, decerebrate rigidity, moribund appearance

TABLE 7-5 —————————————————

CONCOMITANTS OF SUBARACHNOID HEMORRHAGE

Headache
Loss of consciousness
Obtundation
Meningeal signs
Seizures
Nausea
Vomiting
Dizziness
Neck or back pain
Paralysis or paresis
Visual field defects
Cranial nerve palsies III, VI
Fever
GI bleeding
Pulmonary edema
Syndrome of secretion of inappropriate antidiuretic hormone
ECG changes
Visual blurring
Subhyaloid hemorrhage
Papilledema (late)

patients with severe, sudden-onset headaches with normal neurologic exams, about 12% have SAH.

Several symptoms usually found with SAH may be conspicuously absent. Meningeal signs may be absent. Neck or back pain may be the sole complaint, raising suspicion of spinal arteriovenous malformation.

Spontaneous hemorrhage is most commonly caused by an aneurysm, except in patients under age 20, in whom arteriovenous malformations are more common. Other causes for spontaneous hemorrhage are distinctly uncommon. Cerebral thrombosis may cause leakage of blood into the subarachnoid space from infarcted tissue. Embolism and intracerebral hemorrhage can act similarly. Tumors, particularly of the pituitary, may bleed. Rare causes of subarachnoid bleeding include coagulopathies, mycotic aneurysms, and metastatic tumors. Trauma with resultant cerebral cortical contusion or penetrating trauma may cause bleeding into the subarachnoid space. In up to 10% of cases, no cause for the bleed is found.

The diagnostic modality of choice for detection of SAH is an unenhanced CT scan. It will detect most large, recent bleeds, depending upon the amount of blood and other factors discussed above. The concept of spectrum bias, the test being more likely to be positive at the extreme end of the spectrum of disease being investigated, is particularly applicable to CT for SAH. The small bleeds, and those evaluated many hours or days after the event, are the most likely to be missed by CT.

Lumbar puncture should be done if the scan is negative in the clinical setting of suspicion of SAH. If no CT scan is available and no clinical signs are present to suggest mass effect (any decrease in level of consciousness or focal deficit), one may proceed first with lumbar puncture. When clinical suspicion is very low for hemorrhage but one wishes to exclude it in the face of a normal exam, one might proceed directly to lumbar puncture. There may be a place for more definitive vascular imaging, such as cerebral angiography, in selected cases such as those patients with suspected SAH in whom the event was remote in time (weeks), in the presence of an ambiguous or traumatic spinal tap, or in patients who have contraindications to a spinal tap.

In most cases of SAH, many thousands of red cells are seen on microscopic evaluation of the CSF. There is, unfortunately, no particular threshold below which SAH is excluded, and very rare cases with a few hundred cells may occur. Red cells should appear in the lumbar subarachnoid space within the time frame in which clinical and radiographic evaluation can occur. A traumatic tap is particularly problematic in suspected SAH patients, and it may be very difficult or impossible in selected patients to determine whether the red blood cells in the CSF are from spontaneous SAH or the lumbar puncture itself. Xanthochromia may not occur for many hours after SAH and is variably detectable by the laboratory.

Neurologic decompensation following the hemorrhage may be caused by hydrocephalus, cerebral vasospasm, or repeated hemorrhage. Patients with established, common headache syndromes such as migraine may also have intracranial aneurysms, present in up to 7% of the population. Thus, a significant change in the nature of the headache in a patient with recurrent headaches presents a serious challenge to the clinician. Dramatic symptoms such as syncope, seizures, instantaneous onset, or meningismus should prompt further evaluation in such patients.

TEMPORAL ARTERITIS AND OTHER VASCULITIDES

Inflammation of the scalp and intracranial arteries is a cause for headache in the elderly and others with predisposing medical conditions. Left untreated, its consequences, particularly blindness, can be devastating. One should obtain a sedimentation rate in elderly patients with unexplained headaches.

Temporal arteritis usually begins after age 55, is more common in women, and may not have the classical accompanying jaw claudication, fever, malaise, weight loss, anemia, and polymyalgia rheumatica early in its course. Tender, bulging temporal or occipital arteries are not invariable findings, especially early. Elevated sedimentation rates almost invariably occur. Definitive diagnosis by temporal artery biopsy need not always be done in an obvious case and should not delay administration of steroids to prevent the visual loss that can occur suddenly in 50% of cases with visual loss. A brief course of corticosteroids will not obscure the pathologic findings on biopsied temporal artery specimens.

Other conditions associated with vasculitis such as periarteritis nodosa, rheumatoid arthritis, scleroderma, polymyositis, dermatomyositis, erythema nodosum, and Sjögren's syndrome should bring vasculitis to mind as a cause of headache.[14] Other causes of hypersensitivity vasculitis, such as drug reactions, systemic lupus erythematosus, Henoch-Schönlein purpura, and others, should be considered in the appropriate setting.

MENINGITIS AND ENCEPHALITIS

Meningitis, representing as it does a potentially treatable medical emergency, bears consideration in patients with headache. The classic symptoms and signs of malaise, headache, fever, photophobia, meningeal signs, nausea and vomiting, and obtundation may be only incompletely present or conspicuously absent. Bacterial meningitis can occur without stiff neck, particularly in infants but also in older adults.[15] The accompanying mental status changes range from irritability, restlessness, confusion, and hallucination to coma, but all these may be absent. Seizures are not common in adults.[16] In infants, the diagnosis can be difficult because of the lack of meningeal signs and the nonspecificity of manifestations: fever, vomiting, irritability, and anorexia. Drowsiness is common, and seizures are much more usual than they are in adults. In infants, bulging of the fontanel with the patient upright and not crying or straining indicates elevated intracranial pressure and is a sign that should be sought.

The clinical suspicion of meningitis should prompt administration of antibiotic therapy and examination of the spinal fluid. Contraindications to spinal tap, i.e., presence of an intracranial mass, usually will not occur because these patients present different clinical syndromes. The rare patient in whom these two possibilities exist presents a particularly difficult problem and will be discussed later as a separate subject. One should bear in mind that posterior fossa mass with cerebellar tonsillar herniation can cause stiff neck and is a contraindication to spinal tap.

Appropriate antimicrobial regimens for meningitis change with time and drug availability, and current references including local drug sensitivity reports should be used to guide initial therapy. Examination of the fluid for the antigens of *Haemophilus influenza*, *Neisseria meningitides*, and *Streptococcus pneumoniae* may be particularly useful in patients previously treated with antibiotics. Blood cultures may also yield the organism.

Many conditions predispose the patient to meningitis. These include CSF leak, in which *Strep. pneumoniae* is the most common pathogen. Infections near the meninges, such as sinusitis, mastoiditis, and otitis, may lead to meningitis. Defects in the coverings of the nervous system, either surgical or congenital as in dermal sinuses, place the patients at risk. Systemic infections such as bacterial endocarditis and systemic conditions such as sickle cell anemia are predisposing factors, as is splenectomy. Those with systemic malignancy or transplant patients are at risk for a wide variety of unusual infections such as *Cryptococcus*.

Other organisms such as viruses, spirochetes, rickettsiae, fungi, and protozoa may also cause meningitis. Detection of these organisms will depend on special techniques of evaluating spinal fluid. Thus, having clinical suspicion and obtaining sufficient excess spinal fluid remain the best ways to detect less common or less easily diagnosable entities expeditiously.

Pathologically, meningitis or inflammation of the meninges usually also sets up an inflammatory response (encephalitis) in the adjacent brain. The term is then meningoencephalitis. Some disease entities, such as herpesvirus, tend to affect brain tissue primarily and less so the meninges.

Encephalitis presents as headache with dramatic mental changes including drowsiness, delerium, stupor, coma, and irritability. Photophobia, malaise, fever, nausea, and vomiting commonly occur. More details concerning the difference between encephalopathy and encephalitis are discussed in Chapter 3. The etiologies of encephalitis are vast and include many virus infections, parisitic infections, bacterial and rickettsial diseases, and spirochetal disease. Clinical suspicion of herpesvirus encephalitis, one of the few viral encephalitides with a specific treatment, should prompt initiation of antiviral therapy.

Children may present with a clinical picture resembling meningoencephalitis (headache, confusion, irritability, and vomiting) as a result of Reyes' syndrome, a now rare condition. Fever is usually absent.

MIGRAINE

Migraine headache is one of the most common etiologies for headache in an acute care setting and in the population as a whole. One-third of the population will experience migraine in their lifetime. The prevalence of migraines in the general population is 18% among females and approximately 7% among males. In 1999 there were an estimated 28 million people with migraines in the United States.[17] Five percent of the population suffers recurrent migraine.[18] The character of the pain and not the intensity identifies a headache as migrainous, although most patients describe the pain as severe at a physician visit. A pulse-synchronous, often unilateral (about 60%) headache, worse with exertion, accompanied by nausea, vomiting, and photophobia, is commonly seen. In classic or ophthalmic migraine, now termed migraine with aura (about 15% of patients), these symptoms are usually preceded by a neurologic symptom, usually visual. The visual symptom is typically described as having a light of its own, or being bright or scintillating, and typically disappears as the headache begins. The neurologic symptom can come before, during, or after the headache phase, which may also be described as simply pressure and not pounding. Common migraine, now termed migraine without aura, is far more frequent[19]; it lacks the neurologic symptoms, and the pain is less commonly localized. Many patients can have both forms, and the individual characteristics of the headache may change from headache to headache. The diagnosis is solely made by history. The clinical characteristics of migraine are listed in Table 7-6. In hemiplegic migraine, the neurologic symptom is weakness but may also be sensory or speech. Total hemiplegia may occur and may be ipsilateral to the pain. Seizures and vertigo are rare. This variant of migraine is usually familial and occurs in a setting of other forms of migraine. Ophthalmoplegic migraine, with a third-nerve palsy ipsilateral to the pain, is extremely uncommon. Most cases of suspected ophthalmoplegic migraine are in fact due to other pathologic entities, particularly aneurysms. The

TABLE 7-6 —————————————————————————
CLINICAL MIGRAINE CHARACTERISTICS

Visual Aura in Migraine with Aura
Scintillating scotoma, up to 1 hr duration may be followed by visual field loss; contralateral to headache
May have aura without headache

Prodrome
Hours to days prior to headache: psychic symptoms
Irritability, confusion, anxiety, depression, euphoria, alertness, clarity

Headache
Pulse synchronous; may be pressure-like behind eye rarely to face, jaw, neck, back
Peak pain at 1 to 2 hr, possibly days
Nausea and vomiting, rarely diarrhea
Sensitivity to external stimuli (light, sound)
Changing character of headache over time
Temporal arteries tender and dilated, edema of wall may develop
Pain may decrease by occluding temporal artery anterior to ear
Most common age of onset 10 to 30 years, 30% to 50% prior to age 15
Headaches usually decrease after age 40; rarely increase

diagnosis cannot be made without excluding aneurysm and other causes such as tumor, arteritis, and sinusitis.

In childhood migraine, the necessary history may be difficult to obtain. Vomiting is very common, as is motion sickness, and acute crises of abdominal pain, "migraine equivalent," can occur. The headache is usually brief, 1 to 6 hours. Epilepsy is common in patients with pediatric migraine and is unassociated with attacks of headache. Attacks may be triggered by trivial head trauma.[20] Males are more commonly affected. Acute confusional states may occur, simulating a toxic psychosis.

Many factors are felt to contribute to migraine. Some, such as relationship to menstrual cycle, are commonly accepted. Others, such as food sensitivity, are controversial. These factors are listed in Table 7-7.

Migraine of many days' duration, status hemicranicus, may be particularly disabling may and require hospitalization for hydration and analgesia. Other variants of migraine, such as cluster headache, are described in Table 7-8.

Therapy for migraine is the subject of controversy. Some physicians, wary of chronic headache patients as potential substance abusers and seeing such patients at their worst, are reluctant to give narcotic analgesics or use homeopathic doses. Other physicians, secure in their diagnosis and relationship with the patient, recognize the value of full therapeutic doses of narcotic analgesics as rescue medications in the acute painful phase. Longer-acting narcotics such as methadone may be more likely to outlast the headache. The primary goal of therapy is elimination

TABLE 7-7

FACTORS ASSOCIATED WITH MIGRAINE

Menstrual: first day of period or before; decreased headache after third-month pregnancy; rarely increased
Photogenic: flashing lights, glare
Food: alcohol, wine; chocolate, milk, cheese, fruit
Weather: approaching low pressure
Psychic: both "good" and "bad" events
Excessive sleep, lack of sleep
Diseases: chronic renal
Hereditary
Personality

TABLE 7-8

OTHER MIGRANOUS HEADACHES

Cluster Headache
Male predominance
Age of onset 10 to 60 years
Rarely familial
Attacks provoked by alcohol, nitrates
Sudden agonizing unilateral pain deep to eye, restlessness
Conjunctival injection
Lacrimation; rhinorrhea
Small pupil, ptosis (partial Horner's) 10 to 30 min for each attack
Attacks may "cluster" for days or weeks and disappear for years

Basilar Migraine
Rare; patient usually has other sudden visual symptoms of migraine, including cortical blindness followed by a combination of
    Vertigo
    Ataxia
    Dysarthria
    Tinnitus
    Paresthesia
and then gradual decreased level of consciousness or confusional state and severe, pounding occipital headache, nausea, and vomiting; usually females, under 21 years old, with family history of migraine

of the headache, not simply overpowering the pain with opiates. In general, non-narcotic medications such as prochlorperazine, DHE, or triptans are used initially or in combination, with narcotics reserved for rescue in selected cases. However, many migraine medication regimens exist because none are universally effective. Antiemetics are commonly given, and prochlorperazine is particularly effective. All medications are more effective when given early in the course of the headache, but all still have some effect regardless of timing. There seems to be individual preferences among patients for particular medications. Chronic prophylaxis against migraine now includes too vast an array of medications to discuss them adequately here. Steroids, believed to decrease edema around swollen arteries, may be useful for prolonged migraine. Triptans are useful and may be self-administered in some patients. Table 7-9 lists the medications that are useful in migraines.

NONMIGRAINOUS VASCULAR HEADACHES

There are several causes for headaches with "vascular" characteristics, i.e., pounding, worse with exertion, pulse-synchronous. The most common of these is *fever* headache. This pulsatile headache is complained of in a variety of systemic syndromes and is so common that it is usually the feeling that causes people to believe their temperature is elevated. Some systemic illnesses such as shigellosis have headache as such a prominent part of the symptom complex that spinal tap is frequently done to exclude meningitis. Other causes of nonmigrainous vascular headache are listed in Table 7-10. Only a few will be described here. *Carbon monoxide* intoxication is an important cause for headache, which may be episodic or absent on presentation. Carboxyhemoglobin values may also have returned to normal or nondiagnostic ranges while some headache lingers. Checking potential sources of leakage of products of combustion may be reasonable and potentially life-saving.

Hypertension

Hypertension is not a usual cause of headache. This widely seen problem may occur in patients with other common causes of headache. It may not be the etiology even at moderate hypertensive levels (180 mmHg systolic, 110 mmHg diastolic).[6] Hypertensive encephalopathy is a different entity entirely. The place hypertension plays in the generation of headache is controversial; however, many patients and their physicians assume that their headache is caused by hypertension because it may be elevated at the time of the pain. Ambulatory monitoring of moderate elevations of blood pressure, along with headache diaries, fail to establish a cause-and-effect relationship.

Cerebrovascular Accident

The three common etiologies usually encompassed in the nonspecific term cerebrovascular accident (CVA; embolism,[21] thrombosis, and hemorrhage) may all cause

TABLE 7-9

MEDICATIONS FOR MIGRAINES

Phenothiazines
Prochlopromazine
Chlorpromazine

Butyrophenones
Droperidol
Haloperidol

Dihydroergotamine (DHE)

Triptans
Sumatriptan
Naratriptan
Almotriptan
Zolmitriptan

Valproate Sodium IV

Ketorolac

Metoclopramide

Diphenhydramine

Corticosteroids (prolonged migraine)

Opioids
Methadone
Nalbophine
Meperidine
Morphine

Common Analgesics
NSAIDs
Aspirin
Acetaminophen
Caffeine

headache. The neurologic exam will make the diagnosis, but unfortunately the presence of headache will not help to decide among the three given etiologies. Dramatic, sudden headache should suggest SAH.

Posttraumatic Headache

After head trauma, headache is extremely common but usually of brief duration. It may be prolonged in a posttraumatic syndrome (see Chap. 9). Several other entities

TABLE 7-10 ————————————————————————————————————
NONMIGRAINOUS VASCULAR HEADACHES

Fever
Substances
 Carbon monoxide, lead, benzene, carbon tetrachloride, insecticides, nitrites
  ("hotdog headache"), toluene, nitrobenzene, hydrogen sulfide, methanol,
  monosodium glutamate ("Chinese restaurant syndrome"), alcohol
Drugs
 Nitrates, indomethacin, oral progestational, vasodilators
Withdrawal
 Ergots, caffeine, amphetamines, many phenothiazines, alcohol
Other
 Hypoxia, hypoglycemia, hypercarbia, anemia, toxemia of pregnancy, hyper-
  tensive encephalopathy, hypothyroidism, hyperthyroidism, hypoadren-
  alism, vasomotor rhinitis, altitude, effort, CVAs, coital headache

that cause sustained posttraumatic headache are listed in Table 7-11. One should keep in mind that the trauma may not be recalled or may have been trivial, as in chronic subdural hematoma, in which chronic-persistent headache is common.

Uncommon Vascular Headaches

Several uncommon entities should be mentioned. *Coital headache,* a benign, well-described entity,[22] may begin during sexual arousal or at orgasm, or immediately after orgasm. The pain is sudden and usually occipital. Many patients with this condition also have migraine. Subarachnoid hemorrhage can also occur during intercourse. *Effort headache* may occur with athletic efforts, such as running

TABLE 7-11 ————————————————————————————————————
POSTTRAUMATIC HEADACHE

Chronic subdural hematoma
Subdural hygroma
Hydrocephalus
Skull fracture
Meningitis
Brain abscess
Subarachnoid hemorrhage
Muscle contraction (tension)
Neck trauma
Psychogenic

but is also a well-described component of posterior fossa tumors, which may need to be excluded. *Cough headache* is another similar entity, as is the headache that occurs after the exertional effort involved in sneezing and defecating.

HIGH CSF PRESSURE SYNDROMES AND TUMORS

The headache that accompanies high CSF pressure is typically worse in the morning and decreases after arising or vomiting. It may worsen with cough or effort. Although headache is a common early symptom with posterior fossa tumors, it may not necessarily be an early sign with supratentorial tumors, except those lying adjacent to pain-sensitive structures (e.g., meningiomas). Intraventricular tumors, such as colloid cysts, may suddenly occlude the third ventricle by a ball-valve action and cause very sudden headache and possibly syncope. They are a cause of sudden death. Pituitary tumors may cause sudden headache from hemorrhage or necrosis of the tumor. The resultant syndrome (pituitary apoplexy, visual loss, and bloody spinal fluid) may simulate SAH. The reaction in the CSF may also simulate meningitis as an aseptic reaction to tumor contents. Brain abscesses act like tumors and present with similar symptoms and typically no current fever. Children with headache secondary to brain tumor very commonly have abnormalities on neurologic and neuroophthalmologic exam, which is by far the best screening technique. Table 7-12 lists causes of high CSF pressure syndromes.

Pseudotumor Cerebri

Pseudotumor cerebri, a rare condition, is also termed idiopathic intracranial hypertension and refers to a condition characterized by elevated intracranial pressure, headache, and papilledema. Although it typically occurs in obese women in late ado-

TABLE 7-12
HIGH CSF PRESSURE SYNDROMES AND TUMORS

Tumors
    Pituitary, meningiomas, gliomas, posterior fossa
    Metastatic
    Intraventricular
Brain abscess
Subdural hematoma
Vascular malformations
Pseudotumor cerebri
Venous thrombosis
    Adjacent to mastoiditis, postpartum seizures
    Cerebral edema
Hypertensive encephalopathy

lescence or early adulthood, it may also occur in men and children. The headache typically develops over weeks to months and may wax and wane. The condition may last for many months. There are usually no neurologic findings other than papilledema, although sixth nerve palsy may occur. The cause of pseudotumor cerebri is unknown. Many factors have been implicated, often anecdotally, such as menstrual irregularities, weight gain, hypervitaminosis A, oral retinoids, and tetracycline administration. Pseudotumor cerebri is a diagnosis of exclusion. By definition, one must exclude other causes for elevated intracranial pressure, principally mass effect, chronic meningitis, and intracranial venous thrombosis, which can also result in elevated intracranial pressure, and must be excluded. A CT scan should rule out hydrocephalus, and the spinal fluid is typically under pressure of 250 to 400 mm H_2O but should otherwise be normal. Venous magnetic resonance angiography can be performed to exclude dural venous sinus thrombosis.

LOW CSF PRESSURE

The headache of low CSF pressure is worsened by upright posture and relieved by recumbency. The most common cause is postlumbar puncture. Bed rest or head-down position after spinal tap does not decrease the incidence of this problem.[23,24] A syndrome of spontaneously low CSF pressure with the characteristics of a post spinal tap headache has also been described. The cause is unknown, and CSF pressure when measured with the patient supine is low, 0 to 60 mm H_2O. Post spinal tap headaches may respond to caffeine or a blood patch.

TENSION HEADACHE

Sustained scalp and neck muscle contraction may cause pain that outlasts the contraction. Whereas psychic tension may be the underlying cause, muscle tension is the final common pathway to a variety of conditions. It is one of the most common causes of headache. The pain is usually bilateral, dragging, or tight band-like in feeling; it is usually constant and decreases with sleep. It may encompass the entire head or only the back of the head or neck. It is not associated with nausea and vomiting, nor is there a prodrome.

PSYCHOGENIC HEADACHE

Psychogenic headache is usually associated with depression and may be described as a heaviness that prevents thinking and is unrelieved by analgesics. The pain may shift in location and be described in a bizarre fashion, and although tension headache may be a part of it, usually the description is different. This diagnosis may be difficult to make in a single, brief acute care evaluation.

NEURALGIAS

The chief characteristics of the neuralgias are the sudden, brief, lancinating character of the pains, which are usually precipitated by a tactile stimulus. This stimulus may be cold air, touch, or shaving in trigeminal neuralgia (tic douloureaux), or swallowing in glossopharyngeal neuralgia.

ARTERIAL DISSECTION

Nontraumatic carotid or vertebral arterial dissection may cause sudden severe headache, usually in addition to neck pain. Neck manipulation or injury may cause it as well.[25] It is a rare condition and may cause ischemic symptoms, particularly in young patients and especially young stroke patients with significant head/neck pain.[26] The pain, however, may not be intense or different from other headaches, and then the diagnosis can only be suspected once neurologic deficits occur, which may not be for days or weeks.[27] With carotid dissection, local compression on the cervical sympathetic chain may cause an ipsilateral Horner's syndrome.[28] Although most causes of sudden severe headache, especially with neurologic deficit, can be eliminated with a normal CT, lumbar puncture, and very few laboratory tests, arterial dissection cannot, and it may need to be considered in selected cases. Magnetic resonance angiography, ultrasound, or plain angiography can be used to image the problem.

MISCELLANEOUS CAUSES OF HEADACHE

Other causes of headache, some common such as sinusitis and others rare, such as Tolosa-Hunt syndrome, are listed in Table 7-13, along with selected characteristics.

THE PATIENT WITH SUSPECTED MASS OR MENINGITIS

An uncommon but difficult case occasionally arises with clinical suspicion of an intracranial mass and/or meningitis or brain abscess. Whereas in their pure form these syndromes rarely overlap, the real world is full of contradictory examples. For example, a patient may be postictal and have focal deficit, confusion, and lethargy from a mass lesion and fever from an aspiration pneumonia (in retrospect). However, when practicing medicine prospectively, one may not have sufficient information to generate these diagnoses. The sequence could also be one of postictal state and fever from meningitis alone. Stiff neck may arise from posterior fossa tumor and cerebellar tonsillar herniation, or neck injury. Patients may have a coagulation defect, either from medication or a medical condition, which may predispose to a mass lesion such as subdural hematoma, and represents a relative contraindication to lumbar puncture.

TABLE 7-13
MISCELLANEOUS CAUSES OF HEADACHE

Sinusitis
Dental disease
Temporomandibular joint (Costen's syndrome)
Ocular
    Optic neuritis
    Iritis
    Orbital inflammation
    Cavernous sinus thrombosis
    Acute narrow-angle glaucoma
    Pronounced astigmatism
    Poor accommodation
    Hyperopia
    Latent strabismus
Ice cream headache
Post seizure
Cervical spine disease
Pheochromocytoma
    Onset over minutes, bilateral
    Offset usually less than 1 hr
    Throbbing
    Perspiration, palpitation, pallor
    Tremor
    Nausea
    Elevated blood pressure during paroxysm
Tolosa-Hunt syndrome (painful ophthalmoplegia)[16]
    Unilateral pain near eye
    Ophthalmoplegia (pupil usually spared)
    Elevated sedimentation rate
    Optic involvement
    Steroid responsive
    Inflammatory process, etiology unknown

In these cases, one is pulled by opposing factors. Early spinal tap and immediate institution of antibiotics is called for with meningitis, but these measures may be dangerous in the presence of a mass intracranial lesion. CT scans, if rapidly available, should be done to rule out mass lesions. However, they are not always immediately available. One possible solution is to treat the patient as if meningitis were present with antibiotics appropriate to organisms common in that age group after obtaining blood cultures or other (but not CSF) cultures, while awaiting definitive study to rule out mass lesions. Once a mass lesion has been excluded, spinal tap can be done safely, and the CSF characteristics of meningitis will not have been obscured, even after 48 hours of treatment.[29] Otherwise, the value of the CSF culture may be lost. Spinal fluid antigen testing for *H. influenzae, N. meningitides,* and *Strep. pneumoniae* can be done, and blood testing or other cultures may be helpful.

REFERENCES

1. Dickerman RL, et al. Management of non-traumatic headache in university hospital emergency room. *Headache* 1979;19:391.
2. Fitzpatrick R, Hopkins A. Referrals to neurologists for headaches not due to structural disease. *J Neurol Neurosurg Psychiatry* 1981;44:1061–1067.
3. Diehr P, et al. Acute headaches: presenting symptoms and diagnostic rules to identify patients with tension and migraine headache. *J Chron Dis* 1981;34:147–158.
4. Raskin N. Chemical headaches. *Annu Rev Med* 1981;32:63–71.
5. Lipton RB, et al. Migraine diagnosis and treatment: results from the American Migraine Study II. *Headache* 2001;41:638–645.
6. Kattah J. Neurophthalmic signs in headache syndromes. *Am Fam Physician* 1982;25:99–105.
7. Knaus W, et al. CT for headache: cost/benefit for subarachnoid hemorrhage. *AJR* 1981;136:537.
8. Smith W, et al. Acute isodense subdural hematomas: a problem in anemic patients. *AJR* 1981;136:543.
9. Honig P, Charney E. Children with brain tumor headaches: distinguishing features. *Am J Dis Child* 1982;136:121–124.
10. Shinnar S, D'Souza B. The diagnosis and management of headaches in childhood. *Pediatr Clin North Am* 1981;29:79–94.
11. Post K, et al. Ruptured intracranial aneurysms: case morbidity and mortality. *J Neurosurg* 1977;46:290–295.
12. Raskin N, Appenzeller O: *Headache.* Philadelphia: Saunders, 1980, vol 29, *Major Problems in Internal Medicine.*
13. Cougheed WM, Barnett HJM. Lesions producing spontaneous hemorrhage. In: Youmans J, ed. *Neurological Surgery.* Philadelphia: WB Saunders, 1973.
14. Keane JR. Retinal hemorrhages: its significance in 100 patients with acute encephalopathy of unknown cause. *Arch Neurol* 1979;36:691.
15. Marriott H. *Practical Electrocardiography,* 5th ed. Baltimore, Williams & Wilkins, 1972, p 308.
16. Diamond S, Palessio D. *The Practicing Physicians Approach to Headache.* Baltimore; Williams & Wilkins, 1982.
17. Geiseler PJ, et al. Bacterial meningitis without clinical signs of meningeal irritation. *South Med J* 1982;75:448.
18. Saks AL, Joynt RJ. Meningitis. In: Baker AB, Baker LH, eds. *Clinical Neurology.* New York: Harper & Row, 1979.
19. Lipton RB, et al. Prevalence and burden of migraine in the United States: data from the American Migraine Study II. *Headache* 2001;41:646–657.
20. Hartwig H. *Headache and Facial Pain—Differential Diagnosis, Pathogenesis, Treatment.* Chicago: Year Book, 1981.
21. Scheife RT, et al. Migraine headaches: signs and symptoms, biochemistry and current therapy. *Am J Hosp Pharm* 1980;37:365.

22. Haas DC, et al. Juvenile head trauma syndromes and their relationship to migraine. *Arch Neurol* 1975;32:727–730.

23. Norton J. Use of intravenous valproate sodium in status migraine. *Headache* 2000;40: 755–757.

24. Friedman A. Headache. In: Baker AB, Baker LH, eds. *Clinical Neurology.* New York: Harper & Row, 1979.

25. Auerbach S, et al. Headache in cerebral embolic disease. *Stroke* 1981;12:367.

26. Porter M, Jankovic J. Benign coital cepalalgia: differential diagnosis and treatment. *Arch Neurol* 1981;38:710–712.

27. Handler CE, et al. Posture and lumbar puncture headache—a controlled trial in 50 patients. *J R Soc Med* 1982;75:404.

28. Carbaat PAT, Van Crevel H. Lumbar puncture headache: controlled study on the preventive effect of 24 hours of bedrest. *Lancet* 1981;2:1133.

29. Showalter W, et al. Vertebral artery dissection. *Acad Emerg Med* 1997;4:991–995.

30. Zetterling M, Carlstrom C, Konrad, P. Internal carotid artery dissection. *Acta Neurol Scand* 2000;101:1–7.

31. Yoshimoto Y, Wakai S. Unruptured intracranial vertebral artery dissection. *Stroke* 1997;28:370–374.

32. Stapf C, Elkind MS, Mohr JP: Carotid artery dissection. *Annu Rev Med* 2000;51:329–347.

33. Blazer S, et al. Effect of antibiotic treatment on cerebrospinal fluid. *Am J Clin Pathol* 1983;80:386.

ACUTE DOUBLE VISION, BLINDNESS, AND ABNORMAL PUPILS

In emergency and ambulatory care settings, complaints of sudden decrease in visual acuity or diplopia are not common, but when they occur they may be symptoms of both serious and eminently treatable disease.[1] The initial evaluation of such complaints should establish the difference between structural and nonstructural visual system disease and permit the physician to proceed with a rapid, specific diagnosis and appropriate treatment.

HISTORY

The historical features needed to diagnose acute visual problems are specific but few in number (Table 8-1).

Lateralization

The first and most important question is to determine whether the visual problem is monocular or binocular. A patient can usually tell through simple observation whether one or both eyes are involved. As a general rule visual problems such as monocular decreased vision or monocular diplopia represent structural disease lying anterior to the optic chiasm or disease involving the globe itself. Bilateral visual problems usually involve diffuse toxic, infectious, or metabolic processes, posterior circulation, or vascular occlusions. Rarely, structural lesions in the pituitary gland will cause bilateral visual loss.

TABLE 8-1

HISTORICAL FEATURES—
NEUROOPHTHALMOLOGIC SYMPTOMS

Lateralization (right, left, or both visual fields involved)
Associated symptoms
Rate of onset
Drugs and medications
Pain and trauma

Rate of Onset

Decreased vision that occurs within a matter of minutes represents vascular disease or retinal problems.[2] This may be in the form of embolic or hemorrhagic lesions and may involve only the visual system or large areas of the brain. Other disease processes will have time courses that will help to differentiate their various etiologies, i.e., infection, trauma.

Associated Symptoms

Sudden changes in visual acuity or diplopia associated with headache should be considered an urgent neurologic condition.[3] The visual system from the retina moving posterior is essentially insensitive to pain unless meningeal irritation is also involved. Any lesion that will give immediate eye symptoms and severe pain should be considered to be involving the pain-sensitive structures of the eye and head. Pain-sensitive structures from the retina forward to the cornea should be visible and/or testable on physical examination. Other acute painful lesions with visual change should be considered vascular in etiology until proven otherwise.

Trauma

Trauma from the front of the globe to the occipital cortex can affect visual acuity and coordinated eye movements.[4] Along with globe and orbit evaluation, attention should be paid to signs of trauma to the areas of the posterior skull and neck.

Drugs

Heavy use of alcohol and tobacco should be noted along with the patient's over-the-counter medications and prescription drugs, including eye drops. It may be necessary to ask specifically about the use of vitamins, laxatives, pain medications, and tranquilizers.

GENERAL EXAMINATION

The general physical examination of the patient with visual complaints should be centered around the head and neck region and the cardiovascular system (Table 8-2). The general appearance of the patient, with particular attention to focal symmetry, position, and proptosis, should be noted. Evidence of trauma should be evaluated. The position of the eyes within the head and their relationship to the orbital rims (exophthalmus, enophthalmos) should be noted. Palpation of the orbital rims and skull is necessary in traumatic situations.

The neck should be evaluated for signs of trauma or mass lesions. In cases of sudden monocular visual loss, the neck should be examined for bruits. Palpation of the arteries of the head, particularly the temporal arteries, should be performed in elderly patients with a sudden loss of vision.

Ophthalmologic Examination

For a summary of the examination, see Table 8-2.

Visual Acuity

The most important part in examining an eye complaint is visual acuity testing.[2] If corrective lenses are used, the patient should be examined while wearing them in order to obtain the best corrected vision. If the patient has relatively poor visual acuity or the corrective lenses are not available, the pinhole technique can be employed.[7]

Pinhole testing is performed by having the patient read the eye chart while looking through a card with a small hole in the center. Pinhole testing cuts down all extraneous visual input and allows the patient to focus light only on the fovea. Pinhole vision is generally the best vision one can hope to get with corrective lenses. A patient whose vision improves substantially by use of the pinhole has a refractive error and not a neurologic decrease in vision.

TABLE 8-2
EXAMINATION OF ACUTE VISUAL COMPLAINTS

1. General physical examination, including general eye; slit-lamp, and funduscopic examination as appropriate
2. Neurologic examination, including visual acuity, extraocular movements, pupils
3. Specific neuroophthalmologic testing as appropriate:
   a. Marcus Gunn pupil
   b. Optokinetic nystagmus
   c. Red glass test

Visual Fields

In the acute care setting, visual field testing can be done most simply by the confrontation method.[5,6] The patient should look at the examiner while the examiner's fingers are moved simultaneously in the major visual quadrants. Each eye is tested separately. If the patient detects simultaneous movement of two fingers moved on opposite sides of the body, little else need be done. If the patient fails to recognize one of the moving fingers, then the stimuli must be given independently. If the patient can recognize stimuli given independently but cannot detect movement done simultaneously, then he/she is illustrating visual suppression or extinction. This is usually a sign of nondominant parietal lobe disease, as opposed to an involvement of the visual system per se. This finding can be checked by giving other sensory stimuli simultaneously on other portions of the patient's body and noting whether a consistent lateralization of such suppression exists. Sophisticated visual field testing with various-sized objects and tangent screens is not usually available or necessary in the acute care setting. Visual field testing should be reserved for patients with a segmented or partial bilateral visual loss.

Slit Lamp and Funduscopic Examination

Most causes of decreased vision involve the eye itself and are not related to nervous system elements.[2] Careful slit lamp examination, with particular attention to the cornea, anterior chamber, and lens abnormalities, is helpful. Funduscopic examination to view the condition of the vitreous body, retina, and optic nerve head is also important.

Intraocular Pressure

Intraocular pressure recording with either a Schiotz instrument, an applanation tonometer, or other appropriate measuring device should be performed in cases of decreased vision in which glaucoma may be suspected due to pain, conjunctival infection, and decreased movement of the pupil.

Neuroophthalmologic Testing

Basic neuroophthalmologic testing can be done in the ambulatory setting with relative ease and little special equipment. The following three tests will prove particularly useful in the evaluation of acute visual complaints.

Marcus Gunn Pupil

The Marcus Gunn pupil sign, or the swinging flashlight sign, should be elicited in patients with decreased vision.[6] The midbrain nuclei sense the total amount of light received through both eyes to set pupillary size. The Marcus Gunn pupil response tests to see whether a decrease in total light is actually being perceived by an eye.

A strong light is shined in the affected eye, and the size and reactivity of the pupils are noted. The light is then moved to the supposedly good eye, and the pupils are again observed. The light is then moved back to the involved eye, and the size of pupils is checked. As one moves from the eye with poor vision to the eye with normal vision, the pupils should constrict. As the light is moved from the eye with good vision to the eye with poor vision, the pupils should dilate because less total light is actually reaching midbrain nuclei. The Marcus Gunn pupil sign is nonspecific but extremely sensitive. A disease process seriously decreasing vision that is anterior to the optic chiasm should have a positive Marcus Gunn pupil sign. By definition, a positive Marcus Gunn sign is when the light source is moved from the good eye to the eye of decreased visual acuity and both pupils dilate. This test is not helpful if both optic nerves are equally involved.

Optokinetic Nystagmus

Optokinetic nystagmus (OKN) is a simple yet effective test to distinguish cortical from noncortical blindness.[5] OKN can be induced in normal subjects by continuous movement of a series of visual targets across the visual field. This is usually accomplished using paper with narrow lines or a rotating drum with stripes. Normal eyes will fix on a stripe, follow this target for a short distance, and then quickly return to primary gaze, where they will pick up another target to follow. On a repeated basis, this results in nsytagmus. OKN can be induced in any direction. The presence of intact OKN means that the visual input from the eyes has reached the occipital cortex and from there has gone to connections in the brainstem and back to the extraocular control centers of the eyes through the third, fourth, and sixth cranial nerves. These deviations have been monitored by anterior cortical visual centers and corrective instructions sent to the brainstem by the cortex. The presence of OKN virtually ensures that the patient is not blind.

The absence of OKN with preservation of the pupillary light reflex in the face of sudden visual loss is strongly suggestive of cortical blindness involving the occipital lobes.[6,7] Note that a very small group of people who do repetitive spinning and whirling motions (i.e., professional ice skaters, roller skaters, and others) have suppressed their OKN, and so it will not be present.

Red Glass Testing

Red glass testing is done to separate double images in patients complaining of binocular diplopia.[6] The test is performed by having a colored lens placed over one eye with a white light used for testing. The covered eye will then have a colored image, and the uncovered eye will have a white image. Extraocular movement testing is then performed. In all nine regions tested (Figure 8-1) in the normal patient, there will be one image that will represent the fusion of the white and colored light. If these colors are not perfectly fused, separate images will be present, indicating diplopia. If the colored image appears on the same side as the eye being tested, this is considered uncrossed diplopia.[6]

Right		Left
Right Upward Gaze		*Left Upper Gaze*
Right Superior Rectus	Upward Gaze	Left Superior Rectus
Left Inferior Oblique		Right Inferior Oblique
Right Lateral Gaze		*Left Lateral Gaze*
Right Lateral Rectus	Primary Gaze	Left Lateral Rectus
Left Medial Rectus		Right Medial Rectus
Right Downward Gaze		*Left Downward Gaze*
Right Inferior Rectus	Downward Gaze	Left Inferior Rectus
Left Superior Oblique		Right Superior Oblique

FIGURE 8-1   Muscle pairs in extraocular movements.

A sixth nerve palsy would be considered an example of such a diplopia (Figure 8-2).

If the image appears on the opposite side of the white light from that of the eye being tested with the colored lens, this is termed a crossed diplopia, a type seen with third nerve palsies.

It is important to remember that diplopia will be at its maximum when the field of action of the involved nerve or muscle is to be maximally utilized. For example, if a right sixth nerve palsy is present, looking laterally to the left would cause no diplopia, since the right lateral rectus muscle is not involved in this action. Looking laterally to the right, however, which is the principal area of action of the involved muscle, will produce the maximum diplopia.

A second basic rule of the test is that when diplopia exists, the most lateral or outside image is always the false image. One can determine which eye is creating the false image merely by having the patient shut one eye at a time. When one eye is closed and the most lateral image disappears, that is the eye of neurologic involvement.

A third rule of diplopia testing is simply to record what the patient sees in various positions of gaze and then try to relate it to classic patterns. Third, fourth, and sixth nerve palsies have specific patterns of diplopia. If multiple muscles or nerves are involved, testing patterns can be considerably more complex and difficult to analyze.[8]

SPECIFIC COMPLAINTS

Ptosis

Ptosis, drooping of the upper eyelids, is a rare complaint that may be found in a patient presenting with eye problems. Unilateral ptosis may be seen with involvement of third nerve lesions, but pupillary and eye movement motor findings are virtually always seen in conjunction with such a problem. Myasthenia gravis may present unilaterally, and a seventh nerve palsy may on occasion involve the upper lid more than the lower. Unilateral ptosis is almost always a sympathetic chain or third nerve pathology. Although the seventh nerve also innervates the eyelid, isolated ptosis without involvement of other facial muscles is not seen.

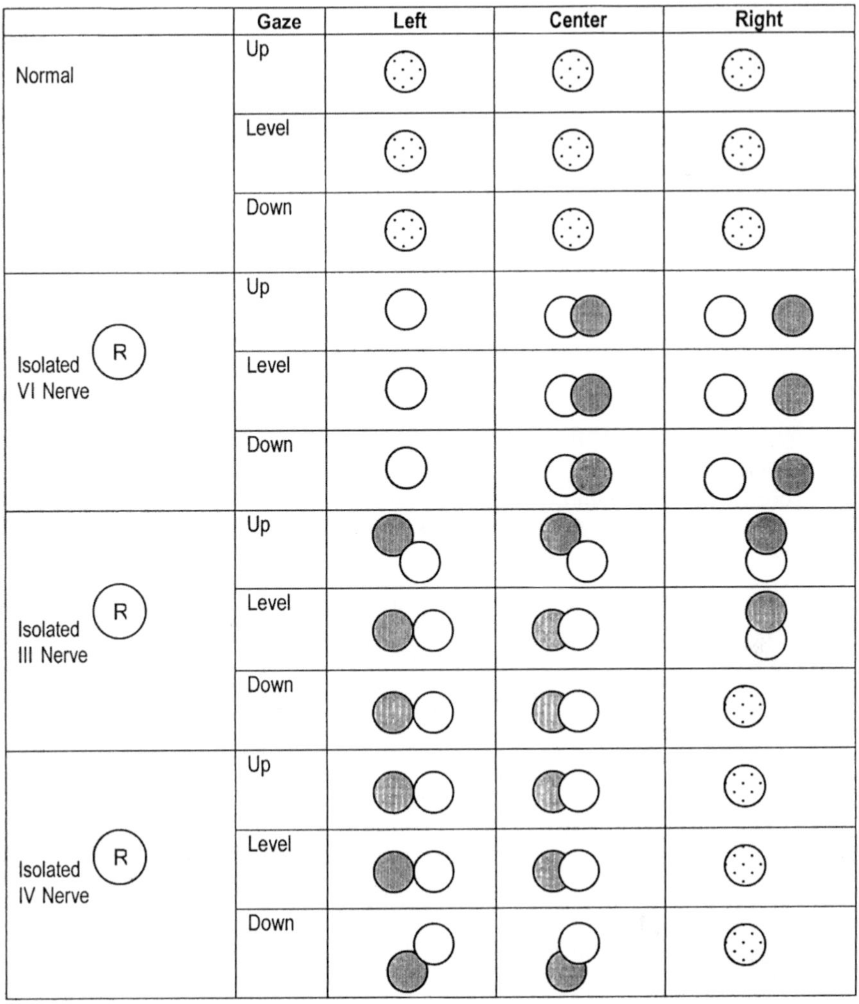

	Gaze	Left	Center	Right
Normal	Up			
	Level			
	Down			
Isolated (R) VI Nerve	Up			
	Level			
	Down			
Isolated (R) III Nerve	Up			
	Level			
	Down			
Isolated (R) IV Nerve	Up			
	Level			
	Down			

FIGURE 8-2   Patterns of specific nerve dysfunctions on red glass testing. Red glass over ® eye in all testing.

Bilateral ptosis is usually from myasthenia gravis or age-related skin changes with redundant tissue. In advanced cases, hypothyroidism, electrolyte abnormalities, and other myopathies can cause bilateral ptosis. Rare sporadic cases of oculopharyngeal dystrophy have been reported, but these are generally slowly progressive problems.

Abnormal Pupils

Pupillary changes, although rarely the presenting complaint of a patient, may be an important part of any neuroophthalmologic problem. Multiple factors can affect pupillary size, because pupils are susceptible to both topical medications and trauma as well as influences through the sympathetic and parasympathetic nervous systems. As a general rule, bilateral pupillary findings such as extremely large or extremely small pupils are on a centrally mediated basis from either structural or chemical causes (drugs and chemicals ingested or placed directly into the eye). An anisocoria (unequal pupils) may represent a lateralized nervous system problem or a local effect on nervous elements supplying that particular eye, or it may be the consequence of topical drugs or local ocular disease (Tables 8-3 and 8-4).[6]

Large Pupils

The unilateral, large, poorly reactive pupil can be the result of parasympathetic denervation, sympathetic excess, or end-organ blockade by drugs instilled into the eyes. Figure 8-3 illustrates a system for deciding the cause of a large pupil.

The first chemical instilled in the eye is 2% mecholyl. This drug stimulates the acetylcholine that should be released by the parasympathetic nerve system. If the pupil constricts with mecholyl, the problem is generally one of parasympathetic denervation. An example of parasympathetic denervation would be compression of

TABLE 8-3

DRUGS AND TOXINS CAPABLE OF PRODUCING CONSTRICTION–DILATION OF PUPILS

Parasympathetic Stimulator (Cholinergics)	Sympathetic Inhibitors (Antiadrenergics)	Parasympathetic Inhibitors (Anticholinergics)	Sympathetic Stimulators (Adrenergics)
Acetylcholine	Guanethedine	Botulinum toxin	Cocaine
Nicotine	Bretylium	Hemicholine	Amphetamine
Tetraethyl	Reserpine	Pentolinium	Ephedrine
ammonium	Alpha-methyl-	Atropine-like	Adrenalin drugs
Bromides	dopa	Scopolamine	Neosynephrine
Physostigmine	Monoamine oxi-	Homatropine	Tyramine
Neostigmine	dase inhibitors	Eucatropine	
Pyrophosphates	Dibenzylines	Over the counter	
Carbachol	Narcotics	sleep medications	
Mecholyl		Toadstool toxin	
Pilocarpine		Jimson weed	
		Wild sage	

TABLE 8-4
CAUSES OF MYDRIASIS (LARGE PUPIL)

Unilateral
1. Topical medications (antiparasympathetic blockade; see Table 8-3)
2. Parasympathetic denervation; uncal herniation, diabetes mellitus, aneurysm
3. Sympathetic excess (stimulation); the "fight-or-flight response"
4. Dilation phase of Adie's pupil
5. Unilateral blindness when the normal eye is covered (Marcus Gunn phenomenon)
6. Ophthalmoplegic migraine
7. Trauma and posttraumatic synechiae

Bilateral
1. Systemic drugs and chemicals (see Table 8-3)
2. Thyrotoxicosis
3. Bilateral parasympathetic paralysis, i.e., bilateral uncal herniation, etc.
4. Blockade at neuromuscular junction, i.e., botulism
5. Neuropathy involving cranial nerve III; diabetes mellitus, diphtheria
6. Cheyne-Stokes respirations
7. Asphyxia

the third cranial nerve. In this case both the pupillary finding (large pupil) and motor finding (eye deviated laterally and slightly down) should be present.

If the pupil does not respond to 2% mecholyl, pilocarpine can be instilled. Pilocarpine will overcome the effects of sympathetic excess in the eye.[9] Sympathetic excess may be due to systemic chemicals or increased outflow from the stellate ganglion. When a pupil does not become smaller with mecholyl or pilocarpine, end-organ blockade with a parasympathetic blocking drug such as atropine (placed in the eye) is strongly suggested.

Small Pupils

The causes of unilateral or bilaterally small pupils are many (Table 8-5). A system is needed to evaluate the unilateral nonreactive small pupil (Figure 8-4). Homatropine can be instilled in the eye. If dilation occurs quickly, a parasympathetic excess from systemic medications or the central nervous system nuclei should be suspected. If the pupil remains small, 4% cocaine may be instilled. The cocaine acts as a sympathetic nervous system transmitter; dilation of the pupil would indicate dysfunction of the peripheral sympathetic system. The small pupil that responds to neither homatropine or cocaine should be considered to have a peripheral sympathetic block such as a pupillary constricting drop that was placed in the eye.

Bilateral midposition pupils that are poorly reactive to either light or dark stimuli in an otherwise awake patient should be considered a normal variant.

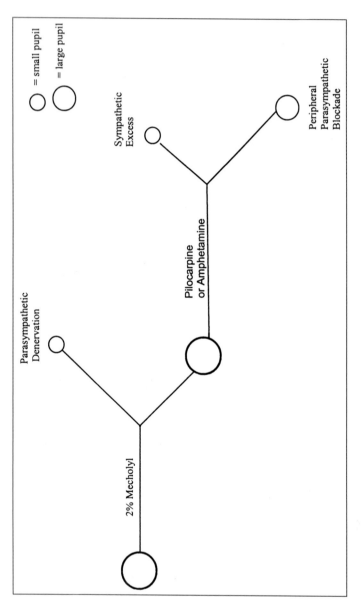

FIGURE 8-3   Evaluation of the large pupil.

TABLE 8-5 —————————————————————————————
CAUSES OF MIOSIS (SMALL PUPIL)

Monocular
1. Topical drugs; peripheral sympathetic blockade (see Table 8-3)
2. Interruption of sympathetic fibers; central sympathetic failure, i.e., lateral medullary syndrome, ciliary migraine (cluster), pontine hemorrhage, disease of the lung (Pancost's tumor), trauma, carotid aneurysm, cavernous sinus fissure, cavernous sinus thrombosis
3. Parasympathetic irritation; purulent meningitis, arachnoiditis, compression of third nerve (very early phase)
4. Syphilis (unilateral Argyll Robertson pupil)
5. Constriction phase of Adie's pupil
6. Histamine cephalgia (cluster headache)
7. Anisocoria
8. Acute or chronic iritis

Binocular
1. Central or topical effects of drugs (see Table 8-3)
2. Pontine hemorrhage
3. Pineal tumor
4. The apneic stage of Cheyne-Stokes respirations
5. Syphilis (bilateral Argyll Robertson pupil)

Adie's Pupil (Myotonic or Tonic Pupil)

Adie's pupil is a syndrome that may be either bilateral or unilateral. In this condition, the pupil is usually dilated, sometimes oval, and apparently fixed to both light and convergence. On other occasions, it may be small and apparently unreactive to light.

Careful testing reveals that patients with this syndrome have a delayed or slow pupillary constriction and dilation phase. Adie's pupil is usually considered to be part of a wider dysautonomia including abnormalities with sweating and orthostatic hypotension. The patients may also manifest decreased reflexes, insensitivity to pain, and generalized slowness in all reactions.[6,10] A patient with the findings of Adie's pupil and no other visual or neurologic complaint should be considered to have a normal variant.

In the evaluation of pupillary size and reactivity, some general rules should be followed. The pupils become smaller at the age extremes of life. The very young and the very old tend to have smaller and less reactive pupils. Pupils generally become smaller when individuals are looking at near objects and dilate when they are looking at far objects, the so-called divergence-convergence response. Large refraction errors of vision may also influence pupil size. Patients with myopia have slightly larger pupils than do patients with hypermetropia.[6]

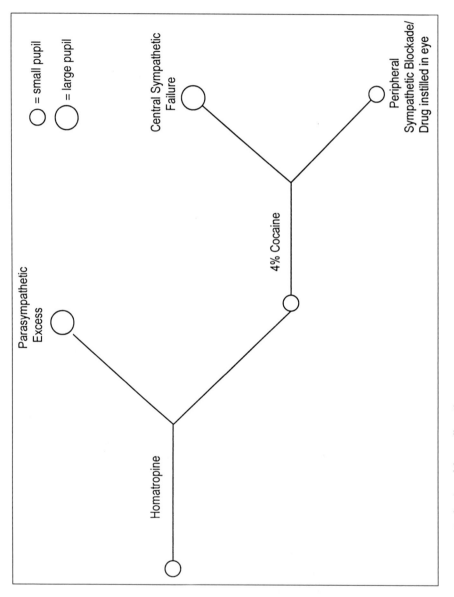

FIGURE 8-4   Evaluation of the small pupil.

ACUTE VISUAL FIELD DEFECTS

The anatomy of the visual system is such that the optic nerves from each eye quickly join at the optic chiasm (Figure 8-5).[7,11] From here the fibers recombine so that the right half of each eye (i.e., the temporal fibers of the right eye and the nasal fibers of the left eye) combine and then again divide into superior fibers passing through the parietal lobe and inferior fibers passing through the temporal lobe to arrive in the occipital cortex[2,12] (Figure 8-6).

Monocular Visual Loss

Monocular losses of vision must be located anterior to the optic chiasm before the fibers have recombined (see section on Visual Loss and Figure 8-7) or in the eye itself (Figures 8-5 and 8-6).

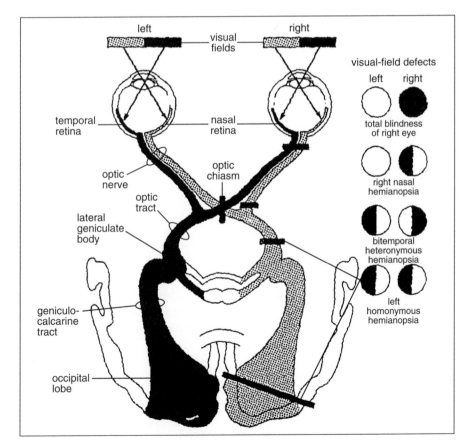

FIGURE 8-5 Lesions in the optic pathways. (From Henry, G: Seeing double or nothing, *Emerg Mag*, Jan 15, 1984, with permission.)

INTERPRETATION OF FIELD DEFECTS		
Defect	Pattern	Possible Diagnosis
1. Monocular Blindness	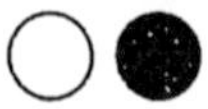	Primary eye disease Optic neuritis Optic neuropathy Retinal arteritis Toxins, trauma
2. Bitemporal, Hemianopsia	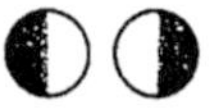	Aneurysm-anterior circulation Tumors-pituitary-meningioma Pituitary infarct or apoplexy Third ventricular cysts, arachoiditis
3. Homonymous Hemianopsia	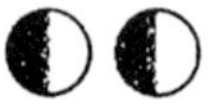	Vascular disease involving parieto-temporal lobe or occipital lobe, large hemispheric mass Trauma, demyelinating disease
4. Homonymous Quadrantanopsia	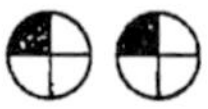	Occipital lobe vascular lesion, temporal lobe vascular lesion, tumor, parietal lobe lesion
5. Altitudinal Defect	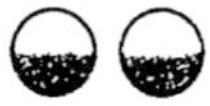	Occipital lobe trauma, inflammatory or destructive process. Both hemispheres above or below calcarine fissure
6. Sparing Central Vision	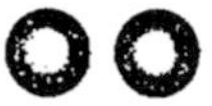	Toxic – metabolic bilateral neuritis, occipital lobe lesions
7. Sparing Peripheral Vision	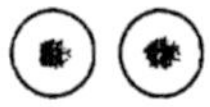	Toxic – metabolic

FIGURE 8-6   Interpretation of field defects.

Bitemporal Hemianopsia

Bitemporal hemianopsia (losing vision in both lateral eye fields), an extremely rare condition, indicates that the medial fibers from each optic nerve are involved[14] (Figures 8-5 and 8-6). The only place that such a lesion can sit is at the optic chiasm. Pituitary lesions, both hemorrhage and tumors, represent the most common causes of bitemporal hemianopsia.[13]

Homonymous Hemianopsia

Homonymous hemianopsia involves the loss of vision in either the right or left visual field in each eye (Figures 8-5 and 8-6).

True, full homonymous hemianopsia must involve the optic tract shortly after leaving the optic chiasm or must include an extremely large lesion affecting both sets of fibers both superiorly and inferiorly passing through the temporal and pari-

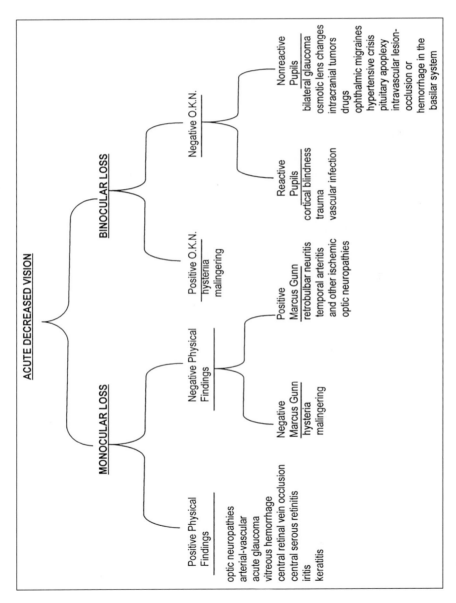

FIGURE 8-7   Acute decreased vision. O.K.N., optokinetic nystagmus.

etal lobes or involve both superior and inferior areas of the occipital cortex. Partial hemianopsia is much more common than full hemianopsia.

Quadrantanopsia

More common than full homonymous hemianopsias are homonymous quadrantanopsias (Figures 8-5 and 8-6). These are the result of involvement by either superior or inferior visual fibers. Minor quadrantanopsias are usually detected as part of the complete neurologic examination in a patient showing other evidence for a cerebral vascular cortical lesion. Frequently the patient is unaware of a quadrantanopsia.

Altitudinal Defects

Altitudinal defects are those that involve the upper or lower half of both visual fields (Figures 8-5 and 8-6). Lesions producing this type of defect most commonly involve the occipital lobes above or below the calcarine fissure bilaterally.[12]

Central Visual Sparing

Preservation of central vision with marked reduction in peripheral vision has usually been associated with quinidine-type drugs or bilateral optic neuritis. Testing needs to be done carefully so as not to mistake this finding for a psychiatric problem (Figure 8-6).

Peripheral Sparing

Certain visual field defects are more likely to be on a metabolic or toxic structural basis. Central visual loss with sparing of peripheral vision may, in rare instances, be caused by lesions in the calcarine cortex (Figure 8-6). Such defects are usually, however, the result of toxins such as methanol.

ACUTE VISUAL DETERIORATION OR LOSS

The etiologies of acute visual loss can in general be divided between entities causing monocular blindness and those causing binocular blindness (Figure 8-7).

It should be pointed out that certain disease entities such as temporal arteritis and retrobulbar neuritis may be present as either unilateral or bilateral processes (Figure 8-7).[2,15]

Monocular Visual Loss

Patients with monocular visual loss basically can be divided into those who have obvious physical findings, i.e., retinal detachments, central retinal artery occlusions, and so on, and those who do not.

Optic Neuropathy

Optic neuropathic processes affect the visual system. Papillitis causes swelling and edema of the nerve head that can be easily mistaken for papilledema[16-18] (Table 8-6.) Unlike patients with papilledema, patients with papillitis generally have a marked decrease in vision without other indications of increased intracranial pressure. Papillitis is also usually a monocular process, whereas papilledema, except in rare instances, is bilateral.[2,16]

Papilledema refers to edema of the optic nerve head from various causes. The current theory about the underlying mechanism of all forms of papilledema relates to axoplasmic transport, or the flow of cytoplasmic material along the nerves themselves, resulting in swelling of the axon. From a practical consideration, papilledema should be thought of as being from one of four causes: (1) increased intracranial pressure, (2) intraorbital disease, (3) intraocular disease, and (4) systemic disease affecting the eyes. Table 8-7 details the multiple causes of papilledema. Except for increased intracranial pressure, all other forms are rare.

Besides papillitis, or inflammation of the optic nerve head, other entities may cause blurring of the optic disk margins, which may be interpreted as papilledema. Table 8-8 details disease entities that may be mistaken for either papilledema or papillitis on general physical examination.[17,18]

Ischemic Optic Neuropathy

Acute ischemic optic neuropathies associated with temporal arteritis, anemia, polycythemia, and carotid artery stenosis are listed in Figure 8-7.[19] The ischemic optic neuropathies should show pale fundi, but the findings may be so subtle as to be nonexistent. Objective evidence of the fact that there is decreased vision in the eye

TABLE 8-6

DIFFERENTIAL DIAGNOSIS OF BLURRED OPTIC DISKS

Finding	Papilledema	Papillitis	Pseudopapilledema
Pupils	Normal	If unilateral + Marcus Gunn	Normal
Vision	Without change	Reduced—variable amount	Normal
Fields	Enlarged blind spot	Central decrease or scotoma	Normal
Other	Hemmorhage occasionally around disk	Frequent hemorrhage	No hemorrhage
Focally	Usually bilateral	Frequently unilateral	Variable

TABLE 8-7
CAUSES OF PAPILLEDEMA

1. Intrancranial
   a. Masses
      (1) Epidural, subdural, intracranial, hemorrhage
      (2) Brain tumor, brain abscess, hydrocephalus
   b. Intracranial hypertension
      (1) Intracranial thrombosis (sinus thromboses)
      (2) Drugs: vitamin A, tetracycline, nalidixic acid
      (3) Pseudotumor cerebri
   c. Hydrocephalus
   d. Meningitis
   e. Arachnoiditis
   f. Cranial suture stenosis
2. Orbital disease
   a. Tumors of the optic nerve
   b. Retroorbital tumor
   c. Thyroid ophthalmopathy
3. Ocular disease
   a. Acute glaucoma
   b. Trauma
   c. Surgery
   d. Uveitis
4. Systemic disease
   a. Malignant hypertension
   b. Anemia
   c. Hypovolemia
   d. Anoxia
   e. Guillain-Barré syndrome
   f. Sarcoidosis
   g. Various poisons

affected, however, is established by the positive Margus Gunn pupil sign and decreased visual acuity. Such patients should receive consultation with an ophthalmologist on an urgent basis.

Arterial Vascular Causes

Arterial vascular lesions, both occlusion and hemorrhage, affect the ophthalmic artery in the same manner as they do all arteries of the internal carotid system. Emboli may occlude the ophthalmic artery from (1) primary cardiac causes such as endocarditis or arrhythmias, (2) carotid artery disease,[20] (3) aortic aneurysms, and (4) arterial thrombus. A sudden loss of vision as a result of an arterial vascular acci-

TABLE 8-8 ————————————————————

CAUSES OF PSEUDOPAPILLEDEMA

More Common
Myelinated nerve fiber
Gliosis
Hyperopia
Hyaline bodies (drusen)

Rare
Occular crescents
Neoplasm of disk
Colomboma

Retroorbital Fibroplasia

dent is virtually always monocular, and the site of the occlusion and areas of decreased arterial flow generally follow the vascular anatomy.[19–21]

Occlusive diseases on an embolic basis tend to involve more than peripheral retinal arteries, causing branch occlusions of the retinal artery. The onset is acute, and usually some vision is preserved. The retina may take on a diffuse cloudiness and paleness in the area of the branch artery that has been occluded.

Central retinal artery occlusion, on the other hand, is generally the result of a thrombosis of the central retinal artery. This usually occurs in elderly patients and may be preceded by amaurosis fugax. It is generally sudden in onset with a complete or nearly complete monocular visual loss. The retina quickly takes on a diffuse paleness while retaining a red center, which is the "cherry red" portion of the macula. After only a few days of occlusion, pronounced optic atrophy will be visible.

Treatment for acute retinal artery occlusions has basically been ineffective.[6] It is believed that treatment delayed beyond 6 hours reduces the likelihood that any meaningful vision will be returned to areas involved. Emergency management of the patient with a branch or central retinal artery occlusion is essentially anecdotal. There are no controlled studies that have tested various hypotheses in the management of such occlusions. In recent years, retrobulbar injection of 2% xylocaine and 200 mg acetylcholine has been tried with limited success. Low-molecular-weight dextran infusions, manual intermittent compression-decompression of the eyeball, and the use of Diamox, carbon dioxide, and steroids have all been advocated but never proved in any series. At this juncture no clear preference for one method or the other can be shown.[6]

Acute Glaucoma

Both narrow- and open-angle glaucoma can result in rapid decrease in vision. Immediate changes in intraocular pressure, however, generally cause pain as well as irritation, with pronounced conjunctival injection. Acute narrow-angle glaucoma is almost always associated with a clouding of the cornea and anterior chamber and relative midposition fixation of the pupil. The sudden onset of decreased vision, eye and head pain, and nausea and vomiting should prompt investigation for glaucoma.

Vitreous Hemorrhage

Hemorrhage into the vitreous body should be readily diagnosable by funduscopic examination. Acute systemic diseases that effect bleeding, as well as intracranial and intraocular problems, can cause vitreous hemorrhage.[22,6] Table 8-9 lists the multiple causes of vitreous hemorrhage.

Central Retinal Vein Occlusion

Multiple underlying disease entities can progress to cause central retinal vein occlusion.[12] This presents a dramatic funduscopic appearance, with multiple areas of hemorrhage and engorgement of the veins of the retina.[23] No specific treatment is available except that of managing the underlying disease[24] (Table 8-10).

Space-Occupying Intracranial Disorders

An intracranial mass lesion lying anterior to the optic chiasm, such as a meningioma or malignant tumor, and causing enough pressure to decrease vision generally has positive neurologic findings. Such disease entities occupying the superior orbital fissure and sphenoid ridge may involve the cranial nerves that pass into the orbit along with the optic nerve. Pressure sufficient to decrease vision usually results in papilledema.[25]

Retinal Detachment

Retinal detachment may present as either a gradual or a sudden deterioration of vision. The disease process involved is actually a separation of the two layers of the retina. The pigmented layer remains attached to the fibrous underlying choroid, and the sensory retina separates and falls away. The amount of vision lost is proportional

---

TABLE 8-9

CAUSES OF ACUTE VITREOUS HEMORRHAGE

1. Clotting disorders
2. Arterial hypertension
3. Venous hypertension
4. Vasculitis
5. Atriovenous malformation
6. Trauma
7. Retinal detachment
8. Neovascularization; bleeding
9. Choroid degeneration
10. Postoperative intraocular surgery
11. Tumor mass of the eyeball

TABLE 8-10 ——————————————————————————————
CAUSES OF CENTRAL RETINAL VEIN OCCLUSION

Diabetes mellitus
Polycythemia
Multiple myeloma
Hyperglobulinemias
Sickle cell disease
Infections
Tuberculosis
Sarcoidosis
Continuous inflammation
Trauma

to the areas of detachment involved. The more central the detachment, the more involvement of macular fibers and the greater the decrease in vision.[2,23] Severe trauma has been associated with both acute and delayed retinal deachments. Patients usually complain of decreased vision over minutes to hours; blurred vision, flashes of light, or hazy clouds are often described. In older patients, so-called secondary retinal detachment may be due not to a primary ocular process but to a metastatic tumor of the choroid layer. Acute retinal detachment is a medical emergency requiring timely involvement of ophthalmology.

Iritis

Iritis may be a unilateral or bilateral disease. Trauma, infectious disease (i.e., sarcoidosis), collagen vascular disease, degenerative processes, and idiopathic ocular disease may all lead to iritis.[6] A typical history includes a deep ocular pain with tearing but no discharge. Unlike conjunctivitis, the pain is not relieved with topical anesthetics. The typical physical findings include perilimbal injection of the iris and the classic finding of cells in the anterior chamber of the eye on slit lamp examination. After the process has become established, proteinaceous material is also seen in the anterior chamber and is referred to as a flair reaction when seen on slit lamp examination. Medical management will depend on the underlying disease entity.

Keratitis

Keratitis, inflammation of the corneal stroma itself, may also be unilateral or bilateral. It may be the result of trauma or an infectious process, but it involves irritation and infiltration of a cloudy proteinaceous material into the layers of the cornea.[2] The differential diagnosis of keratitis is extensive, and an ophthalmologic consultation should be sought before starting therapy.

Retrobulbar Neuritis

In patients with monocular visual loss who do not have an obvious physical finding, a positive Marcus Gunn pupillary reaction is a strong indication that the patient's visual acuity is decreased, from either ischemic optic neuropathy with extremely subtle findings or retrobulbar neuritis. Retrobulbar neuritis is classically considered the disease in which the patient sees nothing and the doctor sees nothing on physical examination of the eye. Such visual loss may come on over hours to days and is usually painless. A young person with monocular visual loss and without ocular findings should be considered to have retrobulbar neuritis. Retrobulbar neuritis may be considered a manifestation of multiple sclerosis.[2,6] Some 70% of young patients with retrobulbar neuritis will carry the diagnosis of multiple sclerosis within 2 years. Steroids have been the mainstay of therapy but should be started in conjunction with either neurology or ophthalmology consultation.

Chorioretinitis

Acute inflammation of the choroid or retinal layers in the region of the macula may cause sudden decrease in vision over a few days. Autoimmune disease, toxoplasmosis, histoplasmosis, bacterial and viral infections, AIDS, and idiopathic inflammation have all been suspected in this disease process. In the majority of cases, no underlying disease etiology is ever found.[6]

The principal symptoms are decreased vision and a feeling of heaviness or fullness in the eye. On slit lamp examination, the anterior chamber of the eye may not show any sign of inflammation. Ophthalmoscopic examination may reveal a cloudy vitreous that may be elevated and may occasionally have small hemorrhages. Treatment of chorioretinitis can be a medical emergency. Specific therapy should be aimed at any underlying disease entities discovered, but the majority of cases are idiopathic.

Psychiatric Causes

Patients who complain of a significant monocular visual loss but who have no positive physical findings and a negative Marcus Gunn pupil test generally have a psychiatric base for their complaint.[6] The differential diagnosis between the hysterical patient and the malingering patient will be based principally on the occupational and social milieu of the patient and the potential secondary gains involved (see Chap. 10).

Binocular Visual Loss

The patient complaining of severely decreased vision or blindness bilaterally may represent a serious medical emergency (Figure 8-7). A patient who lacks OKN is likely to have an organic lesion. Patients complaining of binocular blindness or severe visual loss who maintain normal OKN have a high probability of hysteria or malingering.[5,6]

Pupillary responses become important in determining the location of the lesion. Patients without OKN who maintain normal pupillary light reflexes should be considered to have a cortical type of blindness. Trauma to the occipital lobes and vascular hemorrhage or insufficiency involving the posterior cerebral arteries are the most common causes of cortical blindness.[6,7] Ophthalmic migraine with binocular visual loss should also be considered in this group. Focal infections involving the occipital regions have been (rarely) reported to cause a similar type of cortical blindness.[6] Patients with binocular visual loss, lack of OKN, and decreased pupillary reaction to light stimulus must have as the basis of their disease a process that involves both visual pathways anterior to the optic chiasm or a diffuse metabolic or vascular process.

Bilateral keratitis, iritis, and papapillitis, as well as intraocular bleeding, should all be readily diagnosable by standard ocular examination. Pituitary apoplexy can certainly result in bilateral blindness.[13] Pituitary apoplexy is a catastrophic medical condition caused by hemorrhage into the pituitary gland. This may be on a vascular basis or hemorrhage into a preexisting tumor. Pituitary apoplexy usually causes alterations in consciousness, and other neurologic findings will usually take precedence over the visual loss in determining the diagnostic workup.[7]

Retrobulbar neuritis and the ischemic optic neuropathies may present as bilateral disease, particularly when these entities have only a dimming of vision as opposed to complete blindness. They may represent a complex differential diagnosis. Age of the patient and sedimentation rate may both be helpful in differentiating retrobulbar neuritis from temporal arteritis. Temporal arteritis is suggested in elderly patients with visual loss and elevated sedimentation rates. Retrobulbar neuritis, however, may be essentially indistinguishable from pharmacologic and toxicologic causes of decreased vision.[6]

Acute changes in the lenses may also cause rapid decrease in vision, although not blindness. Diabetics whose blood sugar is significantly elevated may, on an osmotic basis, cause marked shifts in the configuration of the lens, resulting in altered visual acuity. Patients with a bilateral decrease in vision and without obvious physical findings should have a blood glucose obtained along with a sedimentation rate.

The patient with hypertensive encephalopathy may present with decreased vision. These patients generally have other manifestations of their hypertensive problem.[7] Decreased vision should be considered a positive sign of severe involvement of the cerebral vessels and may require a reduction in blood pressure.

Certain drugs and chemicals have long been recognized as toxins to the visual system (Table 8-11). Lead found in improperly distilled alcohols as well as methanol can seriously affect visual acuity, with minimal findings on funduscopic examination. What is not as well understood is alcohol and tobacco amblyopia. Ethyl alcohol in large doses and large quantities of nicotine in patients unaccustomed to their use have been reported to cause severe decreased vision to the point of total blindness.[6] Alcohol-tobacco amblyopia is usually short lived and may completely reverse itself in a matter of hours to days. In preadolescents and adolescents presenting with acute visual decrease, a history of tobacco and alcohol use should be discretely obtained.

ACUTE DOUBLE VISION

The complaint of seeing double can be a confusing symptom because the patient may describe decreased or blurred vision as double vision. Careful history from the patients about exactly what they are indicating is necessary for proper evalua-

TABLE 8-11

COMMON DRUGS AND CHEMICALS AFFECTING VISION

Ethyl alcohol
Methyl alcohol
Quinine and quinidine
Digitalis
Iodoform
Methyl chloride
Methyl bromide
Chloramphenicol
Sulfanilamides
Ergot medications
Salicylates
Ethambutol
Isoniazid
Nicotine

tion. Once it has been determined that the patient is actually seeing split or multiple images, the next step is to separate out monocular from binocular problems (Figure 8-8).

Monocular Diplopia

Patients with abnormalities of their visual axis including the cornea, lens, and retina may get split images that they interpret as double vision.[16,26] Testing with the pen light will appear to these patients as two spots or beams of light in the affected eye. All causes of monocular diplopia lie relatively far forward in the visual system, are rare, and may be diagnosable by careful ophthalmologic examination. Patients complaining of monocular diplopia who have a completely normal ophthalmologic and neurologic examination should be considered to have an underlying psychiatric problem. The ocular lesions that may produce monocular diplopia are varied. With the advent of an inplantable intraocular lens, patients may present who have had dislocations or other problems related to these devices. A dislocated or angulated intraocular lens can cause a split image on the retina. Excimer laser surgery has also been associated with monocular diplopia.[27]

Subluxation of the lens may also cause abnormal light images. Severe trauma has been reported to dislocate the lens. Patients with collagen vascular diseases such as Marfan's syndrome and homocystinuria develop weak supporting structures for the lens, allowing it to dislocate with little or no trauma.

Maturing cataracts may also form irregular opacities that will split the light image and give the impression of double vision. Note also that a mass behind the retina, although theoretically diagnosable by standard ophthalmologic evaluation, may in its

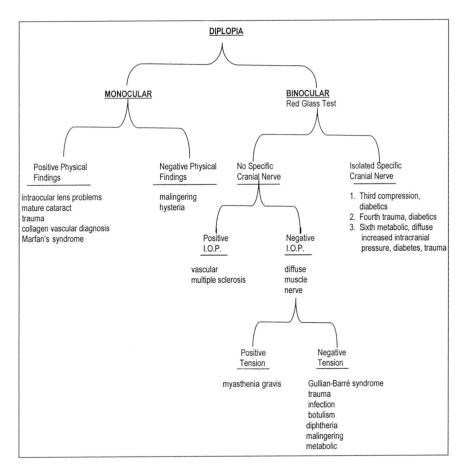

FIGURE 8-8   Evaluation of diplopia. I.O.P., internuclear ophthalmoplegia.

early phases cause mild monocular diplopia by deforming the retina. Such patients should be carefully followed and reevaluated if a retroretinal mass is suspected.

Binocular Diplopia

Binocular diplopia is readily separated from monocular diplopia with a simple cover-uncover test. If the patient sees only one image with each eye independently but has a double image when the eyes are used concomitantly, the patient has a binocular diplopia secondary to abnormalities of alignment of the eyes in various areas of gaze.[7]

The location of the abnormality with limitation of conjugate gaze on command should be thought of in terms of four sites: (1) supranuclear, above the parapontine gaze centers and midbrain; (2) pontine gaze centers; (3) internuclear lesions involving the medial longitudinal fasiculus (MLF); and (4) infranuclear, from the nuclei of the third, fourth, and sixth nerves outward[2,6] (Tables 8-12 and 8-13).

TABLE 8-12 ———————————————————————
CAUSES OF BINOCULAR DIPLOPIA

1. Orbital trauma: muscle entrapment or hematoma
2. Third (III) nerve palsy
3. Fourth (IV) nerve palsy
4. Sixth (VI) nerve palsy
5. Multiple mixed neuritis—vasculitis, mononeuritis, multiple neuritis, infection (herpes)
6. Myasthenia gravis
7. Tolosa-Hunt syndrome
8. Multiple sclerosis
9. Decompensation of existing phoria or tropia (existing disconjugate gaze)
10. Vascular occlusion—brainstem
11. Wernicke's syndrome
12. Viral Guillain-Barré syndrome
13. Bulbar palsy
14. Diphtheria
15. Botulism
16. Tuberculosis
17. Syphilis

Supranuclear Causes

Supranuclear causes of gaze palsies (inability to move the eyes conjugately) are due to lesions in central nervous system structures above the brainstem that send signals through to the eyes, Such lesions can be anywhere from prefrontal lesions to the motor tracts as they descend through the central core of the brain to the brainstem.[6] These patients maintain conjugate gaze on primary position when looking forward owing to brainstem reflexes. They are not able to move their eyes on command.[7] Because the eyes remain conjugate, the patient relates no diplopia in primary gaze, and on gross inspection, no dysconjugate gaze (strabismus) is noted in primary position. Because vestibular nuclei and brainstem centers are all intact, the patient will have normal deviation of the eyes on cold caloric testing. The patient may, however, have problems in the correction phase because of an inability to send information from the cortex. These are extremely rare conditions.

Pontine Gaze Center

Lesions of the pontine gaze center are usually on a vascular basis. In primary position, no disconjugate gaze is noted, and the patient does not complain of diplopia. With voluntary movement of the eyes, the diplopia is elicited. On cold caloric testing, the patient is unable to generate normal conjugate eye movements because the normal flow of information reaching the gaze centers is interrupted.

TABLE 8-13 — COMPARISON OF GAZE PALSY FINDINGS AND LOCATIONS

	Strabismus	Diplopia	Nystagmus	Caloric Response	Examples
Supranuclear	None	None	None	Normal deviation; defective; first phalange	Parietal-frontal tumor; hemorrhage; degenerative disease
Pontine gaze center	None	None	None	Paralysis of conjugate eye movement	Infarct in pons
Medial longitudinal fasciculus (internuclear)	On conjugate gaze	Yes	In abducting (good) eye	Adductor weakness	Multiple sclerosis; brainstem infarct; involving medial longitudinal fasiculus
Infranuclear peripheral lesions	Yes	Yes	None	Defect in pull of involved nerve or muscles	Myasthenia gravis; III, IV, VI nerve injuries

Internuclear Lesions

Normal control of eye movements is through the MLF in the center of the brainstem. Cortical input passes to the gaze centers, which then send signals to the appropriate sixth nerve nucleus and to the opposite third nerve nucleus through the MLF. Internuclear gaze palsies are the result of either multiple sclerosis or brainstem vascular lesions involving the MLF.[7,28] Such lesions are referred to as internuclear ophthalmoplegias (IOPs). Relatively minor trauma and the smoking of crack cocaine have also been associated with transient IOP.[28,29] The patient is able to send information to the pontine gaze center and is usually able to abduct the ipsilateral eye. The patient is, however, unable to adduct the contralateral eye, since it requires information being sent from the sixth nucleus to the third nerve nucleus through the MLF. This produces nystagmus in the abducting eye.

Infranuclear Lesions

Infranuclear lesions are those involving nerves III, IV, or VI, or the muscles of eye movement that they control. Weakness in either the muscle or a specific nerve lesion can cause strabismus even in primary gaze, and the patient will complain of diplopia. Myasthenia gravis, botulism trauma, and the various diseases that affect the third, fourth, and sixth cranial nerves are examples of infranuclear lesions[7] (see specific nerve lesions).

Paralysis of Upward Gaze

A rarely seen entity is paralysis of upward gaze, or Parinaud's syndrome. The lesion in Parinaud's syndrome is generally a mass in the region of the pretectal nucleus, thus preventing conjugate upward gaze.[6] This may, on rare occasions, be seen with shunt malfunctions.

Evaluation of Diplopia

Red glass testing can be performed in patients with diplopia in whom no specific abnormality is readily seen.

Isolated Cranial Nerves

Cranial Nerve III

The muscles intervated by the third nerve move the eye primarily upward and inward. Third cranial nerve lesions present with the involved eye looking laterally and slightly downward.[30] Ptosis may or may not be present depending on the location of the lesion along the nerve. The patient is unable to elevate the involved eye or pull it medially. There is a type of a third cranial nerve lesion that involves only selected motor fibers.[6,7] This is referred to as a pupil sparing or partial third nerve palsy. A complete third cranial nerve lesion involves motor fibers and the fibers of pupillary constriction. Complete third nerve palsies involving motor and pupillary fibers with a dilation of the pupil that is nonreactive to light should initially be considered to be on a compressive basis (Table 8-14). In the trauma patient in coma, a complete third nerve palsy is usually the result of compression of the third cranial nerve by herniation of the uncus of the temporal lobe. A sudden onset of a complete third cranial nerve lesions in nontraumatic patients should be considered to be the result of compression of the third cranial nerve by an aneurysm of the posterior communicating artery. Sudden onset of a complete third nerve palsy, as a result of supratentorial herniation or compression by an aneurysm, represents an emergency. The physician should pay close attention to the patient with an acute headache and complete third nerve palsy. A diagnosis of expanding aneurysm should be entertained until proven otherwise. Incomplete third nerve palsies are those that have motor fibers involved but spare the pupil.[1] Pupil-sparing third nerve palsies are almost always related to the vascular complications of diabetes mellitus with infarction of the nerve. Pupillary sparing is the result of the pupillary fibers having more collateral blood supply than do the motor fibers, so that with lesions of the vasoneurvorum, the pupillary fibers are less susceptible to small vascular lesions. Patients who are diabetic and have a new onset of pupil-sparing third nerve palsy can usually be sent home and managed on an outpatient basis if other medical problems are under control.

Cranial Nerve IV

Acute fourth nerve palsies are rare.[6,31,32] They may be seen with trauma to the nerve itself or to the trochlea (tendon pivot point) of the muscle or vascular involvement of the nerve from diabetic complications. In very rare cases, hypertension, multiple sclerosis, sickle cell anemia, and systemic lupus have been reported to cause isolated fourth nerve palsies. Fourth nerve palsies may be difficult to recognize if the patient's only complaint is double vision when looking down for reading or walking down stairs. Patients are seen to have their head tilted, with the chin toward the affected side and the ear away from the affected side.

TABLE 8-14 ————————————————————————————

CAUSES OF UNILATERAL THIRD NERVE PALSY

1. Diabetes mellitus, usually incomplete, sparing pupil
2. Aneurysm
3. Other neuropathies
4. Cranial and orbital tumors
5. Migraine
6. Trauma
7. Infection: mononucleosis; syphilis
8. Carotid-cavernous fistula
9. AV malformation

Cranial Nerve VI

The sixth nerve has the longest intracranial course of any of the cranial nerves. Because of its course and position, generalized swelling inside the cranial vault can cause stretching of the nerve, resulting in a sixth nerve palsy.[6,31,32] Trauma may affect the nerve directly as it passes through the foramen of the skull. The nerve can be affected indirectly through increased intracranial pressure either focally, such as subdural or epidural pressure, or diffusely, with generalized brain swelling. Like the third and fourth cranial nerves, the sixth cranial nerve is also susceptible to vascular insult from complications of diabetes mellitus.

An acute lack of thiamine in the brainstem affects the sixth cranial nerves preferentially.[4,5] The first sign of an impending Wernicke's syndrome in a nutritionally deficient patient, such as a chronic alcoholic, may be the presence of a sixth nerve palsy.[31,32] Multiple cranial nerves may subsequently be involved, but the sixth cranial nerve is most commonly affected (Table 8-15).

INTERNUCLEAR OPHTHALMOPLEGIA

For diplopias that do not show a specific cranial nerve pattern, the presence of an IOP may be suspected. An IOP is a lesion of the MLF, which connects the various cranial nerve nuclei in the brainstem that control eye movement. Lesions in this area have a characteristic pattern: (1) inability to adduct the ipsilateral eye on the side of the lesion on contralateral horizontal gaze, (2) normal adduction of the involved eye on convergence testing, and (3) nystagmus in the abducting eye.[6,7]

The reason for the findings in an IOP is relatively simple if the anatomy of the visual system is considered. When given a command to look laterally, the eye is moved by its ipsilateral sixth nerve nucleus. To move the opposite eye medially at the same time requires that the signal be sent through the brainstem through the MLF to the opposite third nerve nucleus.[8] A lesion involving MLF fibers will there-

TABLE 8-15 ——————————————————————————
CAUSES OF UNILATERAL SIXTH NERVE PALSY

1. Increased intracranial pressure: trauma, tumor, infection (meningitis)
2. Arteriosclerosis; hypertension
3. Diabetes mellitus
4. Multiple sclerosis
5. Myasthenia gravis, early
6. Gradenigo's syndrome
7. Syphilis
8. Wernicke's syndrome
9. Postlumbar puncture
10. AV malformation

fore not allow adduction of the eye on the side of involvement on contralateral gaze. With convergence, however, the involved eye will adduct because signals for the convergence reflex come up not from the MLF but from a separate center believed to be part of the nucleus of Perlia. Nystagmus in the abducting eye is the result of the brain getting two images and the brainstem moving to align the eyes. The cortex then sends signals to return the abducting eye in its originally ordered direction.

Whenever an IOP is seen, the differential diagnosis is brief. Vascular lesions of the midbrain, including microhemorrhages or infarcts involving the MLF, may produce an IOP. Severe hypertensive crisis with vascular compromise may also produce such lesions.[7] In rare instances a tumor intrinsic to the midbrain may produce an IOP, but it is extremely rare for this to be the only positive neurologic finding. The most common cause of an IOP is multiple sclerosis.[6] In general, young adults with IOPs and without other neurologic findings are manifesting multiple sclerosis. In older adults, an IOP generally indicates vascular disease or a tumor of the brainstem. Other rare but potentially reversible causes of IOP include minor trauma, Wernicke's syndrome, cocaine use, and systemic lupus.[28,31–35]

INFRANUCLEAR DIPLOPIA WITHOUT CRANIAL NERVE INVOLVEMENT

Binocular diplopia without a specific cranial nerve involvement or without evidence of an IOP may represent either involvement of multiple nerves or diffuse neuromuscular disorders.[8] A Tensilon® test can be given to separate out diplopias that are caused by myasthenia gravis. A patient who has a marked positive response to this medication is strongly suspected of having myasthenia gravis (see Tensilon test, Chap. 5).

Trauma

Facial trauma may result in blowout fractures of the infraorbital structures, causing entrapment of extraocular muscles. The most common muscle to be involved is the inferior rectus, and the patient has the greatest diplopia when looking up.[7] Patients with blowout fractures generally have a mild to moderate enophthalmos as orbital contents are pushed into the sinus below.

Trauma may also produce diplopia without blowout fracture by causing swelling of the retroorbital contents or a retroorbital hematoma. Unlike the blowout fracture patients, these patients tend to have a mild exophthalmus and diffuse limitation of motion and may have decreased vision. A patient with decreased vision and exophthalmus following trauma should be considered to have tension on the optic nerve and may need imaging of the orbital and retroorbital structures on an acute basis.

Infection

Retroorbital cellulitis and abscess may also cause diplopia.[6] Such patients generally have signs of infection and extreme pain on movement of the eyes. These patients are at high risk not only of involving the optic nerve but also of spreading the infection posteriorly to involve the cavernous sinus. Diabetics and other patients with compromised immune systems may present with indolent infections involving the cavernous sinus and sagittal sinus regions. Nonspecific diplopia and headache in a diabetic patient should trigger the thought of a fungal infection or some other type of orbital infection. Acute CT scanning of the orbital regions can generally delineate the issue and determine the need for surgery.

Diphtheria may present as an acute syndrome that includes diplopia. These patients generally are toxic with elevated temperature, tachycardia, and oral lesions specifically related to diphtheria.

Botulinum toxin has a predilection for the cranial nerves.[6] The first complaint of a patient with botulism may be diplopia. Although the sixth nerve is most frequently the first involved, by the time the patient presents to a physician, multiple cranial nerves and muscles may be affected, and isolated cranial nerve abnormalities may not be detectable. A specific picture may be difficult to ascertain. Such patients may rapidly go on to other abnormalities of the bulbar musculature and then finally to complete paralysis. The physician needs not only to treat any underlying medical problems but also be prepared to supply airway support.

Guillain-Barré syndrome may also involve the extraocular muscles. These patients generally have diffuse symptomatology and an ascending-type paralysis, but the syndrome may occasionally begin in the cervical and cranial nerve areas. Again, the patient may move rapidly to requiring airway support.

Metabolic Causes

Metabolic causes of nonspecific diplopia are rare. Although Wernicke's syndrome generally begins with the sixth cranial nerves, it may go on to involve multiple cranial nerve nuclei, thus giving a nonspecific diplopic pattern. Patients considered to be at risk for such nutritional deficiencies, i.e., chronic alcoholics, cancer patients, and the elderly, should be given thiamine.

Psychiatric Causes

The psychiatric patient who presents with diplopia may be extremely difficult to diagnose. The best method to use when this is suspected is to repeat the red glass test several times. It is rare that such an individual can remember exactly what patterns were described in previous examinations. Such patients can represent a difficult diagnostic and therapeutic problem (see Chap. 10).

SUMMARY

The vast majority of visual complaints are nonneurologic and relate to the eye itself. The visual system is complex and is intimately related to the nervous system. Separating out structural problems within the eye itself from neurologic disease requires a directed history and physical exam. The neuroanatomy of vision is, however, both precise and specific, and a precise neurologic diagnosis can be made from visual symptoms in the acute care setting.

REFERENCES

1. Simcock PR, et al. Neurological problems presenting to an ophthalmic casualty department. *Acta Ophthalmal (Copenh)* 1992;70.
2. Shingleton B, O'Donoghue M. Blurred vision. *N Engl J Med* 2000;343:556–562.
3. Achesan J, Sander M. *Common Problems in Neurophthalmology.* New York: WB Saunders, 1996.
4. Richardson LD, Joyce DM. Diplopia in the emergency department. *Emerg Med Clin North Am* 1997;15:649–664.
5. Haerer A. *Dejong's The Neurologic Examination,* 5th ed. New York: Lippincott-Raven, 1992.
6. Miller N, Newman N, eds. *The Essentials: Walsh and Hoyt's Clinical Neuroophthalmology.* Philadelphia: Waverly, 1998.
7. Bender M, Rudolph S, Stacy. The neurology of the visual and oculomotor systems. In: Joynt R, Griggs R, eds. *Baker's Clinical Neurology.* Philadelphia: Lippincott Williams & Wilkins, 1998.
8. Cogan D. *Neurology of the Ocular Muscles.* Springfield, IL: Thomas, 1956.
9. Jacobon DM. Pupillary responses to dilute pilocarpine in preganglionic third nerve disorders. *Neurology* 1990;40:804–808.
10. Adie WJ. Complete and incomplete forms of the benign disorder characterized by tonic pupils and absent tendon reflexes. *Br J Ophthalmol* 1932;16:447.
11. Bender M, ed. *The Approach to Diagnosis in Modern Neurology.* New York: Grune & Stratton, 1967.
12. McFadzean R, et al. Representation of the visual field in the occupital striate cortex. *Br J Ophthalmol* 1994;78:185–190.
13. Acheson J. Optic nerve and chiasmal disease. *J Neurol* 2000;247:587–596.
14. Horton JC, Hoyt WF. Quadrantic visual field defects: a hallmark of lesions in the extrastriate (V_2/V_3) cortex. *Brain* 1991;114:1703–1718.
15. Dobbin KR, Saul RF. Transient visual loss after licorice ingestion, *J Neuroophthalmol* 2000;20:38–41.
16. Granandier RJ. Ophthalmology update for primary care practitioner, part I, Update in optic neuritis. *Dis Mon* 2000;46:508–532.
17. Hoyt WF, Pant ME. Pseudopapilledema: anomalous elevation of the optic disk: pitfalls in diagnosis and management. *JAMA* 1962;181:191.
18. Rosenberg MA, et al. A clinical analysis of pseudopapilledderma. *Arch Ophthalmol* 1979;97:65.
19. Benavente O, et al. Prognosis after transient monocular blindness associated with carotid-artery stenosis. *N Engl J Med* 2001;345:1084–1090.
20. Lanske RK. Central retinal artery occlusion. *Am J Ophthalmol* 1965;60:716.
21. Haidenbergh FE. Occlusion of the central retinal artery. *Arch Ophthalmol* 1962;67:556.
22. Bense WE, Spalter HF. Vitreous hemorrhage. *Surv Ophthalmol* 1971;15:297.
23. Jones WL. *Atlas of the Peripheral Occular Fundus,* 2nd ed. New York: Butterworth-Heinemann, 1998.
24. Loong SC. The eye in neurology: evaluation of sudden visual loss and diplopia—diagnostic pointers and pitfalls. *Ann Acad Med Singapore* 2001;30:143–147.

25. Volpe NJ, Gaysas RE. Optic nerve and orbital tumors. *Neurosurg Clin North Am* 1999;10:699–715.

26. Campbell C. Corneal aberrations, monocular diplopia, and ghost images: analysis using corneal topographical data. *Optom Vis Sci* 1998;75:197–207.

27. Hersh PS, Shah SI, Durrie D. Monocular diplopia following excimer laser photorefractive keratectomy after radial keratotomy. *Ophthalmic Surg Lasers* 1996;27:315–317.

28. Diaz-Calderon E, et al. Bilateral internuclear opthalmoplegia after smoking "crack" cocaine. *J Clin Neurophthalmal* 1991;11:297–299.

29. Zee DS. Internuclear ophthalmoplegia: pathophysiology and diagnosis. *Baillieres Clin Neurol* 1992;1:455–470.

30. Brazis PW. Localization of lesions of the oculomotor nerve: recent concepts. *Mayo Clin Proc* 1991;66:1029–1035.

31. Kumar PD, Nartsupha C, West BC. Unilateral internuclear ophthalmoplegia and recovery with thiamine in Weinicke syndrome. *Am J Med Sci* 2000;320:278–280.

32. Brazis PW, Lee AG. Binocular vertical diplopia. *Mayo Clin Proc* 1998;73:55–66.

33. Chan J. Isolated unilateral post-traumatic internuclear ophthalmoplegia. *J Neuroophthalmal* 2001;21:212–213.

34. Dutt I, et al. Unilateral internuclear ophthalmoplegia in systemic lupus erythematous. *J Assoc Physicians India* 2000;48:1210–1211.

35. Flipse JP, et al. Bilateral saccadic eye movements in multiple sclerosis. *J Neurol Sci* 1997;148:53–65.

CHAPTER

9

NEUROLOGIC TRAUMA

Injury to the nervous system is a common cause of death and disability.[1] Injuries to the head often do not occur as an isolated event. Cervical spine injuries are the most significant associated injuries, and extremity injuries are the most common. Associated injuries are at times difficult to detect because of the impaired mental status of the head-injured patient. In this chapter the overall subject of injury to the nervous system is divided into two categories: head injury and spinal cord injury. The focus of the following discussions is on the evaluation and stabilization of patients who have isolated central nervous system injury, with the understanding that trauma management requires a comprehensive, multisystem approach.

TRAUMATIC BRAIN INJURY

Traumatic brain injury (TBI) is a leading cause of death worldwide, particularly in those under the age of 40.[2] Head injury and TBI are two distinct entities that are often, but not necessarily, related. A *head injury* is best defined as an injury that is clinically evident upon physical examination and is recognized by the presence of ecchymoses, lacerations, deformities, or cerebral spinal rhinorrhea or otorrhea. *Traumatic brain injury* refers to an injury to the brain itself and can occur without external signs of trauma.

The Glasgow Coma Scale

Historically, the most often used system for grading severity of brain injury is the Glasgow Coma Scale (GCS) score. The GCS is based upon three factors: eye opening, verbal function (mental status), and motor function; a modified scale exists for nonverbal children (Table 9-1).[3] Created by Teasdale and Jennett in 1974, the GCS was developed as a standardized clinical scale allowing for reliable interobserver neurologic assessments of TBI patients in coma.[4] The original studies applying the

TABLE 9-1

GLASGOW COMA SCALE FOR ADULTS
AND FOR PREVERBAL CHILDREN

Eye Opening	
Spontaneous	4
To speech	3
To pain	2
No response	1
Verbal Response	
Adults	
Alert and oriented	5
Disoriented	4
Nonsensical speach	3
Moans	2
No response	1
Preverbal Children	
Coos, babbles	5
Irritable cry	4
Cries to pain	3
Moans to pain	2
No response	1
Motor Response	
Follows commands	6
Localizes pain	5
Withdraws to pain	4
Decorticate flexion	3
Decerebrate extension	2
No response	1
Grading of TBI	
Mild	13–15
Moderate	9–12
Severe	3–8

GCS score as a tool for assessing outcome required that coma be present for at least 6 hours.[4-6] The scale was not designed to diagnose patients with mild or even moderate TBI, nor was it intended to supplant a neurologic examination. Instead, the GCS was designed to provide an easy-to-use assessment tool for serial evaluations by relatively inexperienced care providers, and to facilitate communication between care providers on rotating shifts.

A single isolated GCS score is of limited value, is insufficient to determine the degree of parenchymal injury after trauma, and does not have prognostic value. On the other hand, serial GCS scores are a valuable clinical tool (when confounding factors such as drugs or alcohol are absent). A low GCS score that remains low, or a high GCS that decreases, predicts poorer outcomes than high GCS scores that remain high, or a low GCS score that progressively improves. In one of the original multi-center studies validating the score, approximately 13% of patients who ultimately were in coma had a GCS of 15 (note that at the time these studies were done, CT was not available to aid in clinical decision making).[6]

The literature refers to "mild" TBI as those patients with a GCS score greater than 12. Some authors have suggested that patients with a GCS of 13 be excluded from the "mild" category and placed into the "moderate" risk group due to their high incidence of lesions requiring neurosurgical intervention.[7,8] The key for the clinican is to not overly rely on a GCS score, but instead to use the GCS score in conjunction with a relevant neurologic exam to assess head-injured patients for TBI.

Epidemiology

In the United States, approximately 1.6% of all emergency department (ED) visits are for a head injury. Approximately 90% of these visits are for mild TBI, and 10% for moderate or severe TBI.[9] TBI is the leading cause of death among people less than 24 years of age.[10] There are 150,000 deaths due to trauma each year in the United States, of which 50% are due to fatal head injuries. The most common cause of head injuries is motor vehicle accidents in the young and falls in the elderly.[1] Approximately 50% of patients who die from TBI arrive at the hospital alive; a number which can potentially be decreased with early and aggressive interventions.[2]

Pathophysiology

When a head injury occurs there are *primary injuries* directly related to the trauma, i.e., skull fractures or blood vessel and parenchymal damage. *Secondary injury* refers to damage that results in neuronal death as a consequence of hypoxia, edema, and initiation of inflammatory cascades. Secondary injury greatly impacts outcome and can be minimized by resuscitative efforts.

Parenchymal brain injury results from a sudden deceleration or rotational acceleration which generates shearing forces within the brain. These forces disrupt small blood vessels and axons at the gray and white matter interface. Injury to small vessels results in petechial hemorrhages or focal edema; disruption of bridging veins results in subdural hematomas; arterial injury, usually laceration of the middle meningeal artery, results in an epidural hematoma. Many patients may have a combination of intracranial injuries.

Diffuse Axonal Injury

Diffuse axonal injury (DAI) is a pattern of white matter changes frequently reported in TBI. It results from trauma-related impairment of intra-axonal neurofilament organization, which in turn impairs axonal transport, leading to axonal swelling, Wallerian degeneration, and transection.[11]

Epidural Hematoma

Epidural hematoma results from arterial bleeding with a rapid change in the patient's neurologic symptoms. The classic history is that of an initial loss of consciousness followed by a lucid interval, during which the patient may either awaken fully or at least show improvement in level of consciousness. The treatment for most acute epidural hematomas is immediate evacuation, ideally done in the operating room by a neurosurgeon. Under rare circumstances where a neurosurgeon is not immediately available, an ED burr hole may be life-saving.

Subdural Hematoma

The pathogenesis of a subdural hematoma is usually that of a tearing of the veins which bridge from the cerebral cortex to the venous sinuses in the dura. The venous bleeding takes place slowly, thus patients frequently present with a less than catastrophic decline in mental status and level of consciousness. However, large lesions can obviously result in profound neurologic damage and require emergent neurosurgical evacuation.

Intracerebral Contusion/Hematoma

An intracerebral contusion is a focal area of damaged parenchyma without significant extravasation of blood. Intracerebral hematomas result from shearing forces in the brain. Neurologic deficits result from the combined compressive forces of the hematoma on the brain and the disruption of neural tissue itself. The history of these patients may be similar to that of patients with the subdural hematoma. They will frequently have focal findings. The decision to evacuate an intracerebral hematoma and the timing of the evacuation is most dependent on size, location, clinical course, and intracranial pressure. Hence, the initial baseline evaluation of the patient will be useful in deciding the course of therapy based on subsequent improvement or deterioration.

Cerebral Perfusion Pressure

Cerebral perfusion pressure (CPP) is the physiologic variable that defines the pressure gradient for cerebral blood flow (CBF). The CPP is the product of the mean arterial pressure minus the intracranial pressure (ICP), thus monitoring of the ICP is a necessity for CPP assessment. It is generally accepted that CPP is best maintained between 70 and 80 mmHg. Under normal conditions, the brain is able to tightly control CBF through the process of autoregulation. Autoregulation is often lost in severe brain injury. A low CPP may jeopardize a region of the brain with preexisting or borderline ischemia while a high CPP may result in progressive cerebral edema and neurologic deterioration.

Prehospital Care of the TBI Patient

The overall goals of prehospital management of head-injured patients include rapid recognition and correction of life-threatening conditions, prevention of secondary brain insults, and transportation to the closest appropriate facility (Figure 9-1).[12] In

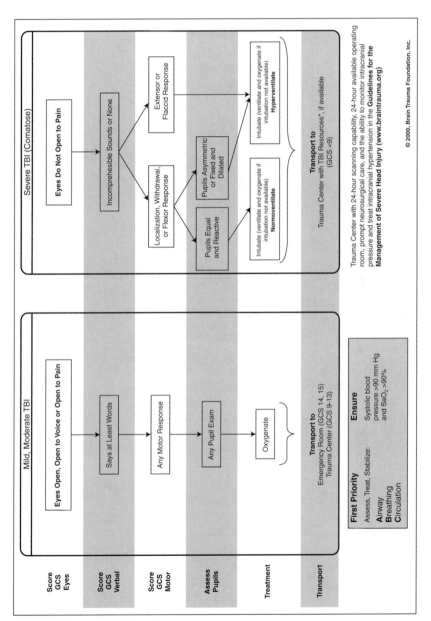

FIGURE 9-1 Prehospital management of patients with traumatic brain injury (TBI). GCS, Glasgow Coma Scale.

PREHOSPITAL TRIAGE FOR THE PATIENT - CONTINUED

Treatment: Ventilation Rates (approximate)

Normal Ventilation Breaths Per Minute

Adults	10 bpm
Children	20 bpm
Infants	25 bpm

Hyperventilation Breaths Per Minute

Adults	20 bpm
Children	30 bpm
Infants	35 bpm

Transport Decisions

The recommended hospital destination may not always be possible given the variability of local and regional resources and transport times. The decision for EMS personnel to follow these recommendations should be based upon discussion and approved by the local EMS Medical Doctor.

FIGURE 9-1   Prehospital management of patients with traumatic brain injury (TBI). GCS, Glasgow Coma Scale. *Continued.*

the case of a moderate or severe TBI patient, transportation ideally should be to a facility with 24-hour availability of neuro-imaging and neurosurgical capabilities, including intracranial pressure monitoring and treatment (Figure 9-2). However, transsport decisions are dependent on a number of factors, including the presence of other injuries and the distance to various facilities.

Prehospital protocols begin with stabilizing the "A, B, Cs," including the cervical spine when indicated. Assessment focuses on determining the GCS score, pupil response, blood pressure, and oxygenation.[12] In patients who appear to have sustained a minor head injury, the only historical parameters proven to be useful in identifying patients with lesions requiring neurosurgical intervention are loss of consciousness (LOC) and amnesia.[13,14] The presence of either of these findings prompts the need for careful serial examinations and consideration for transport to a hospital with neurosurgical capabilities. Although the mechanism of injury is interesting to obtain and may direct additional inquiries, there is no evidence that mechanism alone is predictive of an intracranial injury in blunt head trauma.[15] Patients with a history of a penetrating injury, or the potential for a penetrating injury such as a gunshot to the scalp, deserve special attention and should be transported directly to a trauma center even if the injury appears inconsequential.

Prehospital management of the TBI patient includes assessing for and treating hypoglycemia when present and maintaining oxygenation saturation above 90% and blood pressure above 90 mmHg. Patients who demonstrate signs of increased intracranial pressure are candidates for intubation with hyperventilation (see Table 9-3) until the signs of increased intracranial pressure resolve. There is no proven role for mannitol in the prehospital arena, especially when transport times are relatively short.[12] Agitated TBI patients must be assessed for confounding factors such as pain, hypoxia, or hypoglyemia; they may be treated with a benzodiazepine or a phenothiazine.

Emergency Department Evaluation and Management

Evaluation of the head-injured patient requires a careful assessment of historical information that suggests a brain injury occurred, e.g., loss of consciousness, and an examination that assesses for focal neurologic deficits, including altered mental status. Table 9-2 lists pearls that may be helpful in evaluating TBI patients.

Initial Stabilization

Resuscitation, including brain-specific interventions, occurs simultaneously with the assessment. Since brain injury is a continuum that begins at impact, many secondary insults that enhance the initial damage occur during the ensuing hours and days. Identification of the factors predictive of poor outcome may be helpful in directing management and minimizing morbidity and mortality. These factors include hypotension, hypoxemia; or hypercarbia; abnormal motor response; impaired or absent eye movements or pupil light reflexes, an intracranial hematoma; or an elevation of intracranial pressure over 20 mmHg.

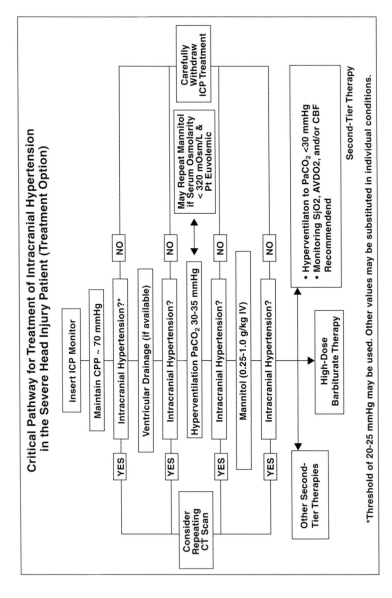

FIGURE 9-2 Hospital management of patients with severe traumatic brain injury. CCP, cerebral perfusion pressure; ICP, intracranial pressure.

TABLE 9-2
CLINICAL PEARLS IN THE MANAGEMENT OF HEAD-INJURED PATIENTS

- Loss of consciousness or amnesia are the best historical predictors that a head-injured patient sustained a brain injury.
- Serial Glasgow Coma Scale (GCS) scores, hypoxemia, and hypotension are the best predictors of outcome in traumatic brain injury (TBI) patients, in the emergency department.
- A single GCS score determination has no predictive value, and thus the GCS must be repeated serially in select patients.
- Clinical signs of increased intracranial pressure include dilated fixed pupil(s) or extensor posturing and are acutely treated with hyperventilation.
- Patients with moderate or severe TBI should be transported to a hospital with neurosurgical capabilities.

BLOOD PRESSURE AND OXYGENATION Multiple studies demonstrate the association of hypoxemia and hypotension with poor outcomes in TBI patients.[16–18] Consequently, the cornerstone of stabilization is to maintain the oxygen saturation over 90% and the mean systolic blood pressure over 90 mmHg.

The airway should be secured with rapid sequence intubation (RSI) in TBI patients who fail to ventilate, fail to oxygenate, or fail to protect their airway, or in those patients at risk of losing their airway, especially if they are leaving the ED. Table 9-3 outlines a sample protocol for RSI in TBI patients. Hypotension should be corrected as quickly as possible to bring the mean systolic pressure over

TABLE 9-3
SAMPLE RAPID-SEQUENCE INTUBATION PROTOCOL FOR THE TBI PATIENT

1. Assess airway for difficulty; ensure ability to bag-valve mask.
2. Preoxygenate with 100% oxygen (do not bag-valve-mask unless necessary).
3. Prepare medications and rescue airway strategies.
4. Premedicate: Vecuronium 0.01 mg/kg
   Lidocaine 1.5 mg/kg
   Fentanyl 3.0 µg/kg
5. Induction: etiomodate 0.2 mg/kg, or thiopental 3–5 mg/kg (if hemodynamically stable).
6. Paralysis: succinylcholine 1.5 mg/kg.
7. Intubate with in-line cervical immobilization.
8. Confirm endotracheal tube placement with capnometry.
9. Consider long-term neuromuscular blockade and sedation.

90 mmHg. Isotonic intravenous crystalloid administration has been the mainstay of initial volume resuscitation.

History

On the initial encounter, it is not possible to determine accurately the degree of brain injury that a head-injured patient has sustained. In patients with blunt trauma who appear to have sustained a minor head injury, the only historical parameters that have proved to be useful in identifying patients with lesions requiring neurosurgical intervention are loss of consciousness (LOC) and amnesia.[13,14,19] A history of headaches, seizures, nausea, vomiting, dizziness, age over 60, or evidence of trauma above the clavicle have not been found to be independent predictors of an intracranial lesion. However, the absence of all of the above has been reported to be 100% sensitive in excluding an injury requiring neurosurgical intervention even when LOC has occurred.[14] The use of anticoagulant therapy or hemophilia are additional historical findings that may be associated with an increased risk for an intracranial event.

Physical Examination

The physical exam begins with a careful set of vital signs and with a general overview of the patient, looking for evidence of scalp trauma, skull fractures, or signs of basilar skull fracture ("raccoon eyes," Battle's sign, or cerebrospinal fluid [CSF] otorrhea or rhinorrhea). Subtle findings such as an external ear canal laceration or hemotypanum may be critical for directing additional testing. Cushing's sign, i.e., hypertension with bradycardia, is a classic descriptor of severe TBI but unfortunately is a late and unreliable finding. Serial evaluations are useful until the clinician is satisfied that the patient is clinically stable. Finally, no decisions can be made until a focused neurologic examination has been completed.

The neurologic exam is necessary to establish the severity of neurologic injury and to establish the baseline with which subsequent exams are compared. The classic sign of an expanding mass intracranial lesion is a unilateral dilated and fixed pupil. This results from uncal herniation compressing the parasympathetic fiber on the outside of the third cranial nerve and is associated with a contralateral hemiparesis. A less common phenomenon, known as Kernohan's notch, refers to a paradoxical motor sign in which there is a unilateral dilated and fixed pupil with an ipsilateral hemiparesis or hemiplegia. In these cases, the brainstem is pushed to the contralateral side of the tentorium and the contralateral cerebral peduncle, and the third nerve is then pushed upon by the edge of the tentorium, resulting in hemiparesis ipsilateral to the mass.

The presence of focal neurologic findings or an altered mental status is predictive of significant lesions,[20,21] although, conversely, the absence of such findings does not eliminate the possibility that an injury has occurred.[22] When performing the neurologic examination, particular attention must be paid to cranial nerves III, IV, and VI. Papilledema is a late finding in increased intracranial pressure (ICP) and thus is not seen in acute head injury. The pupil exam consists of determining pupil size, symmetry, and reactivity to light. Mass effect from edema or an expanding lesion may result in a unilateral fixed and dilated pupil. Bilaterally dilated and fixed pupils are consistent with brainstem injury. Hypoxemia, hypotension, and hypothermia are associated with dilated pupil size and abnormal reactivity, making it necessary to resuscitate and stabilize the patient before an accurate pupillary assessment can occur.[23] Direct trauma to the eye may also result in a dilated pupil, or in an isolated cranial nerve IV or VI deficit that might not be evident until the patient is taken through a careful extraocular range-of-motion exam.[24]

An assessment of cognitive function may be helpful in select cases in that it provides an important baseline in the patient's evaluation. Cognitive function is only superficially assessed in the GCS score through the patient's verbal response. In mild TBI, it has not been shown to be predictive of parenchymal injury demonstrable on head computed tomography (CT).[8,25]

HERNIATION   The signs of cerebral herniation include one or both fixed dilated pupil(s) and extensor posturing (decorticate posturing is not a sign of herniation); in severe TBI patients, a decrease in the GCS score of 2 or more points suggests increasing ICP. Hyperventilation and osmotic diuretics (see below) are the mainstay of medical management and may also be indicated in patients with surgical lesions while preparations are made for operative interventions.

Diagnostic Testing

Laboratory testing is tailored to the individual patient. All patients with altered mental status require an immediate serum glucose determination in order to avoid confusing hypoglycemia with a trauma-related condition.

A noncontrast head CT is the test of choice in evaluating the TBI patient. Moderate and severe TBI patients require an imaging study; the only question is the timing of the scan. In the presence of clinical signs of herniation or progressive neurologic deterioration, the CT scan should be obtained as soon as possible, once the patient has been stabilized. In the absence of clinical signs of herniation or in cases of multiple trauma, CT scanning may be delayed pending the completion of other diagnostic tests. Indications for head CT in mild TBI are discussed below. Although CT is still the gold standard imaging study, MRI has challenged CT in certain nonemergent situations.[26] MRI is more sensitive for brainstem lesions, diffuse axonal injury, and nonhemorrhagic lesions. Its value is even more evident several days after the initial injury when the sensitivity of MRI surpasses CT in detection of nearly all traumatic lesions except for fractures.

Management of Severe TBI

Intracranial Pressure Monitoring

ICP monitoring is used to facilitate maintenance of an adequate cerebral perfusion pressure. The ICP is normally 0 to 10 mmHg; in general, an ICP of more than 20 mmHg is an indication to initiate therapy to lower the pressure.[2] In patients with severe TBI, strong consideration should be given to initiation of ICP monitoring. ICP monitoring is indicated in severe TBI patients with CT evidence of edema, hemorrhage, hematomas, contusions, or compressed basal cisterns. It is also recommended in severe TBI patients who have a normal head CT but who have at least two of the following three features: age over 40 years, unilateral or bilateral posturing, and a systolic blood pressure of less than 90 mmHg.[2] When only one of these features is present and the patient has a normal head CT, the risk of developing intracranial hemorrhage is low, and ICP monitoring is probably not indicated.

Hyperventilation

In the past, hyperventilation, keeping a pCO_2 of less than 25 mmHg, was the cornerstone of both acute and chronic management of patients with increased ICP. Indeed, hyperventilation leads to an initial decrease in the ICP by causing an immediate cerebral vasoconstriction with a resultant rise in cerebral vascular resistance and a fall in cerebral blood flow (CBF). However, there is evidence that cerebral anoxia occurs as the result of the cerebral vasoconstriction, resulting in worsening outcomes when hyperventilation is used past the initial resuscitative phase.[2] Hyperventilation therapy, to a pCO_2 of 30 to 35 mmHg, is recommended only as a temporizing measure in patients with signs of increased ICP and should be discontinued as soon as the signs of increased ICP resolve.

Mannitol

Mannitol, an osmotic diuretic, can reduce ICP by 25% or more within 5 to 20 minutes of its administration to patients with severe TBI. It is administered as intermittent boluses of 0.25 to 1 g/kg.[27] Ideally, mannitol is given once ICP monitoring is in place, although therapy should not be delayed in patients showing signs of increased ICP. ICP monitoring can help avoid the deleterious effects of overadministration of mannitol. When mannitol is used, care should be taken to maintain the patient in a euvolemic state by fluid replacement and to keep the serum osmolarity below 320 mosm to decrease the chances of renal failure.

Mannitol has two proposed mechanisms of action.[28] One is an immediate but transient plasma-expanding effect, leading to improved cerebral perfusion as the result of reduced hematocrit, reduced blood viscosity, and increased CBF, with improved oxygen delivery. The second mechanism is an osmotic effect that is delayed for 15 to 30 minutes while gradients between plasma and cells are established. Smaller and more frequent doses are safe and effective in reducing the ICP while avoiding the risk of osmotic disequilibrium and severe dehydration. After multiple doses or continuous infusions, mannitol may exacerbate ICP by increasing brain swelling, the so-called rebound effect, probably secondary to accumulation in the injured tissue.

Barbiturates

High-dose barbiturates are recommended in hemodynamically stable severe TBI patients with intracranial hypertension that is refractory to maximal medical and surgical ICP-lowering therapy. However, they have not been shown to affect outcome and are not recommended prophylactically.[2]

Analgesia/Sedation/Neuromuscular Blockade

The severe head-injured patient commonly undergoes episodes of agitation and combativeness, both of which tend to increase ICP and complicate patient care. Therefore, treatment protocols should include the use of analgesics and sedatives. These agents should be short acting and are usually narcotic analgesics such as fentanyl and/or a benzodiazepine such as midazolam.

The use of neuromuscular blockade is also helpful in managing severe TBI patients. Neuromuscular blockade should be considered in any patient whose transportation, management, or diagnostic imaging is complicated by uncontrolled agitation or combativeness. The paralytic agents used should be short acting and discontinued as soon as feasible.

Anticonvulsants

Posttraumatic seizures (PTS) are classified as early, occurring within 7 days of injury, or late, occurring 7 days after the injury. Approximately 15% of severe TBI patients have an early PTS; up to 20% will have a late PTS.[29] Phenytoin has been shown to decrease the incidence of early PTS to 4% but has not been shown to impact on the incidence of late PTS. Consequently, prophylactic phenytoin is not recommended after the first week in patients with severe TBI.

Steroids

Evidence suggests that corticosteroids do not lower ICP or improve outcome in severely head-injured patients and therefore they are not recommended.[2]

Penetrating Trauma

When penetrating trauma occurs and penetrating bodies protrude from the head, they should never be removed. While the foreign body is still lodged in the head, it may provide tamponade of bleeding vessels. Release of the tamponade may cause catastrophic bleeding and deterioration of the patient. Penetrating foreign objects should be removed only in the operating room under controlled conditions.

Mild Traumatic Brain Injury

The question of how best to define a mild TBI is of great importance and has been a source of confusion. A small subset of these patients will harbor a life-threatening injury, while many will suffer neurocognitive sequelae for days to months after the injury (see Postconcussive Syndrome section, below). The American Congress of Rehabilitation Medicine has delineated inclusion criteria for a diagnosis of mild TBI. At least one of the following criteria must be met: (1) any period of LOC of less than 30 minutes and GCS score of 13 to 15 after this period of LOC; (2) any loss of memory of the event immediately before or after the accident, with post-traumatic amnesia of less than 24 hours; (3) any alteration in mental state at the time of the accident (e.g., feeling dazed, disoriented, or confused).[30] This definition is extremely broad and contributes to the difficulty in interpreting the mild TBI literature. As already emphasized, the GCS score does not necessarily identify subtle deficits and therefore is not a substitute for a careful neurologic exam. Large studies demonstrate that the absence of LOC or amnesia in patients with blunt head injury are negative predictors of the need for acute intervention after brain injury.[13]

Skull Films

Skull films continue to be used as the first step in assessing mild TBI in many health care facilities, particularly those in which head CT is not readily available. However, a metaanalysis of the literature concluded that, although a fracture demonstrated on plain film increases the likelihood of an intracranial lesion, its low sensitivity precludes its use to rule out the diagnosis of an intracranial hemorrhage; thus plain films are of limited clinical value in risk stratification for brain injury.[31]

CT in Mild TBI

Patients with blunt head injury who do not sustain LOC or posttraumatic amnesia are at almost no risk of significant intracranial injury requiring a diagnosis in the ED and do not need neuroimaging in the ED. On the other hand, approximately 10% of patients with a history of LOC and a GCS score of 15 will have an acute lesion on noncontrast head CT; less than 1% will have a lesion in need of a neurosurgical intervention.[14] The literature does not clearly state which patients with intracranial lesions deteriorate, nor is it clear about the predictive value of intracranial lesions in predicting the development of postconcussive syndrome.

Well-designed studies and evidence-based practice guidelines recommend that patients with blunt head trauma who experienced LOC or posttraumatic amnesia, with a GCS score of 15 and a normal neurologic exam, do not need a head CT in the ED if they do not have headache, vomiting, age over 60, drug or ETOH intoxication, deficits in short-term memory, physical evidence of trauma above the clavicle, or seizure.[14,31] Patients with any of the above findings, and those with a GCS score below 15, should be considered for a head CT.

Concussion and the Second Impact Syndrome

The *second impact syndrome* refers to the cumulative neuroanatomic damage that occurs when the brain is traumatized a second time before it has fully recovered from the first traumatic event. Controversy regarding the proper sideline evaluation and management of sports-related concussions led to the development of practice guidelines (Table 9-4).[32] However, these practice guidelines are consensus-based and await validation by methodologically sound studies.

Intoxication

In some reports as many as 42% of patients with TBI were "legally" intoxicated at the time they presented to the ED.[33] The difficult task of detecting an intracranial injury is compounded by the danger of attributing the mental status change to alcohol. Although observation is an accepted practice for patients suspected of being intoxicated, the clinician must maintain a high level of suspicion and should combine clinical judgment with neurologic evaluations. There should be a low threshold for obtaining a CT in intoxicated patients who have signs of head injury.

TABLE 9-4

MANAGEMENT RECOMMENDATIONS FOR PATIENTS WITH CONCUSSION[a]

Grade I: Confusion but no Loss of Consciousness, no Amnesia
- Remove from activity (e.g., sporting event) and observe. When patient returns to baseline, have him/her exert him/herself by doing exercises; if patient remains asymptomatic, return to full activity.
- Two grade I concussions in one day: no exertional activity for the rest of the day.
- Three grade I concussions: no exertional activities that place the patient at risk for head trauma for 3 months.

Grade II: Confusion and Amnesia, but no Loss of Consciousness
- Remove from activity that places patient at risk for head trauma for the rest of the day.
- Follow-up in 24 hours for reassessment.
- No activity that places patient at risk for 1 week.
- Two grade II concussions: no activity that places patient at risk for 3 months.

Grade III: Loss of Consciousness
- Transport to the ED for evaluation and a CT.
- Return to activities after 1 month of having no symptoms for 2 weeks.
- Two grade III concussions: no activity that places patient at risk for head injury for 3 months.

[a] Modified from recommendations made in the Colorado Medical Society Concussion in Sports Guidelines.

Postconcussive Syndrome

The postconcussive syndrome (PCS) refers to a symptom complex experienced by many patients after mild TBI. In general, PCS is composed of somatic, cognitive, and affective symptoms (Table 9-5). Common symptoms include headache, dizziness/vertigo, difficulty concentrating, and depression. Approximately 30% of patients with mild TBI will have symptoms at 3 months post injury, and up to 15% will continue to be symptomatic at 1 year post injury.[34,35] It appears that well-motivated, young, male patients are at the lowest risk of developing the PCS and that females, those over 55, or patients who experienced prolonged posttraumatic amnesia are at a higher risk of developing PCS.[36] Despite the emerging consensus that somatic and cognitive deficits result from mild TBI, physiogenesis versus psychogenesis of symptoms is debated, especially when symptoms persist for more than 3 months.

When managing patients with mild TBI, it is important to take the time to advise them of the potential sequelae of the injury; such advice may significantly assuage their anxiety about permanent damage. A referral to a specialist with expertise in caring for these patients may be helpful for the patient's prognosis. Recovery appears to be linked not only to the underlying lesion but also to psychosocial issues in the

TABLE 9-5

SYMPTOMS SEEN IN THE POSTCONCUSSIVE SYNDROME

Somatic
Headache
Sleep disturbance
Dizziness/vertigo
Nausea
Fatigue
Oversensitivity to noise/light

Cognitive
Attention/concentration problems
Memory problems

Affective
Irritability
Anxiety
Depression
Emotional lability

patient's life. Consequently, access to a multidisciplinary resource may provide the patient with the most comprehensive support services to assist in recovery.

Mild TBI in Infants and Children

Most injuries in infants are from falls, the vast majority of which are from a relatively short height such as from tables, chairs, and sofas.[37] By early childhood the mechanisms of injury parallel those of adults. When the mechanism of injury is unclear, the possibility of child abuse should be entertained.

The current literature on mild TBI in pediatrics, as in adults, does not provide definitive evidence to make clinical decision making easy. The American Academy of Pediatrics has published recommendations on the management of MTBI in children older than 2 years[38] (Table 9-6). In essence, management is based on a careful neurologic exam, and decisions must take into account the environment to which the child is returning.

Infants are much more difficult to assess clinically in that their presentations are typically subtle and potentially misleading. Infants require careful observation; in falls from less than 3 feet, observation alone is sufficient if the neurologic exam is normal and there is no evidence of scalp trauma.[39] Falls from more than 3 feet or an abnormal neurologic exam should prompt consideration for a CT.

Disposition in TBI

Patients with severe or moderate TBI are usually admitted to the hospital. Patients with mild TBI and a positive CT scan for acute injury also require neurosurgical

TABLE 9-6

SUMMARY OF RECOMMENDATIONS BY THE AMERICAN ACADEMY OF PEDIATRICS FOR THE MANAGEMENT OF MINOR CLOSED HEAD INJURY IN CHILDREN 2 YEARS OR OLDER

- The use of head CT, skull radiograph, or MRI is not recommended for the initial evaluation and management of the child with minor closed head injury and no loss of consciousness.
- The use of skull radiographs or MRI in the initial management of children with minor closed head injury and loss of consciousness is not recommended.
- Skull radiographs have only a limited role in the management of the child with loss of consciousness: CT scanning is the imaging modality of choice.
- The risk-benefit ratio for the evaluation and management modalities of CT scanning or observation is unknown. For children who are neurologically normal after minor closed head injury with loss of consciousness, cranial CT scanning along with observation is an acceptable management option.
- Patients may be discharged from the hospital for observation by a reliable observer if the postinjury CT scan is interpreted as normal.

consultation, if available, and possibly admission for observation. Considerations for admission to the hospital or to an observation unit when the CT is normal include an abnormal mental status or neurologic examination, intractable vomiting, drug or alcohol intoxication, lack of a competent observer, no reliable means of getting home, or suspicion of child abuse or domestic violence.

Neuroimaging has resulted in a decline in the number of mild TBI patients admitted to the hospital for observation without a reported increase in adverse outcomes.[1] In most cases, patients with mild TBI and a negative head CT can be discharged home with a reliable adult. Although the safety of home observation has been established in this subset of patients, patients with TBI may not remember their discharge instructions emphasizing the need not only to give patients written instructions, but also to provide a family member or friend with important information that will impact on the patient during the recovery period.[40]

SPINAL CORD INJURY

An essential part of early trauma care involves the assessment and management of the patient with the potential for injury to the vertebral column and spinal cord. Spinal cord injury can be devastating, with long-term disability, yet it may be preventable if proper stabilization and early interventions are provided. This section focuses on the acute management of the patient with potential spinal cord injury. The emphasis is on diagnostic approaches and initial management.

Epidemiology

The National Spinal Cord Injury Database (NSCID) has been used to compile epidemiologic data on spinal cord injury patients in the United States since 1973; the current database contains more than 21,000 cases.[41] Data from the NSCID estimate 10,000 new cases of spinal cord injury each year. Four times as many vertebral column fractures occur without neurologic sequelae. Most patients with spinal cord injury are victims of vehicular trauma, followed by acts of violence, falls, and recreational sporting activities.

The incidence of cervical spine fracture in most series of blunt trauma patients is between 1% and 6%; fractures of the thoracolumbar spine occur in 2% to 3%. Roughly 65% of vertebral injuries involve the cervical spine, 20% the thoracic spine, and 15% the lumbar spine.[42] The most common site of fracture in the cervical spine is C2 (including the odontoid), which accounts for roughly 24% of fractures. The upper cervical spine (C1 to C3) is more likely to sustain injury in children (younger than 12 years) and in the elderly (older than 50 years), whereas the lower cervical spine (C6 to T1) is more often injured in young adults (12 to 50 years old). Approximately 40% of cervical injuries in patients older than 50 years will involve the atlantoaxial complex.[43] If a patient has one spinal column injury, the chance of a second fracture is significant.

Anatomy and Pathophysiology

The support structures of the spine are composed of 33 individual units grouped into five general divisions according to location and anatomic characteristics. There are 7 cervical vertebrae, 12 thoracic vertebrae, 5 lumbar vertebrae, 5 sacral vertebrae, and 3 to 5 coccygeal vertebrae. Each vertebrae is joined to the next by a flexible intravertebral disc that forms a slightly movable articulation. The intercentral ligaments connecting the vertebral bodies are composed of the anterior and posterior longitudinal ligaments.

In transverse section, the spinal canal consists of (1) a butterfly-shaped central gray substance composed of collections of cell bodies and their processes and (2) a surrounding mantle of white matter composed of bundles of myelinated fibers that are divided into either ascending or descending tracts (see Chap. 1). The posterior columns, fasiculus gracilis (medial) and fasiculus cuneatus (lateral), convey impulses concerned with touch-pressure and kinesthesia (vibratory and position sense). Ascending fibers from caudal segmental levels shift medially and posteriorly as they ascend in the posterior columns, creating a somatotopic organization of the fibers. Fibers ascend to the nucleus gracilis and cuneatus in the medulla ipsilaterally before terminating on relay nuclei whose secondary fibers cross in the medial lemniscus. The lateral spinothalamic tract transmits impulses concerned with pain and thermal sensation. The spinothalamic fibers cross in the anterior white commissure within one or two spinal segments of their origin. This tract is also somatotopically organized, with the sacral and lumbar segments located laterally, and the thoracic and cervical segments located medially.

Descending tracts are concerned with motor function and visceral innervation. The fibers of the corticospinal tracts all originate from the cerebral cortex. At the junction of the medulla and the spinal cord, at the pyramidal decussation, the corticospinal tract undergoes an incomplete decussation, dividing into three tracts: (1) the large lateral corticospinal tract (crossed), (2) the small anterior corticospinal tract (uncrossed), and (3) the smaller uncrossed anterolateral corticospinal tract.

Spinal fractures and dislocations carry a 14% incidence of spinal cord injury. Dysfunction of the spinal cord can result from mechanical impingement on the cord, as by bone, disc material, or hematoma. In the cervical region the incidence of neurologic deficit with fracture is 39%. If there has not been anatomic transection of the cord, a contusion of the cord results in a progressive sequence of changes that begin initially as small hemorrhages centrally in the cord. These are followed in minutes to hours by progressive hemorrhage, edema, and coagulation necrosis.

Initial Stabilization

Most patients with spinal cord injury will manifest impairment at the time of injury. However, manipulation may worsen the injury or cause injury in a patient who has an unstable fracture; thus extreme care must be taken to stabilize the spine.[44] Maximum spinal immobilization is provided by a rigid cervical collar (which incorporates the upper thorax), sand bags or taped blocks, and a long spine board (padded or unpadded).[45] Provisions for vigorous suctioning to prevent aspiration of blood and secretions should be made readily available (see Spine Radiography section below for those patients who do not need spinal immobilization).

In most victims of major trauma requiring urgent airway management, intubation will be done *before* a full assessment of the cervical spine is possible. Rapid sequence intubation protocols incorporating in-line cervical spine stabilization are recommended.[46] There is no evidence that endotracheal intubation with in-line stabilization significantly increases the risk of neurologic injury in patients with unstable cervical spine fractures. Some situations will require alternative airway management techniques such as fiberoptic laryngoscopy, lighted stilets, or an intubating laryngeal mask.

History

The history of the injury should include mechanism (flexion, extension, direct blow, rotation), magnitude of the forces involved (height of fall, speed of accident), timing of the onset of symptoms, and their time course. The presence of spine pain, radicular pain, dysesthesias, and neurologic symptoms (numbness, weakness) should be elicited and particular attention devoted to whether the neurologic deficits were complete or incomplete.

Care must be taken to ensure that distracting injuries do not mask a spinal injury. If the history is unreliable because of intoxication or head injury, the lack of reported spine pain should be ignored, and one should treat the injury as spinal until disproved or until the history can be trusted. A history of osteoporosis, ankylosing spondylitis, or rheumatoid arthritis raises the level of concern that an injury has occurred, even if the injury was minor.

Physical Examination

A systematic neurologic examination is important in the initial evaluation of the patient with a possible spinal injury. Serial examinations are of equal importance in order to identify and document evolving neurologic pathology. Guidelines for motor and sensory evaluations have been established by the American Spinal Injury Association (ASIA; Table 9-7). In the awake, interactive patient, sensation is assessed by dermatome to localize the most cephalad extent of the spinal cord injury; on the anterior chest, dermatome levels abruptly change from C4 to T2 just above the nipple line. Spinal cord level can also be assessed by checking deep tendon reflexes (DTRs; Table 9-8). Pain sensation can be used to test contralateral spinothalamic tract function. Motor function, indicative of ipsilateral corticospinal tract integrity, is assessed on a 0 to 5 scale (see Chap. 2 for information on the neurologic exam). Dorsal column testing, which includes light touch, should not be neglected, as it will differentiate between a complete lesion and an anterior cord syndrome. This is best examined with proprioception or vibration in the distal extremities. Special attention should be paid to rectal tone, sacral sensation, and bladder function to avoid missing injuries to the conus medullaris and cauda equina, as well as documenting complete versus incomplete cord injury.

Spinal shock is a state of complete areflexia following an acute, severe transverse cord lesion. All spinal function and reflexes are lost for up to 6 weeks. Reversal of spinal shock is heralded by the return of the bulbocavernosus reflex. This reflex is easily tested by pinching the glans penis or foreskin, which should elicit a contraction of the bulbocavernosus muscle at the base of the penis and contraction of the rectal sphincter.

TABLE 9-7

AMERICAN SPINAL INJURY ASSOCIATION IMPAIRMENT CRITERIA

Grade A: Complete motor and sensory loss below level of lesion

Grade B: Complete motor loss with some sensory sparing below level of lesion with sacral sparing

Grade C: Motor function intact including key muscles below the lesion level with muscle grade less than 3

Grade D: Motor function intact including key muscles below the lesion level with muscle grade greater than or equal to 3

Grade E: Motor and sensory function normal

TABLE 9-8 —————————————————————————————————————
ASSESSMENT OF DEEP TENDON REFLEXES IN RELATION TO SPINAL CORD LEVEL

Upper Extremities/Torso

Pectoral	C4–C5
Biceps	C5–C6
Triceps	C7 (C8)
Brachioradialis	C5–C6
Upper abdomen	T6–T9
Lower abdomen	T10–T12

Lower Extremities

Patellar	L2–L4
Achilles	S1–S2
Hamstrings	L5–S1
Cremasteric	L1–L2
Bulbocavernosus	S3–S4
Anal wink	S3–S5

Cervical Spine Injury Patterns

Cervical spine injuries are described according to four mechanisms of injury and resultant radiographic alterations: flexion, extension, axial load, and rotational.

Flexion

Flexion injuries cause compression of the anterior column and distraction of the posterior column. This results in varying degrees of crush injury of the anterior aspect of the vertebral body, as well as variable degrees of ligamentous disruption and widening of the posterior column ("crushed in the front and wide in the back"). Simple wedge fractures, flexion teardrop fractures, unilateral facet dislocations, and bilateral facet dislocations represent a progression of severity (and instability) of flexion injuries.

Extension

Extension injuries cause distraction of the anterior column and compression of the posterior column. There is variable disruption and widening of the anterior ligaments, as well as varying degrees of crush injury of the posterior elements ("wide in the front and crushed in the back"). Extension injuries include the hangman's fracture and extension teardrop fractures.

Axial Load

Axial load injuries cause compression of both the anterior and posterior columns. These are the result of forces from above (skull) or below (pelvis) that are applied to the vertebral column in neutral position at the time of impact. Adjacent vertebral bodies are forced against each other with overwhelming force. The resultant vectors cause the vertebral body to shatter outward, resulting in a *burst fracture*. A burst fracture is generally a stable fracture since the ligamentous structures of the vertebral column remain intact. An exception is a burst fracture of C1 (Jefferson's fracture), which is unstable and requires neurosurgical consultation.

Rotation

Rotational injuries occur when one of the facet joints acts as a fulcrum, and rotation with some degree of flexion allows the contralateral facet joint to dislocate by the superior facet jumping superior and anterior to the inferior facet. Thus the superior facet comes to rest in the intervertebral foramen, resulting in a locked-in position and a stable injury (even though the posterior ligaments are somewhat disrupted). The anteroposterior radiograph will show that the spinous process above the injury is angled away from the midline in the direction of the rotational injury. On the lateral projection, a subluxation of the vertebra above the facet dislocation will be present.

Spine Radiography

As with all tests, a positive finding on x-ray has meaning, but a negative result does not disprove injury. There can be significant ligamentous instability or spinal cord injury without radiographic findings. In addition, patients with one spinous fracture frequently have another spine fracture.[47] The National Emergency X-Radiography Utilization Study (NEXUS) was a prospective, multicenter, observational study that included 34,069 patients with potential cervical spine injury.[48] It identified negative predictors of cervical spine injury (Table 9-9). In a follow-up study of 818 patients, 5.5% of patients with a cervical fracture had a distracting injury, and 3% had altered alertness or intoxication as the only criteria that predicted their cervical spine injury.[49]

Similar studies have been conducted for thoracic and lumbar imaging, although they are not as large as NEXUS.[50] Based on these studies, it is reasonable to use criteria similar to those established by NEXUS for imaging the thoracolumbar spine.

Three-View versus Five-View versus Seven-View Cervical Radiography

A single cross-table lateral view of the cervical spine has a sensitivity of between 57% and 85% for identifying a fracture.[51] Addition of the anteroposterior and open-

TABLE 9-9

INDICATIONS FOR CERVICAL RADIOGRAPHY FOLLOWING BLUNT TRAUMA[a]

1. Neck pain
2. Midline cervical tenderness
3. Altered mental status including any evidence of intoxication
4. Focal neurologic deficits or complaints
5. Distracting painful injury

[a] Based on the NEXUS data; cervical radiography is not indicated in the absence of all five criteria.

mouth odontoid views to the cross-table lateral view increases the sensitivity to 99%.[52] Consequently, a minimum of three views should be obtained. Adding two oblique views provides improved visualization of the posterior column (pedicles, articular pillars, neural foramina, and lamina).[53] These views are also useful in visualizing the cervicothoracic junction and may be used instead of the swimmer's view. They are indicated in patients with a poor-quality three-view series or in patients suspected of having a pedicle fracture (Table 9-10).

Flexion and extension views complete a seven-view cervical spine series. They assess for ligamentous injury and are considered in patients who have neck pain but are neurologically intact. Timing of these views is controversial, but in general they are obtained 2 to 3 days after injury since initial muscular spasm can give a false-negative study.[54]

Computed Tomography and Magnetic Resonance Imaging

CT is an excellent modality for identifying fractures of the spine, although it may miss subluxations and simple linear fractures. CT is better than MRI for bony lesions but not as good as MRI for soft tissue and cord lesions. In general, CT is reserved for patients with questionable lesions on plain film radiographs or in patients with persisting pain despite "normal" plain films.[55]

MRI

MRI is playing an increasingly important role in spinal cord injury evaluation. In many centers, it has replaced myelography, except in those patients with indwelling metal.[56] The advantages of MRI include its lack of ionizing radiation, its multiplanar imaging capabilities, and, most importantly, its ability to delineate all soft tissue structures (i.e., cervical discs, anterior and posterior ligamentous structures) as well

TABLE 9-10
INTERPRETATION OF CERVICAL SPINE RADIOGRAPHS

Lateral View
Alignment: anterior, middle and posterior arcs
Bones: uniformity and height of vertebrae and spinous processes
Cartilage: intervertebral disc space height and length
Soft tissue: prevertebral soft tissue width

Anteroposterior View
Alignment of spinous processes
Distance between spinous processes
Uniformity and height of vertebrae

Open Mouth Odontoid View
Spacing of dens and lateral masses
Lateral alignment of C1 and C2
Uniformity of bones

as the spinal cord. Current indications for MRI include complete or incomplete neurologic deficits, deterioration of neurologic function, and suspicion of ligamentous injury despite negative flexion/extension films.

Spinal Cord Lesions

Complete Cord Lesions

Complete transection of the spinal cord is most commonly caused by trauma (other causes include infarction, hemorrhage, and acute disc herniation). Below the level of the lesion there is loss of motor, sensory, and autonomic (including sphincter) function. All reflex function below the level of the lesion is acutely lost secondary to spinal shock. Lesions in the cervical region can interrupt all sympathetic fibers before they exit in the T1 through T10 roots. This results in functional sympathectomy, with a decrease in systemic and pulmonary vascular resistance. Due to the loss of sympathetic tone, there is a relative increase in vagal tone to the heart with concomitant decrease in cardiac contractility and cardiac output. This results in a syndrome of bradycardia with hypotension. Loss of sympathetic tone is accompanied by gastric atony, bowel and bladder dysfunction, and impairment in temperature regulation. Lesions involving C3 to C5 result in loss of phrenic nerve function, diaphragmatic paralysis, and respiratory compromise. Acute lesions below the cervical region usually do not affect sympathetic tone in such a dramatic fashion, but all motor, sensory, and reflex function will be lost below the level of the lesion.

Complete motor-sensory deficit signifies a poor prognosis, especially if it persists for 24 hours post injury; the presence of neurologic sparing represents an incomplete injury with a better long-term prognosis. The perianal region is most commonly spared in both sensory and reflex testing. A complete lesion that persists for 24 hours has only extremely rarely been associated with useful motor recovery.[57] Complete lesions can not be diagnosed until spinal shock has worn off (reflexes are regained), which is usually within 24 hours of injury.

In caring for patients with complete cord lesions, a vigorous search must be made to ensure that hypotension is not due to internal bleeding or drugs. Once spinal shock is diagnosed, treatment is with fluids and vasopressors. These patients also require meticulous supportive care in order to avoid injury such as aspiration and pressure sores.

Incomplete Spinal Cord Injuries

BROWN-SEQUARD SYNDROME   True hemisection of the spinal cord is a rare occurrence; if found, it is usually associated with penetrating trauma. The syndrome, in its pure form, is characterized by ipsilateral loss of motor function and proprioception with contralateral loss of pain and temperature sensation. Since the fibers in the lateral spinothalamic tract move up and down one or two segments before crossing to the contralateral side, analgesia may be noted one or two segments above the lesion. There may be an ipsilateral loss of pinprick at the level of the lesion because the nerves that carry this information have not yet crossed to the contralateral lateral spinothalamic tract. In reality, a "partial Brown-Sequard syndrome" is more often seen with varying degrees of paresis and analgesia.

ANTERIOR CORD SYNDROME   Anterior cord lesions are characterized by loss of motor function, pinprick and light touch, and sensory testing below the level of the lesion. The posterior columns are preserved; therefore light touch, position, and vibratory sense remain intact. This lesion is typically seen following hyperflexion injuries with herniation of dislocated vertebral body fragments or acutely herniated discs compressing the anterior spinal artery and spinal cord.

CENTRAL CORD SYNDROME   The central cord syndrome is the most prevalent of the partial cord syndromes. It is characterized by bilateral motor paresis that is greater in the upper extremities than in the lower. The paresis is often denser distally in the extremities than proximally. There is variable sensory impairment and bladder dysfunction. This syndrome is commonly associated with hyperextension injuries in elderly patients with preexisting cervical spondylosis. A good mnemonic for this syndrome is MUD: *M*otor > sensory, *U*pper > lower, and *D*istal > proximal.

Anatomically, the central cord syndrome is explained by the somatotopic organization of the long tracts of the spinal cord. Since the most central portions of the posterior columns, the corticospinal tract, and the lateral spinothalamic tracts contain fibers from the upper extremities, the degree and location of the neurologic deficits depend on the size of the lesion.

CONUS MEDULLARIS SYNDROME   The conus medullaris is the terminal end of the spinal cord. In adults the conus is located at approximately the L1 vertebral level. Isolated lesions of the conus are rare, but they produce a typical syndrome. Disturbances of urination, specifically a denervated autonomic bladder, are common. Primary sphincteric involvement as well as loss of sexual function are prominent features. Sensory abnormalities may involve only the lower sacral and coccygeal segments or may present as complete saddle anesthesia. There is often a mixed upper and lower motor neuron deficit involving the gluteal musculature and, depending on the extent of the lesion, the lower extremities. The bulbocavernosus reflex is absent.

Spinal Cord Injury in Children

Cervical spine injuries are infrequent in children, and those that do occur frequently involve the occipito-atlantoaxial segment. This is the result of a proportionally heavier head and a higher fulcrum of flexion, laxer ligaments allowing for more mobility at C1 to C2, unfused physes, and horizontally inclined articular facets that facilitate sliding.[58] There are also a number of anatomic characteristics unique to the pediatric cervical spine that may mimic injury. These include pseudosubluxation at either C2 to C3 or C3 to C4; anterior wedging of vertebral bodies; secondary ossification centers that may mimic avulsions; variable interspinous distances; widening of the predental space (up to 5 mm); and lateral displacement of the lateral masses of C1 on C2.

There were 3,065 patients in the NEXUS database who were younger than 18 years old, 30 of whom had sustained a cervical spine injury. Only 4 of 30 injured children were younger than 9 years, and none were younger than 2 years. The decision rule correctly identified all pediatric cervical spine injury victims; however, the small number of infants and toddlers in the study precludes definitive recommendations.

Spinal Cord Injury Without Radiographic Abnormality (SCIWORA)

SCIWORA is a syndrome of neurologic injury without evidence of bony injury or malalignment on plain radiographs or CT. It is common in the pediatric population, making up 4% to 67% of all pediatric spinal injuries; it results from highly elastic ligaments and increased spinal mobility.[59] SCIWORA usually occurs in adults as the result of preexisting spondylitic changes of the cervical spine, resulting in narrow diameters of the cervical canal.

The presentation of SCIWORA ranges from complete paralysis to subjective complaints of numbness. Patients with SCIWORA have positive MRI findings ranging from cord hemorrhage or edema to intervertebral disc herniation or cord transection. MRI findings seem to correlate well with outcome: patients with transient symptoms and a normal MRI have an excellent prognosis, and those with major cord damage on MRI have an extremely poor prognosis.

Spinal Cord Injury Management

Early treatment for any spinal cord injury, incomplete or presumed complete, must address vertebral column alignment and stability and decompression of the spinal cord or nerve roots. Alignment and stability are initially attempted in the cervical region by head-traction devices. When this is not accomplished by closed techniques, operative reduction with internal fixation is considered.[60] In the thoracic region, malalignment is uncommon because of the stabilizing properties of the ribs. Thoracic injury sufficient to cause dislocation usually results in concomitant massive injury to other intrathoracic structures. Thoracic immobilization is usually accomplished by bed rest. Lumbar immobilization is similarly accomplished, but occasionally operative reduction may be necessary.

Intuitively, it would appear reasonable to decompress a compromised spinal cord or nerve root surgically. However, there is no conclusive evidence that early surgery to remove bone and disc fragments provides improved outcomes over conservative management.[60] Consequently, neurosurgical intervention in acute spinal trauma varies from center to center and is dependent on the prevailing experience of the treating physician.

Pharmacotherapy for Acute Spinal Cord Injury

A number of agents have been studied in an attempt to improve neurologic outcome following spinal cord injury, including naloxone, glucocorticoids, nimodipine, tirilazad mesylate, and GM1 ganglioside. Of these, only methylprednisolone has been found to be potentially beneficial. The proposed mechanism is that steroids

TABLE 9-11
METHYLPREDNISOLONE FOR SPINAL CORD INJURY[a]

Must be given within 8 hours of trauma, preferably within 3 hours
Bolus 30 mg/kg over 15 minutes
Continuous infusion 5.4 mg/kg/hr (within 45 minutes of bolus) for 23 hours
  or 47 hours

[a] Use is controversial.

inhibit lipid peroxidation and enhance spinal cord recovery by inhibiting the injury-induced degenerative cascade that follows.

The National Acute Spinal Cord Injury Studies (NASCIS) provided prospective, randomized data showing that patients with spinal injury from blunt trauma receiving methylprednisolone therapy within 8 hours had improved motor recovery at 6 weeks, 6 months, and 1 year[61] (Table 9-11). Contraindications to treatment include penetrating injury, pregnancy, and nerve root involvement only or cauda equina lesions. There is no benefit to initiating treatment more than 8 hours after the injury, and in fact the patients so treated may do worse with steroids than without. Critical reviews of the methodology used in the NSCIS trials have challenged their findings.[62,63] A randomized French trial using an identical treatment protocol failed to show a benefit of corticosteroid therapy.[64] At the present time, the controversy persists, and no standard of care exists.

SUMMARY

Spinal injury should be suspected in all trauma patients. Patients with moderate or severe TBI, altered mental status, or multiple trauma and fractures elsewhere should be carefully assessed for a spine or spinal cord injury. Initial diagnostic evaluation is directed at establishing baseline neurologic function and x-ray signs of spine injury. Particular attention to perianal sensation and reflexes may detect signs of function in a patient who would otherwise be classified as having a complete cord lesion. Early specific therapy is directed at immobilization and reduction of dislocations; the use of corticosteroids remains controversial. Prevention of the complications of paralysis should start at the time of initial diagnosis utilizing a multidisciplinary team approach.

REFERENCES

1. Thurman D, Guerrero J. Trends in hospitalization associated with traumatic brain injury. *JAMA* 1999;282:954–957.
2. *Guidelines for the Management of Severe Head Injury.* New York: Brain Trauma Foundation, 1995.

3. Chameides, L, Hazinski M, eds. *Textbook of Pediatric Advanced Life Support,* vol 8. Dallas: American Heart Association, 1994, p 3.
4. Teasdale G, Jennett B. Assessment of coma and impaired consciousness; a practical scale. *Lancet* 1974;4:81–83.
5. Teasdale G, Jennett B. Assessment and prognosis of coma after head injury. *Acta Neurochir* 1976;34:45–55.
6. Jennett B, et al. Severe head injuries in three countries. *J Neurol Neurosurg Psychiatry* 1977;40:291–298.
7. Stein SC, Ross SE. Mild head injury: a plea for routine early CT scanning. *J Trauma* 1992;33:11.
8. Williams D, Levin M, Howard E. Mild head injury classification. *Neurosurgery* 1990;27:422.
9. Jager T, Weiss H, Coben J, Pepe P. Traumatic brain injuries evaluated in U.S. emergency departments, 1992–1994. *Acad Emerg Med* 2000;7:134–140.
10. White BC, Krause GS. Brain injury and repair mechanisms: the potential for pharmacologic therapy in closed head trauma. *Ann Emerg Med* 1993;22:970.
11. Povlishock J. Pathobiology of traumatically induced axonal injury in animals and man. *Ann Emerg Med* 1992;22:980–986.
12. Brain Trauma Foundation. *Guidelines for Prehospital Management of Traumatic Brain Injury.* New York: Brain Trauma Foundation Press, 2000.
13. Masters SJ, et al. Skull x-ray examination after head trauma. *N Engl J Med* 1987;316:84–90.
14. Haydel MJ, et al. Indications for computed tomography in patients with minor head injury. *N Engl J Med* 2000;343:100–105.
15. Gottesfeld S, Jagoda A. Mild head trauma: appropriate diagnosis and management. *Emerg Med Practice* 2000;2:1–24.
16. Chesnut R, et al. The role of secondary brain injury in determining outcome from severe head injury. *J Trauma* 1993;34:216–222.
17. Stocchetti N, Furlan A, Volta F. Hypoxemia and arterial hypotension at the accident scene in head injury. *J Trauma* 1996;40:764–767.
18. Kokoska E, et al. Early hypotension worsens neurological outcome in pediatric patients with moderately severe head trauma. *J Pediatr Surg* 1998;33:333–338.
19. Stiell I, Wells G, Vandemheen K, et al. The Candadian CT head rule for patients with minor head injury. *Lancet* 2001;357:1391–1396.
20. Shackford SA, et al. The clinical utility of computed tomographic scanning and neurologic examination in the management of patients with minor head injuries. *J Trauma* 1992;33:385–394.
21. Nagurney JT, Borczuk P, Thomas SH. Elder patients with closed head trauma: a comparison with nonelder patients. *Acad Emerg Med* 1998;5:678–684.
22. Vilke GM, Chan TC, Guss DA. Use of a complete neurological examination to screen for significant intracranial abnormalities in minor head injury. *Am J Emerg Med* 2000;18: 159–163.
23. Meyer S, Gibb T, Jurkovich G: Evaluation and significance of the pupillary light reflex in trauma patients. *Ann Emerg Med* 1993;22:1052–1057.
24. Walsh T. *Neuro-Ophthalmology,* 3rd ed. Philadelphia: Lea & Febiger, 1992, pp 145–146.
25. Jeret JS, et al. Clinical predictors of abnormality disclosed by computed tomography after mild head trauma. *Neurosurgery* 1993;32:9–16.
26. Levin HS, et al. Serial MRI and neurobehavioral findings after mild to moderate closed head injury. *J Neurol Neurosurg Psychiatry* 1992;55:255.
27. Mendelow A, et al. Effect of mannitol on cerebral blood flow and cerebral perfusion pressure in human head injury. *J Neurosurg* 1985;63:43–48.

28. Israel R, et al. Hemodynamic effect of mannitol in a canine model of concomitant increased intracranial pressure and hemorrhagic shock. *Ann Emerg Med* 1988;17:560–565.

29. Temkin N, et al. A randomized, double-blind study of phenytoin for the prevention of post-traumatic seizures. *N Engl J Med* 1990;323:497–502.

30. American Congress of Rehabilitation Medicine. Definition of mild traumatic brain injury. *J Head Trauma Rehab* 1993;8:86–87.

31. American College of Emergency Physicians. Clinical policy: emergency department management of mild traumatic brain injury (MTBI) in adults. *Ann Emerg Med* 2002 (in press).

32. Colorado Medical Society Sports Medicine Society. *Guidelines for the Management of Concussion in Sports.* Colorado Medical Society, 1991.

33. Dikmen S, Machamer J, Konovan D, et al. Alcohol use before and after traumatic head injury. *Ann Emerg Med* 1995;26:167–176.

34. Alves W, Macciocchi S, Barth J. Postconcussive symptoms after uncomplicated mild head injury. *J Head Trauma Rehab* 1993;8:48–54.

35. Rimel R, et al. Disability caused by minor head injury. *Neurosurgery* 1981;9:221–230.

36. Rutherford WH, Merret JD, McDonald JR: Symptoms at one year following concussion from minor head injuries. *Injury* 1978;10:225.

37. Green D, Schutzmann S. Infants with isolated skull fracture: what are the clinical characteristics and do they require hospitalization? *Ann Emerg Med* 1997;30:253–258.

38. American Academy of Pediatrics. The management of minor closed head injury in children. *Pediatrics* 1999;104:1407–1415.

39. Gruskin K, Schutzman S. Head trauma in children younger than 2 years: are there predictors for complications? *Arch Pediatr Adolesc Med* 1999;153:15–20.

40. Levitt MA, et al. Biochemical markers of cerebral injury in patients with minor head trauma and ethanol intoxication. *Acad Emerg Med* 1995;2:675.

41. Spinal Cord Injury Information Network (*www.spinalcord.uab.edu*). *Spinal Cord Injury: Facts and Figures at a Glance.* June, 2000.

42. Burney RE, et al. Incidence, characteristics and outcome of spinal cord injury at trauma centers in North America. *Arch Surg* 1993;128:596–599.

43. Goldberg W, et al. Distribution and patterns of blunt traumatic cervical spine injury. *Ann Emerg Med* 2001;38:17–21.

44. Rogers WA. Fractures and dislocations of the cervical spine. *J Bone Joint Surg [Am]* 1957;39A:341–376.

45. Esce PG, Haines SJ. Acute treatment of spinal cord injury. *Curr Treat Options Neurol* 2000;2:517–524.

46. Gerling MC. Effects of cervical spine immobilization technique and laryngoscope blade selection on an unstable cervical spine in a cadaver model of intubation. *Ann Emerg Med* 2000;36:293–300.

47. Bohlman HH. Acute fractures and dislocations of the cervical spine. *J Bone Joint Surg [Am]* 1979;6IA:1119–1224.

48. Hoffman JR, et al. Validity of a set of clinical criteria to rule out injury to the cervical spine in patients with blunt trauma. *N Engl J Med* 2000;343:94–99.

49. Panacek EA, et al. Test performance of the individual NEXUS low-risk clinical screening criteria for cervical spine injury. *Ann Emerg Med* 2001;38:22–25.

50. Terrigino CA, et al. Selective indications for thoracic and lumbar radiography in blunt trauma. *Ann Emerg Med* 1995;26:126–129.

51. Blahd WH, Iserson KV, Bjelland JC. Efficacy of the posttraumatic cross table lateral view of the cervical spine. *J Emerg Med* 1985;2:243–249.

52. MacDonald RL, Schwartz ML, Mirich D, et al. Diagnosis of cervical spine injury in motor vehicle crash victims: How many x-rays are enough? *J Trauma* 1990;30:392–397.

53. Turetsky DB, et al. Technique of use of supine oblique views in acute cervical spine trauma. *Ann Emerg Med* 1993;22:685–688.

54. Pollack CV, et al. Use of flexion-extension radiographs of the cervical spine in blunt trauma. *Ann Emerg Med* 2001;38:8–11.

55. Blackmore CC, et al. Cervical spine screening with CT in trauma patients: a cost-effectiveness analysis. *Radiology* 1999;212:117–25.

56. Orrison WW, et al. Magnetic resonance imaging evaluation of acute spine trauma. *Emerg Radiol* 1995;2:120–128.

57. Stautter ES. Diagnosis and prognosis of acute cervical spinal cord injury. *Clin Orthop* 1975;112–118.

58. Orenstein JB, et al. Age and outcome in pediatric cervical spine injury: 11-year experience. *Pediatr Emerg Care* 1994;10:132–137.

59. Gupta SK, et al. Spinal cord injury without radiographic abnormality in adults. *Spinal Cord* 1999;37:726–729.

60. McDonald J. Spinal-cord injury. *Lancet* 2002;359:417–425.

61. Bracken MB, et al. A randomized, controlled trial of methylprednisolone or naloxone in the treatment of acute spinal cord injury. *N Engl J Med* 1990;322:1405.

62. Coleman WP, et al. A critical appraisal of the reporting of the National Spinal Cord Injury Studies (II and III) of methylprednisolone in acute spinal cord injury. *J Spinal Disord* 2000;13:185–99.

63. Hurlbert RJ. Methylprednisolone for acute spinal cord injury: an inappropriate standard of care. *J Neurosurg* 2000;93:1–7.

64. Pointillant V, et al. Pharmacological therapy of spinal cord injury during the acute phase. *Spinal Cord* 2000;38:71–6.

C H A P T E R

10

PSYCHOGENIC NEUROLOGIC SYNDROMES

The evaluation of patients with presumed psychogenic neurologic symptoms presents a great challenge to the skills of any physician. Because disease affecting the nervous system can manifest in a multitude of ways, differentiation of true organic from functional neurologic manifestations can, at times, be extremely difficult. Psychogenic neurologic syndromes are common, and there may be a psychogenic origin to some aspect of patients presenting symptoms.[1] The term *psychogenic neurologic syndrome* is used to describe a collection of psychologic disorders presenting with neurologic signs and symptoms that have no identifiable organic etiology within the nervous system. They have also been termed pseudoneurologic syndromes[2] or "functional" disorders.

For the purposes of this chapter, some basic definitions are needed.[3] The term *malingering* is used to describe a willful, deliberate imitation or exaggeration of illness that is intended to deceive others for a consciously desired end. Malingering is divided into three types. The first is pure malingering, in which there is not even a presumed organic basis for the symptoms and signs. The second is partial malingering or exaggeration. In this condition, which is a much more common presentation to physicians, there is an expansion of true disability or symptoms that would ordinarily be attributed to a documented organic problem. The third, false imputation, occurs when a patient may indeed have a real disease; however, the symptoms described are not those that could reasonably be attributed to that disease entity.

By contrast, the term *hysteria* has been used to imply that a patient is not conscious of the unreality of their symptoms. This determination can be difficult. The range of possible symptoms is as broad as all of neurology. Although the term "hysteria" is no longer used in a number of official diagnostic classifications, it is in common use in practice and in medical literature.[4] To the extent that the term does not convey the psychiatric nature of the illness, it should be avoided and the term *conversion disorder* used. Signs and symptoms of conversion disorder have been labeled hysteria in the past.[5] Only those syndromes common to the emergency department (ED) or acute outpatient settings are addressed. One should be careful in applying the label of conversion disorder, as patients initially so labeled are not uncommonly later diagnosed with an organic illness.[6] Table 10-1 lists some medical conditions that can easily be mistaken for conversion disorder. When a language or cultural barrier exists, be especially careful. Table 10-2 lists key aspects of the *Diagnostic and Statistical Manual,* 4th ed (DSM-IV) criteria for the diagnosis of conversion disorder.[7] It is helpful not to be biased by the preliminary perceptions of others, as such bias can result in a "chain of presumption" that the problem is not an organic one.[8]

In this chapter, emphasis is placed on a mode of examination and a style of practice that will allow one to gather the information necessary to render an appropriate diagnosis while at the same time establishing a trusting therapeutic relationship with the patient. It may be appropriate in selected circumstances to obtain a psychiatry or neurology referral.[9]

It cannot be overemphasized that the role of any physician faced with patients presenting with possible psychogenic complaints should be that of making the differential diagnosis between two varieties of illness. One must view the differentiation between two legitimate illnesses (psychogenic and organic) in somewhat the same manner as a physician would approach the differential diagnosis between appendicitis and gastroenteritis. The physician's attitude should be that of a caring problem-solver. The communication of this attitude will go far in establishing a relationship with the patient and significant others, which will enable one to do the most good for that patient.

TABLE 10-1

MEDICAL CONDITIONS WITH FEATURES SUGGESTING CONVERSION DISORDER

Guillian-Barré syndrome
Multiple sclerosis
Nonconvulsive status epilepticus
Pure sensory stroke
Ciquatera poisoning
Hypoglycemia
Electrolyte disorders
Brain/spinal abscess
Dystonic-type medication reaction

TABLE 10-2

DIAGNOSTIC CRITERIA FOR 300.11 CONVERSION DISORDER

A. One or more symptoms or deficits affecting voluntary motor or sensory function that suggest a neurologic or other medical condition

B. Psychological factors are judged to be associated with the symptom or deficit because the initiation or exacerbation of the symptom or deficit is preceded by conflicts or other stressors.

C. The symptom or deficit is not intentionally produced or feigned (as in Factitious Disorder or Malingering).

D. The symptom or deficit cannot, after appropriate investigation, be fully explained by a general medical condition, or by the direct effects of a substance, or as a culturally sanctioned behavior or experience.

E. The symptom or deficit causes clinically significant distress or impairment in social, occupational, or other important areas of functioning or warrants medical evaluation.

F. The symptom or deficit is not limited to pain or sexual dysfunction, does not occur exclusively during the course of Somatization Disorder, and is not better accounted for by another mental disorder.

Specify type of symptom or deficit:
With Motor Symptom or Deficit
With Sensory Symptom or Deficit
With Seizures or Convulsions
With Mixed Presentation

GENERAL APPROACH

Physicians must communicate to patients, through actions and words, that they are the patients' advocate. A physician's attitude must be one of trying to do the best that can be done for the patient. As in other parts of medicine, this will be accomplished by firmly establishing a diagnosis while at the same time developing a trusting relationship.

Open-ended questions can be the most productive. Specifics must be elicited, all of which will be covered under specific subject headings later in the chapter. Frequently, when patients are allowed to respond to an open-ended question, they reveal data that would not otherwise have been elicited. Asking what the circumstances were and what was going on in the patient's life at the time the symptoms occurred will allow patients the option of expressing what is uppermost in their minds, thereby furnishing facts that might have gone unsuspected.

A functional neurologic diagnosis should be based on the demonstration of positive signs. The patient must demonstrate neurologic signs and symptoms that are inconsistent with the functioning of the nervous system,[2] thereby allowing examiners to best differentiate organic from nonorganic illness. This presupposes a relatively detailed knowledge of the anatomy and physiology of the nervous system. It also presupposes that patients lack the sophisticated knowledge of the nervous system that physicians possess. At times such might not be the case, because some patients can be extremely sophisticated in their knowledge. Because knowledge of anatomic and physiologic mechanisms in neurologic illness is incomplete and current methods of objective verification have limitations, a general attitude of caution is preferable in diagnostic evaluation.

Early in the encounter with the patient, the examiner must assess this level of sophistication in order to pursue an appropriate line of questioning and examination. The positive signs that are inconsistent with the functions of the nervous system will be the academic substance of this chapter. The method of obtaining these signs has more to do with the art of medicine.

For the examiner to convince the patient and everyone involved that a careful opinion has been rendered, a focused history and a detailed, relevant, professional neurologic exam are important. It is only when the patient is taken seriously that the family will recognize that the physician is carefully pursuing the problem.

The physician must constantly ascertain the level of certainty of the information obtained. For example, the sensory examination is primarily subjective. There are limitations to asking nonmedical first-hand observers to describe what may be a relatively sophisticated neurologic event. At times, first-hand observers and witnesses, such as emergency medical technicians, paramedics, and bystanders, may render information that is much more important than is any neurologic test. Phone calls to relatives, other physicians, and so on may provide a great deal of useful information, as can a review of past records.

The neurologic examination should be conducted with attention to certain details. The reasons for this are many. For most patients the neurologic exam is something outside their usual experience. It is common for them to realize that injured extremities will be palpated and chests will be auscultated. However, the neurologic exam is something different. The tapping of reflexes, observation of coordinated motor acts, and ophthalmologic exam are unusual experiences. It is a legitimate use of this aspect of the neurologic exam to communicate to the patient that the examiner does truly possess a sophisticated knowledge of the nervous system, which will in turn lead to trust and confidence in the examining physician.

Although the subject matter of this chapter is that of neurologic syndromes, one must always be alert to exclude organic, but unrelated, medical conditions. When an organic medical condition is discovered, the patient may simply drop all the functional complaints, having adopted a genuine focus of medical attention.

The best attitude for the physician to adopt is one of intellectual humility. The most experienced and concerned physician will at times label a syndrome as functional only to find it attributed to an organic problem at a later date. Diseases of the nervous system and their presentations are so variable that 100% accuracy is impossible. One must remember the words of William Beaumont, "Even if the story we are told is a tangle of impossibility, copied from the repertoire of the father of lies, and worthy of the mother of invention, it may have a genuine pathological basis."[10]

The examiner should be aware of the limitations of the clinical neurologic exam. Testing of coordination, motor function, and strength is done on a relatively crude basis. These modalities are not tested in a repetitive, strictly reproducible fashion. Confrontation visual field testing, for example, is crude by comparison with that obtained by a tangent-screen apparatus. The sensory exam is likewise a highly subjective examination, and all exams are done at one moment in time in the course of a patient's illness.

Most experienced examiners have encountered patients with large nervous system lesions who had a normal exam relative to the functional area of the nervous system involved.[5] This is not to say that the neurologic exam is a poor starting point for neurologic evaluation. There is nothing more informative, cost-effective, or valuable to the physician than a carefully obtained history and properly performed neurologic examination.

One final point relative to the neurologic examination is worth emphasis. In general, patients who are malingering will wish no or very few examinations. They are consciously trying to imitate a neurologic deficit, which involves intense concentration for reproducibility. Therefore, if one gets a sense from a patient that he or she does not wish to be examined, this may be the first indication of malingering. This is in contrast to the patient with a conversion disorder, who, because they lack knowledge of the unreality of their symptoms, are not aware that they may sometimes present with conflicting and shifting neurologic deficits (Table 10-3).

PSYCHOGENIC NUMBNESS

Numbness is a difficult neurologic symptom to evaluate. It is subjective and frequently vague. Each patient has his or her own idea of what it means. By numbness, most physicians mean an area of altered sensation. Examiners clearly separate the sensory functions from the motor functions. Patients, however, frequently do not separate these two functions. Examiners must be certain early on in the interaction that they and the patient have the same perception of altered sensation and not some other neurologic symptom.

Patients with numbness on an organic basis are usually specific about the modality involved and the location, as opposed to patients with psychogenic complaints, in

TABLE 10-3

CLUES TO PSYCHOGENIC ORIGIN

Indifferent attitude
Bizarre symptoms
Fluctuating, suggestible, or alternating deficits
Past history of psychogenic symptoms
Role model for symptoms
Temporal psychological proximity for stressor

whom the area of numbness may be vague or shifting, or not clearly defined in the patient's mind. One must establish whether the patient feels the area of numbness is that of complete anesthesia, or of analgesia (meaning lack of painful sensation), or some other alteration of sensory modality. Precise definition of the involved area is essential. There are several classic psychogenic locations of numbness (Table 10-4).

In taking the history, one should note the time course of the symptom and what actions were taken by the patient. An indifferent attitude to the sudden onset of large areas of numbness, possibly associated with other neurologic symptoms, can be seen in functional patients. The mode of onset and particularly a history of trauma should be elicited. It is during this time that one asks about the circumstances under which the event took place, thereby allowing the patient a means of expressing feelings related to an event that may have caused psychological trauma. Asking how a problem has affected the patient will give further clues to a psychogenic complaint. Patients may say that it kept them from caring for a child or performing a specific task. Without asking such specific questions, physicians might be unaware of the significance of a psychogenic complaint. Asking relatives similar questions is a valuable tool, because relatives might be able to relate how this deficit has impaired the patient's ability to interact with others.

The key to the neurologic exam is observation. One first notes the affect of the patient. What is the attitude expressed toward what could potentially be a significant neurologic illness? As mentioned before, an indifferent attitude, seen frequently in conversion disorder, can be a clue.

The neurologic examination, excluding the sensory exam, should be performed first, to isolate the complaint and allow one to examine the sensory system indirectly without drawing attention to the exam. The examiner realizes that motor and sensory exams are linked as a functional unit and in areas such as reflex arcs. The examiner, but not the patient, realizes that many sensory functions have been found to be normal prior to a more formal sensory exam. Certain classic neurologic findings, which one should begin to elicit and document, are inconsistent with the normal functioning of the nervous system. Although split vibratory sensory loss, with the lack of reporting of vibration on one side of a bilateral structure such as the cranium, has been classically associated with psychogenic illness, infrequently patients with organic disease report this phenomenon.[11]

TABLE 10-4

SIGNS OF PSYCHOGENIC NUMBNESS (see text)

Split vibratory senses
Touch response when not touched
Motion but not position sense
Pin withdrawal
Glove-and-stocking anesthesia stopping at joint lines
Hemigenitalia-hemirectum anesthesia
Crossed interlocked finger test

Extremely unsophisticated patients can be examined with a technique in which they are asked to close their eyes and respond when they feel they have been touched with a "yes" and a "no" when they feel they have not been touched. The examiner then proceeds to touch various parts of the body. Patients with a psychogenic complaint may promptly report "no" immediately after an area has been touched, indicating that they had some sensation there but are not yet willing to say they felt it. This obviously suggests that one is dealing with a very unsophisticated patient, so the test must be done rather quickly and not repeated very often, for even the most unsophisticated patient will realize its contradictory nature.

A more sophisticated variety of this touch-response test can be done when testing position sense. Classically, when position sense is tested, the proximal interphalangeal joint of the finger is fixed, and then the examiner either elevates or depresses the distal interphalangeal joint of the finger. With their eyes closed, patients are instructed to respond with an "up," a "down," or an "I don't know" with respect to the movement of the distal phalanx. If they respond promptly "I don't know" to every position change of the distal phalanx, they are at least reporting that they have intact motion sense and touch.[12] Motion and position sense are very closely aligned in the nervous system, so the patients have demonstrated that they do have motion sense.

Withdrawal to a pinprick is another test. The patient's withdrawal from a brief prick at least demonstrates that the reflex arc is intact. If there is associated verbalization of pain, then that sensation has at least reached consciousness. Some altered sensation may be present, but at least one has documented the presence of some sensation; at this point the patient may realize that sensation has been demonstrated and reverse the complaint.

One other classic pattern of sensory loss is that of the glove-and-stocking distribution. Although glove-and-stocking distribution sensory loss is commonly seen with peripheral neuropathies, these are not of acute onset, and they do not stop abruptly at joint lines, as they often do with psychogenic complaints. There is no anatomic sensory boundary at the elbow, wrist, or shoulder. Acute vascular insufficiency to an extremity could give this pattern, but it should be obvious clinically.

Physicians should tailor their sensory exam to what they predict will be the most productive modalities to test, since it is impossible to test all of them all the time. It is sometimes useful to do sensory testing on the interlocked crossed fingers[13] (Figure 10-1). The midline sensory supply of the trunk can be tested. There is some crossover to either side of the midline, and patients with organic lesions will usually have some preservation of sensation over the midline and then gradual diminution after that. Sensory loss directly at the midline is uncommon in organic lesions.

PSYCHOGENIC WEAKNESS AND PARALYSIS

A psychogenic complaint of weakness is common. The examiner should be careful to differentiate between weakness and numbness and should be aware of the patient's

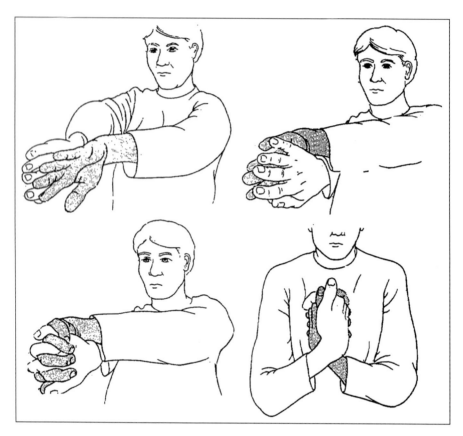

FIGURE 10-1 Crossed fingers test.

meaning. Although the physician may initially think of weakness in terms of specific anatomic locations, or nerve distributions, patients may have a concept of weakness as a generalized loss of energy, or neurasthenia. They may feel there is a lack of energy throughout the body.

The history from a patient complaining of weakness should be obtained in a way similar to that described for numbness. The physician should first attempt to find out what the patient means with respect to the paralysis, i.e., was it complete or partial, what the time course was, and what functions were lost and what functions were preserved. Frequently patients with weakness on a psychogenic basis are unable to perform certain acts (for instance, picking up a pen and writing one's name or picking up a child to care for them), whereas other motor actions that require use of the same muscles are preserved. Questioning the patient concerning trauma and especially emotional trauma is important.

Observation of the patient is again the key to the neurologic examination. Watching the patient undress, sign the chart, move about the room, or gesture during the exam is clearly superior to the formal muscle strength testing that is a usual part of the neurologic exam, because the patient is somewhat distracted by questions and routines.

A classic sign of psychogenic weakness is that of *giveway weakness* (Table 10-5). It is difficult to imitate the true mild decrease in muscle strength that accompanies a true organic deficit. The patient may try to simulate something less than full strength. When formal muscle strength resistance testing is done, one feels a cogwheel or ratchet-type loss of strength. If examiners vary resistance continually over a wide range, they will find at times that their most powerful effort cannot overcome the patient's muscle; at other times, a very weak effort can overcome it. This is what is meant by giveway weakness. One commonly sees a giveway weakness in a painful limb as an organic cause. Frequently, when the extremity is dropped, such as back down to the patient's lap or examining table, it falls at less than the speed that would be dictated by gravity alone. It also will sometimes fall into a very natural position into the lap.

There are means of testing cooperation and effort and not specifically the degree of power in the muscle. The first is the abduction test. To perform the test as diagrammed (Figure 10-2), patients are asked to abduct their legs while lying supine. This is a bilaterally innervated function, and if they are truly trying to move the supposed weak leg, the examiner will feel the supposed normal leg making an effort. This is also the basis of Hoover's sign. In this test, the examiner's hands are placed beneath the heels of the patient, as in Figure 10-3, and the patient is asked to raise the supposedly weak leg. The examiner should feel increased pressure under the good leg as the patient presses down to counterbalance an effort to raise the supposed weak leg. Failure to feel this is a sign that the patient is not making a conscious effort. It must be emphasized that the most these tests reveal is that the patient is not cooperating with the exam. Whether the patient is truly weak in addition to this cannot be determined by these tests.

Other motor signs are occasionally seen in the patient who complains of weakness and/or difficulty with coordination. They are referred to as astasia-abasia: the patient's loss of coordination represents a wild flinging motion of the arms and possibly the legs. The patient tries to walk or stand on one foot with large flinging motions of the arms but does not fall. This actually demonstrates superior bal-

TABLE 10-5 ———————————————————————————

SIGNS OF PSYCHOGENIC WEAKNESS

Weakness of motion but not specific muscles
Giveway weakness
Abduction test
Hoover's sign
Astasia-abasia
Falling toward safety
Contraction of antagonist

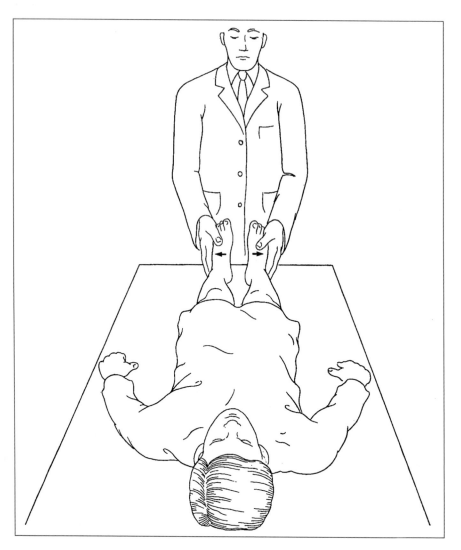

FIGURE 10-2 Abduction test.

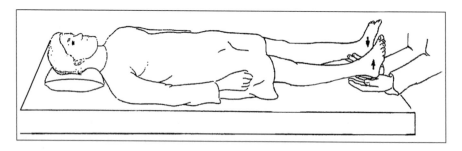

FIGURE 10-3 Hoover's sign.

ance, muscle strength, and coordination, as opposed to the poor results the patient may have wished to demonstrate. Psychogenic gait problems are characterized by exaggerated efforts, extreme slowness, variability, and unusual or uneconomic postures.[14]

Frequently a patient with a psychogenic weakness will fall only to the side of the examiner or a supportive relative or friend. Falling only toward the stretcher or toward the door of the examination room is also seen. When placed in the middle of the room, such patients seem to walk well until they approach a "safe" object, and then they fall and grasp the object. The fall may be theatrical.

Another sign seen in patients with supposed weakness in one leg is that of actually dragging a foot as if it were made of lead. It is as though the patient were pressing the foot very tightly to the floor.

Testing the action of the sternocleidomastoid muscle in turning the chin to the opposite side has somewhat limited applicability. A patient with a hysterical paralysis involving the right side of the body may not realize that the right sternocleidomastoid turns the head to the left. Motion in that direction may be strong, and motion in the other direction may be weak.

An important sign that can be demonstrated when doing individual muscle strength testing is that the patient is actively contracting the antagonistic muscle to the action being requested. By palpating the antagonistic muscle, the examiner can demonstrate good strength in the opposing muscle. If one then asks for the antagonistic action to be performed, the patient will contract the muscle that was supposedly weak.

The examiner must obviously be selective in choosing which one of these signs to try to elicit. The signs should be elicited once or at most twice and not repeated, because their usefulness tends to decline with time as the patient becomes more familiar with the tests. The tests should be performed with an attitude that they are routine, not to somehow trick the patient but simply to reveal the nature of the problem.

PSYCHOGENIC COMA AND DISORDERS OF CONSCIOUSNESS

Coma and alterations of consciousness are common as psychogenic problems (Table 10-6). The disorders are often an embellishment on a mild organic deficit, or they may occur in the setting of other, serious diseases. For example, mild alcohol or other drug intoxication may be embellished to the point of coma when in reality it may produce minimal lethargy. There is no other area in which first-hand observers are as helpful in obtaining a history, especially if the patient has awakened upon arrival in the ED. One should obviously search for a history of diabetes, drug ingestion, seizure disorder, and trauma, both physical and emotional. There is also no other time when one can lose rapport faster with the patient than when conducting the coma examination unless meticulous care is exercised. The patient and significant others must place trust in the examiner as a caring physician in order to arrive at a reasonable disposition. Efforts to "awaken" the patient that involve

TABLE 10-6

SIGNS OF PSYCHOGENIC COMA

Trance-like states
Normal postures and tone
Voluntary eyelid closure
Bell's phenomenon
Normal involuntary movements
Fixed downward gaze on opening the eyes

painful stimuli or other degrading or humiliating procedures only serve to weaken whatever limited therapeutic relationship existed at the start. The examiner must obviously ensure the patient's airway and circulation prior to other examination, because what on first brief encounter may appear to be a functional deficit could in fact turn out to be a true coma.

Several important clues to disorders of consciousness can alert the examiner to a psychogenic possibility. Patients may be in a trance-like state in which their eyes are open. They seem to be unresponsive and may have alternating laughing and crying spells. They may have unresponsiveness but purposeful movements. If one suspects embellishment on a true deficit and feels that laboratory analysis may be in order for toxocologic screens, glucose, or other laboratory work, it is expeditious to obtain these tests very early in the evaluation, because later the patient may not be cooperative. It cannot be emphasized strongly enough that using painful stimuli and other provocative procedures, such as ammonia capsules, Foley catheters, needle punctures, and so on to awaken the patient with psychogenic unresponsiveness is unproductive and jeopardizes the caring relationship that the physician should wish to establish. Noxious procedures may turn a patient who was benignly comatose into a belligerent and physically aggressive person. It may also be interpreted by the family as lack of respect and sensitivity toward the patient.

In many patients, unresponsiveness on a psychogenic basis can be established by pulling open the eyelids and observing the eyes. Once the patient has made eye contact with the physician, he or she may begin to respond and talk. Sometimes only the sclera is seen, thus demonstrating Bell's phenomenon. This voluntary eyelid resistance to opening causes the eyes to turn up in the head, and one can then see only the sclera. If this has not occurred, the physician can examine the pupils and check extraocular movements. It is frequently with this maneuver alone that patients can no longer maintain unresponsiveness; once they establish eye contact, they will proceed to become "responsive." Patients may always look to the side away from the examiner. This has been described as the eye's consistently being deviated toward the side of the bed.[13] Also, the slow, very gradual, and often incomplete eyelid closure that occurs in truly comatose patients when the lids are released from the open position cannot be simulated.

Observation alone may alert the physician that the patient may not be truly unconscious. Patients may have purposeful motor movements when being transferred from stretcher to bed or x-ray table. They may grasp at personal objects. They may cross their legs, set their hands behind their head, or assume other voluntary postures. If the examiner feels certain that there has been no trauma to the cervical spine, sitting patients up may cause them to become responsive. Dropping the hand onto the face is a relatively poor test. Patients may in fact allow the hand to strike the face. A better test is to see that they actually have voluntary limb resistance, or that the hand, when dropped, falls too slowly. Although intact slow- and fast-phase nystagmus on ice-water caloric testing indicates that the patient is physiologically awake, it is usually very uncomfortable and unnecessary.

Simply talking to patients in a normal conversational tone and establishing oneself as a physician is important. Asking them to cooperate so that you might help them establishes the fact that you are on the side of the patient and that you understand they are not unconscious. Moreover, it illustrates that you know they are troubled and that you are there to try to help with whatever kind of problem they have, regardless of its nature.

Minimally provocative tests, such as nasal tickle, will provoke patients to use their extremities in a coordinated and purposeful way and to open their eyes. Once eye contact has been made, patients can be further examined. Frequently a brief discussion with patients whose eyes are closed about the fact that the physician is aware they may be having some problems is useful. This can be followed by a brief period of observation, which will allow patients the dignity of reversing their "coma." Allowing patients their dignity while performing all these maneuvers strengthens the therapeutic alliance with the physician.

If there is sufficient doubt about whether the embellishment on a mild deficit may be organic or not, one should treat patients as if they have true coma or disorders of consciousness. As mentioned above, laboratory specimens can be obtained early and then held should the examiner find it necessary to analyze them. Performing a general physical examination sufficient to exclude a true unrelated medical problem such as the result of trauma is important.

Even in the best of hands of the most caring physician, some patients deprived of their "comatose" state may become uncooperative and leave the ED without the physician's having had the opportunity to document the fact that such patients had no physical evidence of a serious condition.

PSEUDOSEIZURES

Patients who present with pseudoseizures have varying levels of sophistication and knowledge of what constitutes a true seizure. Frequently pseudoseizures, also termed nonepileptic seizures or psychogenic nonepileptic seizures,[15] are an embellishment on a true seizure disorder, which makes evaluation even more difficult. Ten to fifty percent of patients with pseudoseizures have an underlying seizure disorder.[16] The neurologic literature is clear on the point that many varieties of abnormal behavior can be attributed to a seizure disorder. Conversely, there are almost no manifestations of true epilepsy that cannot be simulated in conversion disorder or malingering.

Usually, however, pseudoseizures are very unsophisticated and easy to diagnose. There are certainly patients, usually with an underlying seizure disorder, who present with pseudoseizures that are difficult even for the most experienced examiner to differentiate. The vast majority of all pseudoseizures, however, are very unsophisticated and are easy for an examiner with sufficient experience in observing true seizure disorders to differentiate.

It is important for the physician to observe the episode. Without direct observation, it is difficult to make the differentiation. If one must resort to a first-hand observer, there are several areas to be questioned. The nature of the shaking movements is the most important. The position of the eyes in the head and other associated events such as verbalizations are also important subjects to cover. It may be difficult for observers to either describe or imitate the motions of a seizure. Frequently there is embarrassment at trying to imitate what seems to be a bizzare act, but given some encouragement and possibly a brief demonstration of what the physician is looking for will allow the observer to differentiate the nature of the shaking movements. The true tonic-clonic movements seen with a major motor seizure are frequently not very well imitated. The nature of the shaking movement may be such that there is a wild flinging of the arms; frequently there are purposeful movements and goal-oriented behavior. Partially treated organic seizure disorders, on the other hand, may be somewhat "abortive." There is no goal-oriented behavior in a true seizure disorder. Grabbing the physician or other medical personnel is not a manifestation of an organic seizure disorder. Also, assaultive behavior is not a seizure disorder. Asynchronous movements of the extremities and pelvic thrusting are unusual in organic seizures,[17] as is weeping[18] and side-to-side head movements.[19] Although it is true that temporal lobe seizures can result in stereotyped and somewhat aggressive, repetitive behavior, goal-directed behavior is not a true seizure (Table 10-7).

Shaking movements in pseudoseizures are at times tremulous, such as those of impending DTs or those with a fever. Observation of the eyes with pseudoseizures does not reveal the usual pupillary changes that may accompany true seizures. During a pseudoseizure patients will frequently look directly at the observer or examiner. At other times they will speak on request during the seizure. Although it is true that focal motor seizures can present without loss of consciousness and without impairment of mentation and speech, it is impossible for any generalized tonic-clonic seizure to have preservation of speech or to have speech very shortly after brief

TABLE 10-7

SIGNS OF PSEUDOSEIZURES

Purposeful movements
Flinging movements
Harmful movements
Theatrical movements
Preservation of voluntary speech

episodes of shaking. It is somewhat difficult to describe the exact nature of a pseudo-seizure, but one is usually aware of a theatrical quality to the spell. It usually happens only when there are observers present. A pseudoseizure frequently may involve something that will look potentially harmful to the patient, such as slamming the arm against the wall. It frequently happens at the time of emotional upset, and questioning observers about this can be extremely important. Also, patients may not be aware that consciousness is usually impaired during a seizure. Simply talking to them, telling them that the seizure will soon abate, or asking them to perform coordinated motor action during a seizure reveals the true nature of the spell. Patients with pseudoseizures may bite their tongue or become incontinent of urine. Accidental injuries do not rule out pseudoseizures. They are usually done by patients with organic seizure disorders who know that after a true seizure they sometimes have a small bite mark on their tongue or have been incontinent of urine. Incontinence of stool is extremely unusual in pseudoseizures, because patients do not have very much voluntary control over the passage of stool. Cyanosis is obviously a strong sign of organic seizure, but brief breath-holding spells may be found with pseudoseizures.

As with the other disorders previously described, one should consider a true, unrelated emergent medical condition. Although simultaneous electroencephalography (EEG) and video recording is outside the provenance of initial evaluations, it may be helpful in difficult cases of suspected pseudoseizures.[20] If the patient is on anticonvulsants, it may be necessary to check the anticonvulsant level and to discuss care and follow-up with the patient's personal physician.

PSYCHOGENIC VISUAL COMPLAINTS

Psychogenic visual complaints are unusual as an isolated event. The physician should establish whether the patient means that the visual loss is complete or partial and whether it involves one or both eyes, because the examination will be different depending on such initial history. Malingered blindness is usually unilateral, and hysterical blindness is usually bilateral (Table 10-8).

Psychogenic visual complaints are frequently embellished on a partial deficit. The patient may have decreased vision owing to some organic problem and then "lose" vision completely. The best and easiest test is again observation. Patients who

TABLE 10-8
SIGNS OF PSYCHOGENIC BLINDNESS

Intact optokinetic nystagmus
Threat response
Looking away from examiner
Lack of concern to protect self from harm
Inability to write name legibly
Inability to touch finger to finger

are truly blind in both eyes will protect themselves from harm. They will not walk purposely into doors, will not walk quickly about a room, and will act as any other person would when awakened from sleep in a dark room, i.e., take a wide-based stance with hands out protecting themselves from harm and seek other sensory input to get about in their environment. They will look directly at someone when talking to them, using the tracking function of the auditory system, which is so good that a truly blind patient can almost look one in the eye. A truly blind person can look at his or her own hand. The classic finding of someone feigning blindness is that of walking into objects to cause oneself minimal harm.

There are patients with denial of blindness on an organic basis, so-called Anton's syndrome, who may initially present like those with a psychogenic syndrome. This is a cortical blindness. If a patient is complaining of a partial deficit, the tests cannot be used as well. However, noticing whether the patient gazes in the direction of the examiner can still be used as a sign. Threat response, elicited by moving the examiner's hand toward the eye, can be used to demonstrate some intact vision.[21] However, one should be careful that they are not eliciting a corneal reflex by a gust of air on the patient's cornea. Optokinetic nystagmus testing is more sophisticated and can be extremely useful. To perform the test, a striped object or revolving drum is placed in front of the patients' eyes; if they have intact vision, their eyes will have nystagmoid jerks. This cannot be faked and essentially cannot be suppressed except by a very select group of individuals, such as ballerinas and ice skaters, who perform rotatory movements and can at the same time suppress optokinetic nystagmus.

Other highly sophisticated tests can be done for the hysterical patient's or malingerer's visual complaints; these are beyond the scope of a preliminary examination. It is, however, useful to know that these can be done in the eventual evaluation. Different-colored lenses are placed over both eyes, and reading material is presented in two different colors. The patient is then asked to take a test based on the facts presented. There are other similarly sophisticated tests with prisms to isolate the images of the two eyes, in addition to EEG tests of visual-evoked response.

The examination should include the pupils and the position and motion of the eyes. It is unusual for a truly blind eye to have a direct response to light; however, one can have a cortical lesion and be blind on a cortical basis with preservation of pupillary reflexes. Pupillary responses may be altered by instillation of drops in malingerers. Drug-induced mydriasis is virtually the only cause for a dilated pupil not to respond to pilocarpine. Patients with psychogenic loss of visual acuity may be able to read only the top line on the Snellen chart regardless of how far they stand from it.

Psychogenic diplopia may present as monocular diplopia, which is found only in extremely unusual organic lesions,[6] such as dislocation of the lens, either artificially implanted or natural.

Psychogenic Hearing Loss

Psychogenic hearing loss is an uncommon problem in an acute care setting. It may be part of a "pansensory" or "hemisensory" loss. These occur when patients have loss of feeling, smell, vision, taste, hearing, and movement on one side of the body. This obviously cannot happen on an organic basis. Psychogenic hearing loss is a common malingerer's problem and has been common in both military and civilian circumstances. Again, there are highly sophisticated tests to determine the extent of hearing loss, which would not be done in an initial exam, but several general principles can be applied in the examination. Truly deaf people try to develop some sensory input from their environment. They will attend to the examiner's face and lips. Whether they can lip read or not, they will try to get sensory input. Patients who cannot hear, and who stare in another direction and appear to be ignoring someone, are not trying to get that sensory input. Unilateral hearing loss usually results in turning of the good ear toward the examiner. This is such a natural phenomenon that the lack of it may be a clue that there is no hearing loss. Patients with true long-standing hearing loss may raise their voice.

There are sophisticated tests in which the two ears are isolated with stereophonic headphones, information is presented to either or both ears, and the patient is then asked to take a test based on that information. It is sufficient to know that the tests exist and can be performed, if needed, in the evaluation of the patient.

SMELL AND TASTE

Aberrations of or loss of smell and taste are extremely uncommon as an isolated psychogenic complaint. Irritating substances, such as ammonia or acetic acid, do not test smell but are really perceived by the fifth cranial nerve because they are an irritant in the nose. Complete lack of taste requires bilateral seventh, ninth, and tenth nerve deficits, which is clearly a devastating neurologic insult. The most common cause of decreased taste is decreased smell, because most of our perception of taste is associated with smell. This will not be dealt with further because of the rarity of its presentation.

SPEECH

Disorders of speech are common in psychogenic syndromes, particularly in conversion disorders. As mentioned in the motor system examination discussion, patients may have a concept of the nervous system malfunction that simulates a lack of energy, or neurasthenia. They feel that they cannot speak in a full voice, but only whisper, as seen in soap-opera death-bed scenes. There is no neurologic deficit that results in patients' whispering; it actually involves no less energy to whisper than it does to speak.

Hysterical patients may move their mouth, but no sound will come out or they may only whisper. Sometimes it can be mentioned to the patients that the physician perceives that they have some difficulty with speaking and that perhaps if they talked in whispers he or she might be able to help them further. The examiner can then obtain an entire history in whispers. Sometimes there will be no speech, or there will be a very abrupt onset and termination of the ability to speak. Occasionally there is stuttering, which again does not have an organic neurologic deficit as its cause.[22] The speech may be very slow or garbled or sound like baby talk. Although it is sometimes difficult to differentiate these disorders of speech from true dysphasia or aphasia, for the most part it is not a difficult differentiation. The patient with a true aphasia will try to speak.

DISPOSITION

Once a diagnosis of a psychogenic complaint has been made (which may be easy), the most difficult part of the encounter with the patient begins: the disposition. It must be emphasized that the diagnosis must be based on positive findings that are inconsistent with known knowledge of the nervous system. One must have established a relationship of trust and caring with the patient and their family so that opinions, once rendered, will be taken seriously. The opinion that will be rendered is frequently unpopular with both the patient and the family.

One can separate the disposition into several categories based on the reason for the psychogenic complaint. Obvious malingerers can sometimes be allowed to simply reverse their story without losing face. A brief mention of some contradictory facts or a demonstration during the examination to such patients of a contradictory fact will allow them to realize that the complaint is on a nonorganic basis. The examiner usually need not confront such patients. Simply suggesting the fact that the symptom will be resolved very quickly or that it will not be a problem will allow patients to reverse their story and preserve their dignity. Sometimes a brief period of observation is all that is required, with the encouraging report of the physician that all seems to be well, thus allowing patients to then reverse the problem on their own terms. If this is insufficient, it is not inappropriate to seek an opinion from another physician. It is extremely important to let patients know that all the records obtained during any encounter will be available to anyone who will see them so that they are given the feeling that the medical system is maintaining records and that nothing about the encounter, no matter how contradictory, will ever be lost to anyone who is looking into the problem. This alone may discourage the patient from pursuing a malingered complaint.

Frequently one must simply explain what has been observed, without drawing a conclusion. You must state that as a careful physician and a concerned examiner, you have examined your patient and to the best of your ability cannot document a problem that might cause a complaint. If a physician has established rapport with a patient and has done a careful exam, then the truth of the matter (that he or she is unable to document a problem) is all that can be said. It is obviously clear to both the physician and the patient that this does not mean it is impossible for the problem to exist. A problem may exist that the physician is simply unable to uncover with an honest attempt. Such problems are frequently difficult to deal with in disposition, and it is not uncommon that a second examination by a different examiner must be obtained before a diagnosis is accepted or an organic one made.

Embellishment on true deficit is one of the most common settings seen and the most difficult one in which to establish a diagnosis. Patients are seeking to have a disease, and once they are given one they may let go of all the parts that do not fit that disease. Sometimes a brief discussion of what can be explained on the basis of their illness and what cannot be explained will encourage them to simply drop the embellished symptoms and pursue the true organic parts of their illness. Treat what can be treated and call to the attention of the patient what specific symptoms will be treated. Mention should be made of the fact that there are components to the complaint that cannot fit known knowledge of the nervous system. Again, seeking consultation, arranging for follow-up, and letting patients know that all records will be available to other examining physicians are important parts of the disposition. The obviously non-organic patient is sometimes the easiest to diagnose. The diagnosis of functional neurologic complaint can be made at times within seconds. However, the disposition becomes extremely difficult. Patients may agree to a combined workup that is neurologic and psychiatric. It is rare that patients with acute conversion disorder will have their disposition settled and their problem sufficiently evaluated on a brief outpatient basis. Hospitalization is sometimes necessary in some settings, to arrive at an equitable disposition for such patients. Patients who are in coma on a psychogenic basis and allow various humiliating procedures to be performed upon them truly have a serious illness. The illness may not be an organic one as we currently understand it, but it is serious and it probably will not be resolved by allowing them to leave the care of the physician.

TREATMENT

Treatment of psychogenic neurologic disorders is beyond the scope of this text. It is rare that a psychogenic neurologic disorder is the sole manifestation of a patient's problems. It may be appropriate to refer a patient to certain resources to deal with other problems, i.e., social, psychiatric, substance abuse, and so on. These resources vary with location and medical setting but may include psychiatrists, psychologists, social workers, and counselors, in addition to the patients' physicians. Even though the psychogenic syndrome seen may be only one facet of the patients' spectrum of problems, they may be most amenable to intervention following an acute episode, so that efforts to direct them to therapy may be rewarding. A precise psychiatric diagnosis is rarely made in the acute care setting and is rarely necessary.

SUMMARY

Psychogenic complaints need a systematic evaluation. They are frequently embellishments on true, established organic problems. The examiner must approach the patient with humility and must never lose the rapport and trust of the patient while performing the examination and gathering data. The most important part of the examination is that of skilled observation.

REFERENCES

1. Lempert T, et al. Psychogenic disorders in neurology: frequency and clinical spectrum. *Acta Neurol Scand* 1990;82:335–340.
2. Shaibani A, Sabbagh MN. Pseudoneurologic syndromes: recognition and diagnosis. *Am Fam Physician* 1998;57:2485–2494.
3. DeJong RN. *The Neurologic Examination,* 3rd ed. New York: Harper & Row, 1970.
4. Mai FM. "Hysteria" in clinical neurology, *Can J Neurol Sci* 1995;22:101–110.
5. American Psychiatric Association. *Diagnostic and Statistical Manual of Mental Disorders,* 4th ed. Washington, DC: American Psychiatric Association, 1994, p. 452–457.
6. Moene FC, et al. Organic syndromes diagnosed as conversion disorder: identification and frequency in a study of 85 patients. *J Psychosom Res* 2000;49:7–12.
7. Schuepbach WM, Adler RH, Sabbioni ME. Accuracy of the clinical diagnosis of 'psychogenic disorders' in the presence of physical symptoms suggesting a general medical conditions: a 5-year follow-up in 162 patients. *Psychother Psychosom* 2002;Jan–Feb:71.
8. Glick TH. Suspected conversion disorder: foreseeable risks and avoidable errors. *Acad Emerg Med* 2000;7:1272.
9. Dula D, DeNaples L. Emergency department presentation of patients with conversion disorder. *Acad Emerg Med* 1995;2:120–123.
10. Beaumont WM. Malingering in relation to sight. In Jones, Llewellyn (eds). *Malingering or the Simulation of Disease,* London: Heinemann, 1917.
11. Gould R, et al. The validity of hysterical signs and symptoms. *J Nerv Ment Dis* 1986; 174:593.
12. Magee KR. Hysterical hemiplegia and hemianesthesia. *Postgrad Med* 1962;31:339.
13. Bowlus WE, Currier RD. A test for hysterical hemianalgesia. *N Engl J Med* 1963;269:1253.
14. Hayes MW, et al. A video review of the diagnosis of psychogenic gait: appendix and commentary. *Mov Disord* 1999;14:914–921.
15. Rosenbaum M. Psychogenic seizures—why women? *Psychosomatics* 2000;41:147–149.
16. Benbadis SR, Agrawal V, Tatum WO 4th. How many patients with psychogenic nonepileptic seizures also have epilepsy? *Neurology* 2001;57:915–917.
17. Boon PA, Williamson PD. The diagnosis of pseudoseizures. *Clin Neurol Neurosurg* 1993;95:1–8.
18. Walczak TS, Bogolioubov A. Weeping during psychogenic nonepileptic seizures. *Epilepsia* 1996;37:208–210.
19. Groppel G, et al. Clinical symptoms in psychogenic seizures. *Wien Klin Wochenschr* 1999;111:469–475.
20. Krumholz A. Nonepileptic seizures: diagnosis and management, *Neurology* 1999;53(5 Suppl 2):S76–S83.
21. Peguero E, et al. Self-injury and incontinence in psychogenic seizures. *Epilepsia* 1995;36:586–591.
22. Mahr G, Leith W. Psychogenic stuttering of adult onset. *J Speech Hear Res* 1992;35: 283–286.

11
SEIZURES

Seizure is frequently the presenting symptom that precipitates the patient's entrance into the medical care system. This chapter deals with the evaluation and stabilization of the seizure patient in the acute care setting. The focus is on a differential diagnostic approach as well as clinical decision making. Status epilepticus and febrile seizures are discussed in detail.

Ictus refers to the period during which a seizure occurs. An *aura* is actually a partial seizure; thus its manifestation depends on the area in the brain that is affected. A focal seizure can remain focal or spread into a generalized event; a corollary to this is that patients with a primary generalized seizure disorder do not have an aura (see discussion below). *The postictal period* is the time after a seizure ends but before the patient returns to baseline. *Epilepsy* is a condition of recurrent unprovoked seizures. *Status epilepticus* refers to those seizures that last more than 30 minutes, or recurrent seizures without a return to baseline mental status between events.

CLASSIFICATION AND ETIOLOGIES

A seizure can be the result of an acute process, in which case it is referred to as an *acute symptomatic seizure;* it can result from a past intracranial insult such as stroke, trauma, or anoxia, in which case it is referred to as a *remote symptomatic seizure;* or it can be *idiopathic,* i.e., no etiology identified. A seizure's manifestation depends on the area of the brain that is discharging and whether or not the abnormal discharges are focal or generalized throughout the cerebral cortex. Consequently, the clinical spectrum of seizures includes focal or generalized motor activity, altered mental status, sensory or psychic experiences, and/or autonomic disturbances. The classification of seizure types is presented in Table 11-1. In essence, generalized seizures are always associated with altered mental status.

TABLE 11-1

CLASSIFICATION OF SEIZURES

Partial Seizures
Simple partial
  Motor
  Somatosensory
  Autonomic
  Psychic
Complex partial
  With focal onset prior to alteration in consciousness
  Without focal onset prior to alteration in consciousness

Generalized Seizures
Primary generalized nonconvulsive
  Absence
Primary generalized convulsive
  Tonic-clonic
  Clonic
  Tonic
  Myoclonic
  Atonic
Secondary generalized
  Convulsive
  Nonconvulsive

Status Epilepticus
Convulsive generalized
  Primary generalized
  Secondary generalized
Convulsive focal
Nonconvulsive
  Primary generalized (absence)
  Partial with or without secondary generalization (complex partial)

Acute symptomatic seizures are associated with acute or progressive neurologic insult or physiologic stressors. Clinicians are challenged with identifying those patients with potentially reversible etiologies (Table 11-2). Hypoglycemia is the most common metabolic cause of seizures, while hyponatremia and hypocalcemia are rare.[1–3] The metabolic encephalopathies such as nonketotic hyperglycemia and uremia can cause both focal and generalized seizures.

Alcohol is the most common toxin associated with seizures followed by tricyclics, cocaine, amphetamines, antihistamines, theophylline, and isoniazid.[4] Drug withdrawal, including noncompliance with anticonvulsant medications in a patient with a known seizure disorder, is a leading cause of recurrent seizures.[5]

TABLE 11-2 ——————————————————————————

ETIOLOGIES OF SECONDARY SEIZURES

Tumors

Vascular Event
  Subarachnoid hemorrhage
  Subdural hemorrhage
  Epidural hemorrhage
  Stroke
  Vasculitis

Infection
  Meningitis
  Encephalitis
  Abscess

Metabolic
  Hypoglycemia[a]
  Hyponatremia[b]
  Hypomagnesemia[c]
  Hypocalcemia

Toxic (Consider the following in overdose):
  Cocaine and sympathomimetics
  Tricyclic antidepressants
  Anticholinergics
  Theophylline
  Isoniazid

Eclampsia

[a] The most common metabolic cause of seizures.
[b] A rare cause of seizures except in infants < 6 months olds.
[c] Rarely an isolated cause of seizures; possibly facilitates seizures, especially in malnourished patients, e.g., alcoholics.

Infections can result in physiologic stress and lower the seizure threshold. Acute central nervous system (CNS) infections are responsible for 4% to 12% of acute isolated seizures and up to 28% of cases of refractory status epilepticus. Aside from those seizures caused directly by HIV, toxoplasmosis and cryptococcal meningitis make up the majority of infection-related seizures in AIDS patients.[6]

Epidemiology

Seizures account for an estimated 1% of emergency department (ED) visits.[7] The prevalence of active epilepsy is approximately 6 in 1,000, whereas approximately 25%

to 55% of patients with epilepsy continue to have recurrent seizures despite therapy.[8] Under the best of circumstances, excluding noncompliance and other variables, it is estimated that 5% to 10% of patients will have intractable epilepsy despite optimal medical management. The cumulative incidence of all epilepsy is estimated to be 1.2% of the population through age 24, increasing to 4.4% by age 85.[9]

There is a projected annual incidence of status epilepticus of 50 in 100,000 population, with an overall mortality of 22%—3% for children and 26% for adults.[10] More than half of the patients presenting to the ED in status epilepticus have no prior seizure history. Mortality in patients with status epilepticus is linked to the duration of the seizures and the underlying etiology.

PATHOPHYSIOLOGY

Seizures result from either recurrent excitatory connections in the cerebral cortex or a loss of synchronization between aggregates of neurons. The excitability can be due to positive feedback loops or lack of inhibitory pathways. At the neuronal level, hyperexcitability can occur from hypoxic or hypoglycemic impairment of the Na-K pump. Glutamic acid is an excitatory transmitter and γ-aminobutyric acid (GABA) an inhibitory transmitter; disturbances in the balance between these two transmitters result in seizures. For example, vitamin B_6 is necessary for the syntheses of GABA, and deficiency may result in seizures; this explains the intractable seizures related to isoniazid overdose, which depletes vitamin B_6. The mechanism of action of anticonvulsants is primarily through selective blockade of high-frequency action potentials or potentiation of the inhibitory effect of GABA.

There are a number of pathophysiologic consequences of a seizure. There is often a period of transient apnea and hypoxia during a convulsion. Early in a motor seizure, there is an increase in blood pressure, followed later by a fall in the blood pressure. Serum lactate and serum glucose levels increase, and there is often an increase in the white blood cell count (but with no increase in bands). Body temperature is frequently elevated, with up to 43% of patients who have a generalized convulsion experiencing a rise in temperature above 100°F.[11,12] Acidosis due to elevated lactate occurs within 60 seconds of a convulsive event but should normalize within 1 hour after ictus. A transient cerebrospinal fluid (CSF) pleocytosis of up to 20 white blood cells (WBC)/mm^3 has been reported to occur in 2% to 23% of patients with seizures.

If the seizure lasts for more than 30 minutes, the body's homeostatic regulating mechanisms begin to deteriorate. Cerebral blood flow autoregulation may be lost and, combined with alterations in blood pressure, cerebral perfusion may be compromised. The addition of increased neuronal metabolism to this picture may result in significant neuronal damage. Even if systemic factors such as acidosis and hypoxia are controlled, prolonged status epilepticus results in neuronal damage secondary to the release of neurotoxic excitatory amino acids and influx of calcium into cells.

DIFFERENTIAL DIAGNOSIS

A number of conditions can mimic or be misinterpreted as an epileptic seizure. These include convulsive syncope, with or without cardiac dysrhythmias; decerebrate posturing; psychogenic events; and migraine headaches. Careful consideration of these mimickers is clearly important since misdiagnosis may have significant impact on patient management. Neither tetanus nor strychnine poisoning result in altered mental status, thus they are rarely confused with a seizure.

Syncope

Based on observational studies in blood donors, up to 40% of patients who have syncope will have some component of motor activity, most commonly involving tonic extension of the trunk or myoclonic jerks of the extremities.[13] This will usually occur if the patient is kept in a sitting position. These events are termed convulsive syncope and are not usually associated with tonic-clonic movements, tongue biting, cyanosis, incontinence, or postictal amnesia.

Cardiac Dysrhythmias

Cardiac dysrhythmias can cause hypotension with CNS hypoperfusion, resulting in symptoms that can be confused with convulsive or nonconvulsive seizures.[14] A careful history will often identify preceding cardiac symptoms such as palpitations, lightheadedness, or diaphoresis (see Chap. 12, Syncope). The diagnosis frequently requires careful coordination with the patient's primary care physician for Holter monitoring, continuous cardiac loop monitoring, and head-up tilt table testing.

Decerebrate Posturing

Decerebrate posturing has been mistaken for tonic seizures, resulting in misdiagnosis and delay in providing potentially life-saving interventions for increased intracranial pressure.[15] It should be remembered that tonic seizures are rare in adults, and when they do occur they are usually of short duration with upper extremity abduction. Decerebrate posturing results in both upper and lower extremity extension.

Migraines

Migraines are typically diagnosed by characteristic symptom patterns associated with a unilateral throbbing headache. However, rare migraine variants have been associated with transient loss of consciousness or confusion as the primary complaint, making it difficult to distinguish this form of migraine from complex partial seizures, postictal vascular headaches, drop attacks, or transient ischemic attacks.

Psychogenic Seizures

See Chapter 10, Psychogenic Neurologic Syndromes.

Dystonia

Dystonia is muscle rigidity with autonomic instability. Seizures can be excluded since there is no alteration of mental status or postictal confusion.

ANTIEPILEPTIC DRUGS

The "traditional" antiepileptic drugs (AEDs; phenytoin, phenobarbital, carbamazepine, valproic acid, and ethosuximide) suppress the repetitive, high-frequency neuronal firing characteristic of seizure activity through one of three general mechanisms: (1) blockade of voltage-dependent sodium channels, e.g., phenytoin; (2) potentiation of GABA-mediated postsynaptic inhibition, e.g., phenobarbital; and (3) blockade of calcium channels, e.g., ethosuximide. Traditionally, the first-line treatment for partial seizures, with or without secondary generalization, has been carbamazepine, valproic acid, phenytoin, and phenobarbital (listed in order of preference). For primary generalized convulsive epilepsy, valproic acid and phenytoin are recommended, whereas ethosuximide is used for absence seizures. Over the past decade, several new AEDs have been introduced that have greatly expanded the drug armamentarium available for treating epilepsy (Table 11-3).

PREHOSPITAL MANAGEMENT/INITIAL STABILIZATION

Prehospital management of the convulsing patient centers on securing the airway, maintaining oxygenation, obtaining intravenous access, and protecting the patient from injury. Fortunately most seizures are of short duration and in most cases little else needs to be done. The use of a padded tongue blade is contraindicated since it may induce emesis or break a tooth; a nasal trumpet may be helpful. Seizing patients require an immediate blood sugar determination or, if not available, dextrose can be given empirically. If the seizure continues for more than several minutes, lorazepam 2 mg IV every minute up to a maximum of 10 mg can be administered; diazepam 5 mg IV every minute up to a total of 20 mg can also be used, but its shorter duration of action makes it less desirable than lorazepam. Intramuscular midazolam and rectal diazepam are alternatives when intravenous access is not available.

Patients who have had a first-time seizure should be transported to the ED via an advanced life support unit, when available. Patients who have a known seizure disorder, who experience a "typical" event, and who are asymptomatic do not necessarily require transport to the hospital if they have capacity and are familiar with

TABLE 11-3

THE ANTI-EPILEPTIC DRUGS (AEDs)

Drug	Trade Name	Route	Seizure Type	Loading Dose (mg/kg)	Daily Dose (mg) in Adults	Therapeutic Range (µg/mL)
Phenytoin	Dilantin	PO, IV	P, GC	20	300–400	10–20
Fosphenytoin	Cerebrex	IV, IM	P, GC	20		10–20
Carbamazepine[a]	Tegretol	PO	P, GC	—	800–1,600	6–12
Valproate[b]	Depakene	PO	All	—	1,000–3,000	50–120
Divalproex sodium	Depakote	PO	All	—	1,000–4,800	50–120
	Depacon	IV	All	10–20		50–120
Phenobarbital		PO, IV, IM	P, GC	10–20	90–150	15–35
Primidone	Mysoline	PO	P, GC	—	750–1,250	6–12
Clonazepam	Klonopin	PO	A, M	—	1.5–20	0.02–0.08
Ethosuximide[c]	Zarontin	PO	A	—	750–1,250	40–100
Lamotrigine	Lamictal	PO	All	—	200–600	—
Felbamate[d]	Felbatol	PO	P, GC	—	1,800–4,800	—
Gabapentin[e]	Neurontin	PO	P, GC	—	1,200–4,800	—
Topiramate	Topamax	PO	P, GC	—	200–600	—
Tiagabine		PO	P, GC	—	32–48	—
Diazepam[f]	Diastat	Rectal	All	0.2–0.5	—	—

Abbreviations: P, partial seizure, GC, generalized convulsive seizure; A, absence seizure; M, myoclonic seizure.
[a] Drug of choice for partial seizures, with or without secondary generalization.
[b] Drug of choice for primary generalized tonic-clonic seizures.
[c] Drug of choice for absence seizures.
[d] Associated with aplastic anemia in 1 in 5,000 patients; hepatic failure in 1 in 30,000.
[e] Only anticonvulsant that is renally metabolized; recommended in patients with multiple medical problems.
[f] Used primarily in children to control clusters of breakthrough seizures.

their disorder. These patients should be advised to contact their primary care provider as soon as possible. All other asymptomatic patients who have had a seizure should be transported to an ED for evaluation.

EMERGENCY DEPARTMENT EVALUATION

In approaching the seizure patient, the physician is often constrained by the paucity and questionable reliability of historical information, and by the limited resources available to some patients in obtaining the follow-up care that their condition might require. Consequently, multiple factors must be carefully weighed when deciding on the best approach to the diagnostic testing and therapeutic interventions initiated in the ED.

History

The history begins with a careful description of the event and its surrounding circumstances, with documentation of the preliminary symptoms, progression of the clinical pattern, the duration of the event including the postictal period, and the presence of incontinence or biting of the tongue (Table 11-4). Efforts should be made to obtain a clear description of the event(s) from witnesses. In patients with epilepsy, any changes in the character of the seizure such as frequency or clinical features should be investigated. Noncompliance with anticonvulsants is the most common cause of recurrent seizures in this group of patients. The use of anticonvulsants and other medications should be ascertained, if possible. Initiation of new medications may have on impact the bioavailability of the AEDs a patient with epilepsy may be using. Seizure disorders may be exacerbated by a number of stressors, such as fatigue, pregnancy, or systemic infection. Identification of the stressors may explain an event and become the focus of management.

Physical Examination

Seizure activity tends to prompt aggressive interventions, but it is critical to stress the importance of taking the time to carefully observe the patient and perform a physical exam. Obtain an accurate set of vital signs including a rectal temperature. Assess the mental status, skin color, and pupil position and reactivity. If the patient is actively convulsing, describe the motor activity. Look for "automatisms," which are repetitive actions such as lip smacking, swallowing, chewing, or fumbling. Automatisms are frequently seen in complex partial seizures and may be the only indicator that there is ongoing seizure activity.

Seizures resulting from drug overdose may be suggested by the presence of a toxidrome, as is seen in anticholinergic, sympathomimetic, or tricyclic ingestions. Hypertension with bradycardia may indicate an intracranial catastrophe, whereas fever may be the manifestation of a central nervous system (CNS) infection (although seizures may independently result in elevated temperatures from muscular hyperactivity or central deregulation). Irregular heart rate or carotid bruits may suggest a stroke as the seizure etiology, a common cause of new-onset seizures in the elderly.

Evaluate the patient for both soft tissue and skeletal trauma, especially head trauma and tongue lacerations. Seizure activity has been reported to directly cause both dislocations and fractures. However, seizure-induced fractures are rare, occurring in less than 1% of events; they most commonly involve the humerus, thoracic spine, and femur.[16]

Perform a complete neurologic examination identifying focal deficits that may represent an old lesion, new intracranial pathology, or reversible postictal neurologic compromise (Todd's paralysis). In cases of a new Todd's paralysis, consider the presence of a new structural lesion. Other physical findings suggesting that a seizure has occurred include hyperreflexia and extensor plantar responses, both of which should resolve during the immediate postictal period.

TABLE 11-4 ———
——————————————— ELEMENTS OF THE HISTORY AND PHYSICAL EXAMINATION

History
Description of the event including:
  Initial symptoms
  Sensory or autonomic symptoms
  Motor activity: focal versus generalized
  Altered consciousness or awareness
  Timing of event (wakefulness versus asleep)
  Duration
  Postictal period
  Incontinence
Provoking conditions
  Pregnancy
  Sleep, e.g., deprivation
  Systemic infection
  Drugs or medications
  Environment
Current medications
Past history of similar events
Past medical history including:
  Malignancy
  Immunocompromise
  Vascular disease
  Trauma
  Febrile seizures
Family history

Physical Examination
Vital signs
Evidence of head trauma
Eye exam including:
  Pupil reactivity and size
  Fundi
  Deviation
  Nystagmus
Mouth exam for evidence of intraoral trauma
Neck/spine for meningismus/tenderness
Extremity exam for evidence of trauma
Neurologic exam:
  Level of consciousness/mental status
  Abnormal movements/eye deviation
  Automatisms
  Cranial nerves
  Focal weakness
  Hyperreflexia/upgoing toes
Skin for evidence of trauma or intravenous drug use

Document the patient's mental status, recruiting the assistance of persons familiar with the patient. Postictal confusion usually resolves over several hours, and the failure of gradual improvement to occur should prompt a search for other causes (Table 11-5). In particular, nonconvulsive status epilepticus can present with subtle behavioral changes that may be discounted unless the clinician maintains a high index of suspicion (see Nonconvulsive Status Epilepticus section, below).

Laboratory Studies

The laboratory tests indicated in the ED for patients presenting after a first-time seizure who are alert, oriented, and have no clinical findings include a serum glucose level, electrolytes, and a pregnancy test in women of child-bearing age[17,18] (Figure 11-1). A drug of abuse screen should be considered. All other tests are of very low yield in this group of patients. Patients who are on dialysis, malnourished, or taking diuretics or who have underlying significant medical disorders usually require comprehensive testing including a complete blood count (CBC), blood urea nitrogen (BUN), creatinine, calcium, phosphate, and magnesium, as well as a urinalysis. Rhabdomyolysis is a rare consequence of a seizure and is diagnosed if the urine tests positive for blood in the absence of red blood cells on the microscopic exam. Serum creatine phosphokinase (CPK) levels are not useful in differentiating seizures from other causes of loss of consciousness.

Patients with a known seizure disorder who have a "typical" event but who are asymptomatic, alert, and oriented in the ED are only in need of a serum anticonvulsant level (if they are taking their medication) unless they have other underlying disease such as diabetes that could result in a metabolic derangement. It is important to consider potential precipitants such as infections or new medications that might have contributed to the event.

Patients in convulsive status epilepticus, as well as patients who are not actively convulsing but who are persistently postictal, require comprehensive diagnostic testing, which may include serum glucose, electrolytes, urea nitrogen, creatinine, magnesium, phosphate, calcium, CBC, pregnancy test in women of child-bearing

TABLE 11-5

DIFFERENTIAL DIAGNOSIS OF ALTERED MENTAL STATUS IN THE PATIENT WHO HAS SEIZED

Postictal state
Nonconvulsive status or subtle convulsive status
Hypoglycemia
CNS infection
CNS vascular event
Drug toxicity
Psychiatric disorder

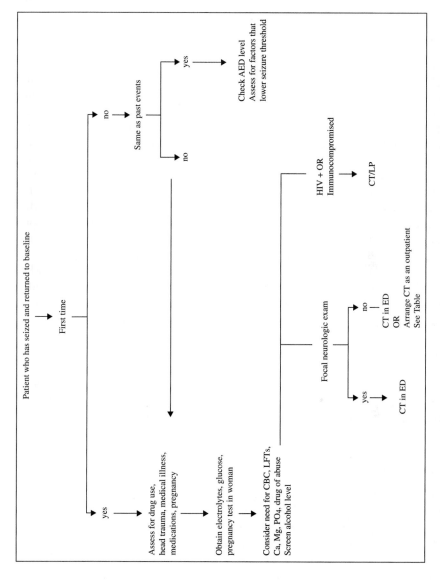

FIGURE 11-1 Approach to a patient who has seized and returned to baseline. AED, antiepileptic drug; CBC, complete blood count; CT, computed tomography; LFT, liver function test; LP, lumbar puncture.

age, AED levels, liver function tests, and a drug of abuse screen. An arterial blood gas analysis (ABG) obtained in a convulsing patient will show an anion gap metabolic acidosis that is usually secondary to lactic acidosis. The anion gap acidosis should resolve within 1 hour after the seizure ends; persistence after 1 hour suggests the presence of one of the other causes of an anion gap acidosis.

Lumbar Puncture

A lumbar puncture is considered in patients who are in status epilepticus of undetermined etiology, who have an unresolving postictal state, fever, headache, meningeal signs, or positive HIV history, or who are otherwise immunocompromised. There is no evidence to support the performance of a lumbar puncture as part of the diagnostic evaluation in the ED on patients who are alert, oriented, asymptomatic, and not immunocompromised, even if the seizure was a first-time event.[19]

Neuroimaging

The indications and timing of head computed tomography (CT), especially in patients with a first-time seizure, are controversial. Three percent to 41% of patients with a first-time seizure have an abnormal head CT.[2,20] An estimated 20% of patients with a first-time seizure and an abnormal CT have a normal neurologic exam. A head CT should be performed in the ED whenever a seizure patient has a suspected acute intracranial process, a history of acute head trauma, malignancy, immunocompromise, fever, persistent headache, anticoagulation, or a new focal neurologic examination[21] (see Table 11-6 for neuroimaging recommendations).

Electroencephalography

An urgent electroencephalogram (EEG) in the ED may be useful for those patients with persisting altered mental status in whom subtle convulsive or nonconvulsive status epilepticus is suspected (see below). An EEG may also be useful when a patient's motor activity has been suppressed by either paralysis or barbiturate coma and there is a need to assess ongoing seizure activity.

MANAGEMENT OF CONVULSIVE STATUS EPILEPTICUS

Management of status epilepticus must take into consideration potentially treatable etiologies (Table 11-2), since it will be difficult to control the seizures unless the precipitating causes are addressed. Therefore a comprehensive approach must be taken that concomitantly ensures oxygenation and intravenous access, obtains diagnostic studies, and initiates pharmacologic interventions (Figure 11-2).

Oxygenation is monitored with pulse oximetry. If at any time breathing appears compromised, rapid-sequence intubation is recommended. Long-acting paralyzing agents are relatively contraindicated until bedside EEG monitoring becomes avail-

TABLE 11-6

AAN/ACEP/AANS/ASN RECOMMENDATIONS FOR NEUROIMAGING IN EMERGENCY PATIENTS PRESENTING WITH SEIZURE[a]

First-Time Seizure

CT in the ED (guideline): new focal deficit, persistent altered mental status, fever, recent trauma, persistent headache, history of cancer, history of anticoagulation or suspicion of AIDS, fever

CT in the ED (option): age over 40 years; partial onset seizure

Arrange CT as outpatient or consider scan in ED if follow-up uncertain (option): normal exam and no cause identified for the seizure

Recurrent Seizure in Patient with Known Epilepsy

CT in the ED (guideline): new focal deficit, persistent altered mental status, fever, recent trauma, persistent headache, history of cancer, history of anticoagulation, suspicion of AIDS

CT in the ED (option): new seizure pattern or new seizure type, prolonged postictal confusion or worsening mental status

Arrange CT as outpatient or consider scan in ED if follow-up uncertain (option): no clear-cut cause of seizure is identified

[a] There are no "standards" since no high quality studies with outcome data are available; "guidelines" are recommendations based on studies whose designs preclude definitive conclusions; "options" are recommendations that are concensus based and have limited or no studies to support them.

able, since they mask clinical findings that guide pharmacologic interventions. Intravenous access is best secured with a nondextrose solution since dextrose will precipitate phenytoin if administered concurrently. A rapid bedside serum glucose determination should be obtained and dextrose given if the level is less than 80 mg/dL; if a rapid dextrose determination is unavailable, administer 50 mL of 50% dextrose intravenously in adults, or 2 mL/kg of 25% dextrose in children. Thiamine, 100 mg, is recommended with dextrose boluses in patients who appear malnourished or abuse alcohol. In certain situations in which infection is suspected, early consideration must be given to empiric antibiotic treatment, since head CT and lumbar puncture will most likely be delayed pending patient stabilization. Likewise, early administration of activated charcoal, 1 g/kg, is recommended in cases of suspected overdose.

Benzodiazepines are the first-line drugs in managing status epilepticus and have been shown to be equal to phenobarbital alone and superior to using phenytoin alone.[22] Diazepam, 0.2 mg/kg at 5 mg/min, and lorazepam, 0.1 mg/kg at 2 mg/min, are equally effective in terminating seizures; lorazepam has the advantage of a much smaller volume of distribution, with anticonvulsant benefit lasting up to 12 hours versus 20 minutes for diazepam. In patients with no intravenous access, intramuscular or intranasal midazolam is an excellent alternative since it is water-soluble, nonirritating, and rapidly absorbed.

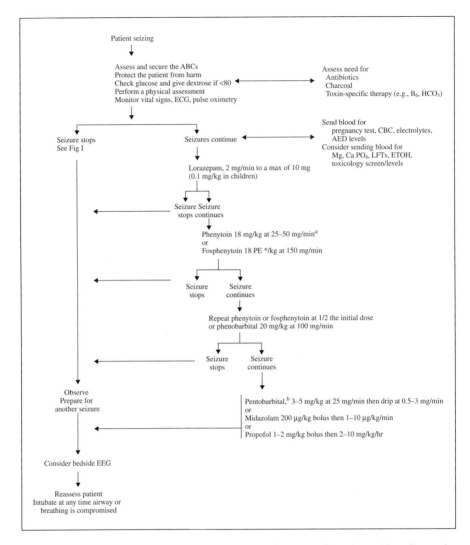

FIGURE 11-2   Approach to a patient who is undergoing a seizure.[a] Slower rates for patients with cardiovascular disease. Infusion should be through a large-bore intravenous drip.[b] Watch for hypotension and treat initially with fluids; give dopamine if needed. ECG, electrocardiogram; EEG, electroencephalogram; PE, phenytoin equivalent. For other abbreviations, see Figure 11-1 legend.

When diazepam is used as the initial AED, intravenous phenytoin loading, 18 to 20 mg/kg, should also be started; 18 mg/kg is the dose found to give serum drug levels that remained above 10 mg/dL for 24 hours. The dose of phenytoin can be increased up to a total of 30 mg/kg if the seizures do not stop after the initial load.[23] Phenytoin loading can result in infusion site irritation, hypotension, confusion, and ataxia; it will rarely result in progressive distal limb edema discolorations and ischemia. Infusions are best administered through a large vein to minimize sclerosis from the alkaline pH. The infusion rate should be no faster than 25 mg/min in patients with cardiac disease, to minimize cardiovascular complications, and 50 mg/min in other patients.

Fosphenytoin, a phosphate ester of phenytoin, has a safety profile that makes it preferable to phenytoin in certain situations. It is water-soluble and nonirritating and thus can be given intramuscularly with 100% bioavailability. It has fewer cardiotoxic effects than phenytoin, although hypotension can occur. The loading dose is 18 to 20 phenytoin equivalent units (PE)/kg. In emergencies, when given intravenously, the recommended infusion rate is 150 mg/min.

An alternative to phenytoin, particularly in patients who have seized secondary to subtherapeutic valproic acid levels, is intravenous valproic acid. A loading dose is 20 mg/kg, which can be infused at 150 mg/min.

Phenobarbital, 20 mg/kg at 100 mg/min, has been used as a first-line drug in status epilepticus, although it is generally reserved for patients who continue to seize despite benzodiazepine and phenytoin loading or who are seizing from drug withdrawal. Resuscitation interventions should be continually reassessed to ensure that the patient is properly oxygenated and is not hypoglycemic, that intravenous lines are functioning, and that phenytoin was not administered in a dextrose solution.

After phenobarbital, there are three options for cases of refractory status epilepticus, i.e., cases that do not respond to first- and second-line AEDs: pentobarbital, propofol, and a benzodiazepine infusion. Pentobarbital, 5 mg/kg, followed by an infusion of 0.5 to 3 mg/kg/hr, is effective in suppressing electrical discharges. Pentobarbital can compromise cardiovascular status, and its use necessitates EEG monitoring since motor activity will be suppressed. Pentobarbital-induced hypotension is initially managed with fluid boluses followed by dopamine in resistant cases. Other drugs that have been used include lidocaine, propfol, etiomate, and paraldehyde.[24]

NONCONVULSIVE STATUS EPILEPTICUS

Nonconvulsive status epilepticus (NCS), like convulsive status epilepticus, is a state of continuous or intermittent seizure activity lasting for more than 30 minutes without a return to baseline function. The hallmark of NCS is altered mental status, which can range from subtle behavioral changes to paranoia to coma. Therefore, unless it is suspected, the diagnosis can be easily missed. Although the distinction is not clear in the literature, NCS in general should be distinguished from subtle generalized convulsive status epilepticus. This is the end stage of generalized convulsive status when the patient is in continuous coma with only subtle motor convulsions; unlike NCS, this entity has a very poor prognosis. The literature reports many patients presenting with altered mental status who were initially labeled as psychiatric and only at a later time in their evaluation was the correct diagnosis identified, either by EEG or by onset of a convulsive component to the status.[25,26] Nonconvulsive status can be either a primary generalized process, in which case it is absence status, or secondarily generalized, i.e., complex partial status. NCS can occur on a continuum with convulsive seizures. Up to 15% of patients with a prolonged postictal period after convulsive status epilepticus are in NCS.[27]

When NCS is suspected, an EEG should be obtained. NCS is highly responsive to the benzodiazepines, either diazepam or lorazepam; thus some clinicians recommend a trial of a benzodiazepine when EEG monitoring is not available; this is generally best done in coordinatation with the neurologist who will be assuming the patient's care.

ALCOHOL SEIZURES

The risk of an unprovoked seizure is increased with increased alcohol intake, but, interestingly, studies have questioned the existence of "alcohol withdrawal seizures" as a distinct entity.[28] The alcoholic who has seized must be approached with caution in order to avoid bias influencing clinical decision making. In a study of 259 patients with suspected alcohol withdrawal seizure, 58% had an abnormal CT; 16 of these patients (6%) had a clinically significant lesion.[29] Phenytoin does not have a role in managing withdrawal seizures or controlling recurrent alcohol-related seizures.[30] Two milligrams of IV lorazepam is effective in decreasing recurrent seizures related to alcohol use and decreases the need for hospitalization in these patients.[31]

SUBTHERAPEUTIC AED LEVELS IN THE ED

Many patients with a history of seizures present to the ED with low serum AED levels. Serum levels can be brought up to therapeutic range by oral, intramuscular, or intravenous supplementation depending on the urgency of the situation and the AED. When oral loading is used, 19 mg/kg in men and 23 mg/kg in women provide therapeutic serum levels of AED within 4 hours in the majority of patients. Single-dose loading has been shown to be safe, although patients should be watched for ataxia and dizziness.[32,33] Intramuscular fosphenytoin, intravenous phenytoin, or fosphenytoin are other options. Valproic acid and carbamazepine (Tegretol) cannot be orally loaded with a single dose. Intravenous valproic acid is available and provides physicians with an alternative when rapid therapeutic levels are needed.

SEIZURES IN PREGNANCY

Faced with a pregnant patient having a seizure, physicians must determine whether the seizure is associated with an existing disorder, is of new onset, or relates to eclampsia. Patients whose gestation has progressed beyond 20 weeks should be checked for hypertension, proteinuria, and edema. Patients whose seizures are associated with eclampsia are treated with magnesium sulfate, which has been shown to be superior to phenytoin and diazepam in eclamptic seizures.[34] Once eclampsia has been ruled out, precipitating etiologies such as sleep deprivation, infections, and drug toxicities should be considered. In patients with a history of seizures, compliance with therapy should be explored. Pregnancy changes the "free" AED level of those AEDs that are protein bound. "Free AED levels" are required to accurately assess the true serum drug level. Fetal monitoring is a consideration in patients in the second half of pregnancy, and an obstetrics consultation should be obtained.

Pediatric Seizures

Several seizure types are seen primarily in pediatrics, including absence, infantile spasms, Lennox-Gastaut syndrome, and febrile seizures.

Absence Seizures

Primary generalized nonconvulsive seizures, also called petit mal or absence seizures, are typically characterized by a sudden onset of unresponsiveness that is not preceded by an aura or succeeded by a postictal period. Absence seizures account for approximately 15% of all cases of childhood epilepsy. They are seen primarily in the young, usually beginning between the ages of 5 and 10 years, and are rare after the mid-teens. The average duration of an absence event is 10 seconds. Atypical absence seizures (possibly complex partial seizures with rapid generalization) are events that last longer, have more complex automatisms or associated motor activity, and often have a postictal period. Patients are generally not cognizant that the seizure has occurred. The treatment of choice is ethosuximide unless the child also has motor seizures, in which case valproic acid is recommended.

Febrile Seizures

A febrile seizure occurs between 6 months and 5 years of age, is associated with fever, and has no identifiable underlying cause.[35] Simple febrile seizures are generalized tonic clonic events with no focality, last less than 15 minutes, and have a short postictal period. Complex febrile seizures last longer than 15 minutes or occur in a series, or have a focal onset or a prolonged postictal period.

Two to four percent of all children will have a simple febrile seizure. Children who have had a febrile seizure have a 25% to 50% chance of having a second event associated with a fever, usually within a year. Children at highest risk for recurrence are those with a first-degree relative who has had a febrile seizure, those who had a complex first febrile seizure, or those who were younger than 1 year when the first event occurred. Ten percent to 50% of cases of status epilepticus in children are associated with febrile seizures, and status epilepticus in this group is a consistent predictor of increased risk for subsequent seizures.

Simple febrile seizures are a benign process; when they occur in children older than 18 months who have not been on antibiotics, they do not require any diagnostic workup, even for a first-time event.[35] Management focuses on a careful history and physical exam and on parental education. Diagnostic studies are guided by general fever protocols. In patients between 6 and 12 months, the physical exam is un-reliable for meningitis, and lumbar puncture is recommended; between the ages of 12 and 18 months, clinical signs of meningitis may be subtle, and strong considera-tion should be given to obtaining CSF for analysis. Electrolytes, calcium, phospho-rus, magnesium, blood sugar, CBC, or neuroimaging are not routinely necessary in patients with simple febrile seizures. Complex febrile seizures necessitate a complete diagnostic workup looking for underlying precipitating etiologies. Because simple febrile seizures are a benign entity, AEDs as a preventive therapy are unwarranted.[36]

DISPOSITION

Patients who were in status epilepticus or who have persisting altered mental sta-tus or a new neurologic deficit require a period of observation. Initiation of AED therapy in the ED is best coordinated with the patient's primary care provider. In general, this decision can only be made on the basis of the underlying cause of the seizure, which requires the results of laboratory testing, a neuroimaging study, and an EEG. All these data are rarely available prior to ED discharge. Consequently, decision making (whether to admit to the hospital and whether to initiate AED ther-apy) must be based on the predicted risk for seizure recurrence, with the under-standing that even if an AED is initiated, seizure recurrence may not be changed.[9]

The chances of a patient having a recurrent event after one unprovoked sei-zure varies depending on patient age and the underlying etiology of the seizure. Seizure etiology and EEG findings are the best predictors of recurrence. Patients who have structural lesions on CT or patients with focal seizures that secondarily generalize have a risk of recurrence of up to 65%; this is the group of patients that will probably benefit from initiation of AED therapy. Patients with a new-onset seizure who have returned to baseline and who have a normal neurologic exam, a normal head CT, and normal electrolytes and glucose can be safely sent home on no therapy. Follow-up with a primary care provider or neurologist should be discussed with the patient.

SUMMARY

The approach to the seizure patient begins with a careful assessment of the event with consideration given to the various disorders that can mimic epileptic seizure activity. History, physical exam, and diagnostic tests are obtained to elucidate the seizure's etiology and to guide management. When possible, care should be coor-dinated with the patient's primary care physician or neurologist. Disposition from the ED must take into consideration the patient's social situation, resources, and compliance. All patients who have had a seizure must be advised not to drive and to avoid placing themselves or others in potentially dangerous situations. All states have laws regulating driving and epilepsy, although few states actually have manda-tory reporting requirements.

REFERENCES

1. Turnbull T, et al. Utility of laboratory studies in the emergency department patient with a new-onset seizure. *Ann Emerg Med* 1990;19:373–377.
2. Henneman P, DeRoos F, Lewis R. Determining the need for admission in patients with new-onset seizures. *Ann Emerg Med* 1994;24:1108–1114.
3. Sempere A, et al. First seizure in adults: a prospective study from the ED. *Acta Neurol Scand* 1992;86:134–138.
4. DeLorenzo R, et al. Seizures associated with poisoning and drug overdose. *Am J Emerg Med* 1993;11:565–568.
5. DeLorenzo R, et al. A prospective, population-based epidemiologic study of status epilepticus in Richmond, Virginia. *Neurology* 1996;46:1029–1035.
6. Wong M, Suite N, Labar D. Seizures in human immunodeficiency virus infections. *Arch Neurol* 1990;47:640–642.
7. Krumholz A, et al. Seizures and seizure care in an emergency department. *Epilepsia* 1989;30:175–181.
8. Hauser W. The natural history of drug resistant epilepsy: epidemiologic considerations. *Epilepsia* 1992(suppl 5):25–28.
9. Hauser W, et al. Seizure recurrence after a first unprovoked seizure: an extended follow-up. *Neurology* 1990;40:1163–1170.
10. Wachtel T, Steele G, Day J. Natural history of fever following seizure. *Arch Intern Med* 1987;147:1153–1155.
11. Aminoff M, Simon R. Status epilepticus: causes, clinical features and consequences in 98 patients. *Am J Med* 1980;69:657–666.
12. Aminoff M, et al. Cerebrospinal fluid analysis in children with seizures. *Pediatr Emerg Care* 1995;11:226–229.
13. Lin J. Convulsive syncope in blood donors. *Ann Neurol* 1982;11:525–528.
14. Linzer M, et al. Cardiovascular causes of loss of consciousness in patients with presumed epilepsy: a cause of increased sudden death rate in people with epilepsy. *Am J Med* 1994;96:146–154.
15. Haines S. Decerebrate posturing misinterpreted as seizure activity, *Am J Emerg Med* 1988;6:173–177.
16. Finelli P, Cardi J. Seizures as a cause of fracture. *Neurology* 1989;39:858–860.
17. American Academy of Neurology. Practice parameter: evaluating a first nonfebrile seizure in children. *Neurology* 2000;55:616–623.
18. American College of Emergency Physicians. Clinical policy for the initial approach to patients presenting with a chief complaint of seizure who are not in status epilepticus. *Ann Emerg Med* 1997;29:706–724.
19. Green S, et al. Can seizures be the sole manifestation of meningitis in febrile children? *Pediatrics* 1993;92:527–534.
20. Tardy B, Lafond P, Convers P. Adult first generalized seizure: etiology, biological tests, EEG, CT scan, in an ED. *Am J Emerg Med* 1995;13:1–5.
21. American College of Emergency Physicians, American Academy of Neurology, American Association of Neurological Surgeons, American Society of Neuroradiology. Practice parameter: neuroimaging in the emergency patient presenting with seizure (summary statement). *Ann Emerg Med* 1996;27:114–118.
22. Treiman D, et al. A comparison of four treatments for generalized convulsive status epilepticus. *N Engl J Med* 1998;339:792–798.

23. Lowenstein D, Alldredge B. Status epilepticus. *N Engl J Med* 1998;338:970–976.

24. Jagoda A, Riggio S. Refractory status epilepticus. *Ann Emerg Med* 1993;22:1337–1348.

25. Krumholz A, et al. Complex partial status epilepticus accompanied by serious morbidity and mortality. *Neurology* 1995.

26. Tomson T, Lindbom U, Nilsson B. Nonconvulsive status epilepticus in adults: thirty-two consecutive patients from a general hospital population. *Epilepsia* 1992;33:829–835.

27. Delorenzo R, et al. Persistent nonconvulsive status epilepticus after the control of convulsive status epilepticus. *Epilepsia* 1998;39:833–840.

28. Ng S, Hauser A, Brust J, Susser M. Alcohol consumption and withdrawal in new onset seizures. *N Engl J Med* 1988;319:666–673.

29. Earnest M, et al. Intracranial lesions shown by CT scans in 259 cases of first alcohol related seizures. *Neurology* 1988;38:1561–1565.

30. Rathlev N, et al. The lack of efficacy of phenytoin in the prevention of recurrent alcohol-related seizures. *Ann Emerg Med* 1994;23:513–518.

31. D'Orofrio G, et al. Lorazepam for the prevention of recurrent seizures related to alcohol. *N Engl J Med* 1999;340:915–919.

32. Ratanakorn D, et al. Single oral loading dose of phenytoin: a pharmacokinetics study. *J Neurol Sci* 1997;147:89–92.

33. van der Meyden CH, et al. Acute oral loading of carbamazepine-CR and phenytoin in a double-blind randomized study of patients at risk of seizures. *Epilepsia* 1994;35:189–194.

34. Lucas MJ, Leveno KJ, Cunningham FG. A comparison of magnesium sulfate with phenytoin for the prevention of eclampsia. *N Engl J Med* 1995;333:201–205.

35. American Academy of Pediatrics. Practice parameter: the neurodiagnostic evaluation of the child with a first simple febrile seizure. *Pediatrics* 1996;97:769–775.

36. American Academy of Pediatrics. Practice parameter: long term treatment of the child with a simple febrile seizure. *Pediatrics* 1999;103:1307–1309.

C H A P T E R

12
SYNCOPE

Syncope, from the Greek word *syncope* meaning a cessation or pause, is the sudden loss of consciousness and postural tone with spontaneous rapid return to normal. Syncope, commonly called fainting, is a nonspecific symptom that can be the final common pathway for a number of underlying conditions. Although syncope may be due to other disorders, it most commonly results from conditions that cause a 35% reduction in cerebral blood flow, or a transient (as short as 8 to 10 seconds) episode of absent cerebral blood flow. Syncope, like coma, is characterized by lack of self-awareness, yet, unlike coma, it is very brief. Presyncope, near-syncope, or faintness is the sensation of severe lightheadedness or impending loss of consciousness that may precede frank syncope, or occur without syncope. These symptoms occur along a continuum of severity. Its causes are generally the same as syncope, with the major difference being the magnitude of the physiologic derangements. Although syncope has a very narrow definition, other conditions may simulate syncope or cause transiently altered consciousness. Clinically, the most common syncope mimic is seizure.

OBJECTIVES

The primary emergency department (ED) objective in evaluation of the syncopal patient is to try to make a determination as to whether the cause for syncope represents a life-threatening condition or not. Syncope is a common problem and represents up to 3% of emergency department visits. In general, patients under age 30 and those over 70 with vasovagal, psychogenic, or unknown causes for syncope have a relatively benign prognosis, and those over age 60 with cardiac syncope or poor left ventricular function tend to have higher risk for subsequent morbidity and mortality.[1] It is difficult to prognosticate for many patients.[2]

There are several challenges to the clinician in the evaluation of syncope. The transient and episodic nature of syncopal episodes make a firm diagnosis a challenge. In evaluating the patient who has recovered from a syncopal episode, the conditions prevailing at the time of the event are, almost by definition, no longer present. To discover with certainty what happened during the episode (but not present currently) can be a great challenge. Even if a current abnormality can be found, establishing cause and effect can be difficult. Causes for syncope range from benign to life-threatening, and a cause cannot be found, at times despite numerous investigations, in 38% to 49% of patients.[3,4]

Syncope is a common symptom, occurring in 12% to 48% of young adults at some time in their life and 30% to 50% of adults; it precipitates 1% to 6% of hospital admissions, and up to 3% of ED visits.[3] It is a particularly common symptom in the elderly, and it increases in incidence with advancing age.

PATHOPHYSIOLOGY

In order for consciousness to be lost, the factors that sustain consciousness must be briefly, but reversibly, interrupted. Loss of consciousness, as can be seen from the chapter on coma, involves loss of normal, organized electrical activity of both cerebral hemispheres or brainstem centers, or acute loss of substrates, primarily glucose and oxygen, which are necessary for cerebral metabolism. Such losses usually occur because of inadequate cerebral perfusion. Cerebral blood flow of approximately 55 mL/100 g brain tissue/min is necessary for an adequate supply of oxygen and glucose; if it falls to 20 mL/100 g brain tissue/min, then syncope occurs. The brain does not store energy resources and is dependent on a continuous supply of substrate. Isolated deficiencies of glucose or possibly oxygen rarely occur and reverse rapidly enough to simulate syncope. The process of cerebral hypoperfusion must be rapidly reversible, or death would ensue. The two prerequisites of rapidity of onset and rapid reversibility limit the number of etiologies to be considered.

Although much individual variation exists in the magnitude of decrease in cerebral blood flow that can cause syncope, systolic pressures below 70 mmHg or mean arterial pressure as low as 40 mmHg may result in syncope,[3] depending on the individual's general state of health, existence of impaired cerebral circulation and capabilities for compensation, and prior blood pressure levels. Several pathophysiologic changes may combine in a given patient to produce syncope, when none of these changes by themselves are of sufficient magnitude. Regardless of the exact mechanisms involved, virtually all syncopal episodes occur in the upright posture and are generally terminated with attaining supine positioning.

Response to Change from Supine to Upright Position

When a person changes from the supine to upright position, there is a shift of approximately 300 to 800 mL of blood to the lower extremities. This results in less venous return, less ventricular filling, decreased cardiac output, and reduced arterial pressure. Such a drop in pressure stimulates baroreceptors in the carotid sinus and aortic arch to reduce inhibitory control of the medulla's vasomotor center. This results in enhanced sympathetic tone and diminished parasympathetic tone. Catecholamines, vasopressin, and other neurohumoral substances increase systemic vascular resistance, myocardial contractility, and heart rate, resulting in restoration of blood pressure or blunting of the decrease in blood pressure. Interruptions in any part of this regulatory pathway can impair the body's ability to maintain normal arterial pressure and cerebral perfusion and thus cause or contribute to syncope.

CLASSIFICATION

There are a number of ways to classify syncope, some of which are listed in Tables 12-1 and 12-2. Grouping disorders that result in similar pathophysiologic changes is a common method of categorization. Considerable overlap exists in mixed organ system

TABLE 12-1
CAUSES OF SYNCOPE

Common
Ventricular or supraventricular tachycardia
Orthostatic hypotension (blood loss from ruptured ectopic pregnancy, GI bleed, ruptured abdominal aortic aneurysm)
Vasodepressor/vasovagal syncope
Situational syncope (cough, micturition, defecation)
Sick sinus syndrome, bradycardia
Seizure disorder
Unknown etiology
Drug-induced

Less Common
Pulmonary embolism
Supraventricular tachycardia
Complete heart block
Aortic, subaortic, or mitral stenosis
Myocardial infarction
Pacemaker malfunction
Psychogenic
Breath-holding spells in children
Subarachnoid hemorrhage
Bradycardia

Rare
Aortic dissection
Basilar migraine
Glossopharyngeal or trigeminal neuralgia
Subclavian steal syndrome
Pulmonary hypertension
Atrial myxoma

TABLE 12-2 ——————————————————————————————————

PHYSIOLOGIC CAUSES OF SYNCOPE

Generalized Low Cardiac Output

Pump Failure
Acute MI
Cardiac tamponade
Aortic dissection

Decreased Venous Return
Hypovolemia
Orthostatic hypotension
Drug-induced
Autonomic neuropathies

Cardiac Arrhythmia
Bradyarrhythmias
   Carotid sinus sensitivity
   Sick sinus syndrome
   Second- and third-degree AV blocks
   Pacemaker malfunction
Tachyarrhythmia
   Supraventricular tachycardia
   Ventricular tachycardia
   Runaway pacemaker
   Drug-induced torsades de pointes
   Long QT syndromes

Obstruction to Flow
Left ventricular outflow obstruction
   Aortic stenosis
   Hypertrophic cardiomyopathy
   Left atrial myxoma
   Mitral stenosis
Right ventricular outflow obstruction
   Pulmonic stenosis
   Pulmonary embolism
   Pulmonary hypertension
   Right atrial myxoma

Combinations
Vasovagal (neurally mediated, neurocardiogenic vasodepressor)
Pulmonary embolus, situational (micturition, defecation, cough, swallow)
Carotid sinus syndrome

and pathophysiologic classification schemes. Frequently, several factors, none of which would cause syncope by themselves, combine to transiently impair cerebral blood flow to the point of loss of consciousness. Compensatory mechanisms then reverse one or more factors, and cerebral blood flow and consciousness are restored.

It is uncommon that blood flow solely to parts of the brainstem critical for maintenance of consciousness occurs in a rapidly reversible fashion without affecting other brainstem structures. It is likewise uncommon that the availability of the substrates of oxygen and glucose is suddenly but rapidly reversibly diminished to the point of loss of consciousness.

GENERAL APPROACH TO THE SYNCOPAL PATIENT

One of the primary tasks of the ED clinician in the evaluation of possible syncope is to try to establish whether, indeed, the patient had what is defined as syncope. The largest practical distinction that is usually made is between syncope and seizure. The patient may not be sufficiently aware of certain characteristics of the incident, there may be no witnesses, and usually there is no physiologic monitoring in place during the incident. If any of these can be found, they can be very helpful. Attention may need to be directed at the consequences of the incident, such as trauma from a fall. The starting point for evaluation of the potential syncopal patient is the history and physical exam, which will be used to guide further evaluation. When a cause for syncope can be found, as it is in 50% to 70% of cases, the history and physical examination alone will provide the answer in 50% to 80% of patients.

Cardiac arrhythmia is one of the most common overall categories for the etiology of syncope. Typically the prodromal symptoms are brief (less than 5 seconds) or absent. An arrhythmia may occur in isolation (ventricular tachycardia), or in combination with other factors (vasovagal). In the unusual circumstance in which syncope and an arrhythmia capable of inducing syncope occur in a monitored patient, a definitive diagnosis can usually be established. Other rhythm electrocardiographic (ECG) monitoring, in the absence of a concurrent syncopal episode, may or may not be helpful in establishing a diagnosis. Ventricular tachycardia is the most common of the cardiac causes for syncope[4,5] and represents one of the greatest potential threats to life. An ECG, recorded during a syncopal episode, an uncommon occurrence, is invaluable in establishing a diagnosis. Even the pulse taken by a bystander can be useful.

TYPICAL SYNCOPE SYNDROMES

Neurocardiogenic Syncope

The mechanism for neurocardiogenic syncope (vasovagal, neurally mediated, neurocardiogenic, vasodepressor) is not completely understood. It can be initiated by venous pooling, leading to decreased central blood volume and stroke volume, causing a compensatory increase in sympathetic activity. In susceptible patients, this increase in sympathetic activity can trigger the Betzold-Jarish reflex, leading to bradycardia and/or hypotension. This reflex occurs because cardiac sensory receptors in the posterior inferior left ventricle become stimulated (by stretch, cardiac distention, forceful cardiac contraction with a relatively empty ventricle, or chemical substances) and send signals to the vasomotor center in the medulla. This leads to increased parasympathetic activity, decreased sympathetic activity, and bradycardia, which can be inhibited by atropine.[4] The response to elevated blood pressure, not diminished blood pressure, is then stimulated. Hypotension, exacerbated by decreased venous return from pooling of blood in the limbs, or the Valsalva maneuver occurs. Alcohol impairs vasoconstriction and may thus exacerbate the loss of compensatory adjustments.[5] Catecholamine release itself (as with fear, panic, and other stimuli) may trigger the ventricular contraction and thus the Betzold-Jarish reflex.

Clinically, patients with neurocardiogenic syncope will maintain normal blood pressure and cerebral perfusion immediately upon standing or upon another precipitating event, only to experience a sudden drop in blood pressure with bradycardia. They may feel lightheaded and may experience autonomic prodromal symptoms such as nausea, vomiting, pallor, diaphoresis, and epigastric discomfort.

Orthostatic Syncope

Orthostatic syncope occurs when the normal compensatory mechanisms that counter the effects of gravity (as discussed under the Response to Change from Supine to Upright Position section above) are impaired. Clinically, patients with orthostatic syncope have a gradual decrease in blood pressure over time after standing from a lying or sitting position, rather than the abrupt decrease seen in neurocardiogenic syncope, They may lack the autonomic responses (nausea, vomiting, pallor, diaphoresis, and epigastric discomfort) often seen in neurocardiogenic syncope. Patients tend to be elderly, diabetic, and/or receiving cardiovascular medications. Orthostatic syncope can occur in the setting of volume depletion, such as blood or other fluid loss, or with vasodilation; it can be exacerbated by alcohol or by medical disorders affecting autonomic regulation (Shy-Drager syndrome or diabetes mellitus) Prolonged bed rest may result in cardiovascular deconditioning and syncope due to diminished responses to upright posture.

Situational Syncope

Situational syncope, often referred to as "swooning" in previous times, may be mediated by neuroautonomic mechanisms similar to those causing neurocardiogenic syncope, but it is precipitated by a triggering event. Events such as injury, pain, hunger, fear, crowding, sight of blood, prolonged standing, or anxiety may result in a catecholamine surge that stimulates cardiac mechanoreceptors, resulting in the same feedback loop described for neurocardiogenic syncope.[6] Other causes for situational syncope, such as urination, defecation, coughing, sneezing, and swallowing, may be found in the setting of decreased venous return (as from the Valsalva maneuver) and enhanced vagal tone.

Carotid Sinus Syndrome

This has been defined as syncope or presyncope when carotid sinus massage produces asystole (cardioinhibitory) for 3 or more seconds or hypotension (vasodepressor: more than 30 mmHg when accompanied by symptoms, or more than 50 mmHg when asymptomatic), or mixed when both cardioinhibitory and vasodepressor responses occur.[7] Although neck movement or tight collars have been described as precipitating factors, syncope generally occurs without warning and is only rarely precipitated by neck movement.[8]

Seizure

Seizures are discussed in Chapter 11, but a few points are worth noting. The loss of consciousness in seizure is usually abrupt in onset, and an aura may not be present or remembered. The return to consciousness is slow, however, and confusion after an unexplained episode of unconsciousness points strongly toward seizure, as does transient focal neurologic deficit (Todd's paralysis). Patients may appear confused after a syncopal episode, but usually for no more than 20 to 30 seconds. Transient cerebral anoxia may cause a brief (usually less than 6 to 8 seconds) episode of seizure activity (convulsive syncope) and may be difficult to distinguish from a true underlying seizure disorder. Other discriminating factors are discussed below.

Psychogenic Syncope

Up to 20% of patients with unexplained syncope may have psychogenic syncope.[9] Syncope may be one of the manifestations of anxiety, panic, somatization, and conversion disorder.[10,11] However, this is a difficult diagnosis and should be considered a diagnosis of exclusion.

Syncope in Children and Adolescents

Syncope in children and adolescents is a common and generally benign event,[10] and the tendency to faint in childhood may be familial.[11] It is common during acute illness, as a response to other noxious emotional or psychologic stimuli, or related to medications or alcohol. Orthostatic syncope is common.[12] Serious causes are rare (hypertrophic cardiomyopathy, prolonged QT syndrome, myocarditis, anomalous origin of left coronary artery, and Wolff-Parkinson-White syndrome). Exertional syncope, a positive family history suggestive of long QT syndrome, sudden death at a young age, or a cardiac murmur on exam can be red flags for possibly serious etiologies.

Breath-holding spells may cause syncope. The term breath holding, implying a voluntary prolonged inspiration, is a misnomer. Breath holding usually occurs during expiration and is involuntary.[13] There are two types: cyanotic and pallid. In cyanotic breath-holding spells, the child holds the breath at the end of a bout of crying and becomes cyanotic and limp with loss of consciousness. There is rapid return of normal color, respirations, and consciousness. In the pallid variety, the child seems to be responding to a mild irritation, and breath holding may not be obvious. The child usually, but not always, becomes pale and has a sudden syncopal episode. The pathophysiology of breath-holding spells is felt to involve carotid sinus hypersensitivity and brief cerebral anoxia on the basis of brief cardiac asystole.[14] The condition has been associated with iron deficiency anemia.[15] Some children may have these on a daily basis, and a breath-holding spell may rarely precipitate an anoxic seizure. Breath-holding spells are usually benign, and most children outgrow them by age 5.[16]

Drug-Induced Syncope

A number of drugs, usually those with cardiovascular effects, may precipitate syncope. Some common examples are nitrates, β-blockers, vasodilators, calcium channel blockers, angiotensin-converting enzyme inhibitors, phenothiazines, and alcohol.[17] Some drugs that can precipitate arrhythmias, including torsades de pointes, are quinidine, procainamide, disopyramide, flecanide, amiodarone, sotalol.

DIAGNOSIS

History

A detailed history of the event, if available, can be the most helpful part of the evaluation. A reliable witness can be invaluable, and it may be worthwhile to pursue first-hand observers of the event. A history of events leading up to and immediately following the suspected syncopal episode is particularly helpful. History combined with physical examination may reveal 56% to 85% of the causes of syncope.[17] Aspects of the history that may be useful, if available, are listed in Table 12-3. The duration of a warning period of minutes, sometimes several minutes, points to vasovagal syncope; very short warning, 10 seconds or less, points to cardiac syncope.[18] The duration of any postevent alteration of consciousness is particularly helpful, as it is usually brief with true syncope and prolonged with seizure. Headache accompanying a syncopal episode, if not owing to injury from a fall, can suggest subarachnoid hemorrhage.

In many cases, a major branch point in diagnosis is to distinguish a cardiogenic from a neurogenic cause. The most common neurogenic cause is seizure. Another neurogenic cause, brainstem ischemia, may cause "drop attacks," but involvement of other brainstem centers results in a variety of neurologic signs and symptoms (vertigo, diplopia, dysarthria, ataxia, limb numbness or weakness, or facial paresthesias), as is more fully described in the section on transient ischemic attacks (TIAs). TIAs that are related to carotid artery disease virtually never cause syncope.[6] Factors strongly favoring seizure include cyanosis, frothing at the mouth, lateral tongue biting, disorientation, sore muscles, sleepiness after the event, and unconsciousness lasting for more than 5 minutes.[19] Factors that more strongly favor syncope are sweating, nausea before the event, and being oriented immediately after the event. It should be kept in mind that cardiac syncope may have brief tonic or

TABLE 12-3 ————————————————————————————
ELEMENTS OF SYNCOPE HISTORY

Body position at time of event
Activity: physical and emotional
Prodromal feelings: warmth, nausea, diaphoresis, visual loss, odors, heart rate
    and rhythm, pain, lightheadedness
Physical result of event: fall, injury, pain
Current illness
Incontinence
Tongue biting
Duration
Motor activity during event
Skin color, warmth
Pulse, respiratory activity, shortness of breath
Rate of return to normal level of consciousness
Alcohol use
Medication use
History of similar events
Medical history

tonic-clonic muscular activity at onset, and some forms of partial epilepsy may have bradycardia associated with them.[20] In trying to distinguish syncope from seizure, incontinence and trauma from the event are not especially discriminating.

Physical Examination

Some elements of the physical and neurologic exam tend to be more helpful than others. On cardiac exam, murmurs reflecting valvular heart disease (particularly aortic stenosis and idiopathic hypertrophic subaortic stenosis) or arrhythmias can point one in the direction of cardiac syncope. Findings suggesting congestive heart failure may correlate with higher risk of sudden death in the syncope patient. Orthostatic hypotension is a finding that requires a great deal of clinical interpretation. It can be misleading, as patients with other causes of syncope have blood pressure declines of 20 mmHg or more upon changing from the supine to the upright posture; also, orthostatic hypotension is common in the elderly[21] and in ED patients without syncope, especially the elderly.[22] The recurrence of presyncope or even syncope upon standing is probably more significant than any particular numeric blood pressure change. Focal neurologic findings may be a result of seizure, if they are not preexisting. The tip of the tongue may sustain a laceration when the patient with syncope falls for any reason and strikes the chin, but a laceration of the side of the tongue is extremely suggestive of a seizure.[23] as is disorientation after the event. Although testing for carotid sinus sensitivity is rarely done in the emergency setting, it may be diagnostic. Carotid sinus sensitivity is a rare cause for syncope[24]; it may be found in many normal people. Testing for carotid sinus sensitivity itself carries with it a small risk of adverse neurologic outcome (stroke or TIA). Contraindications include carotid bruit, stroke, recent myocardial infarction, or history of serious cardiac dysrhythmia.[25]

Laboratory Evaluation

Laboratory evaluations are rarely helpful in diagnosing the cause of a syncopal event. Although a low hemoglobin may precipitate orthostatic syncope, the history is usually more suggestive, and orthostasis can occur without low hemoglobin. The elderly may be more prone to silent blood loss. Although elevation of creatine phosphokinase (especially if drawn more than 3 hours after the event) has been described more commonly in patients with seizures than in those with vasovagal syncope, it is unlikely to be more valuable than history and physical exam in most cases, and it is neither sensitive nor specific.[26,27] A pregnancy test may be useful in selected patients. Electrolytes, although commonly obtained, rarely lead to an etiologic cause for syncope. Abnormal electrolyte levels may be consistent with etiologies discovered by other methods but are unlikely to be differentially diagnostic by themselves.

Neuroimaging and Other Studies

Electrocardiography/Rhythm Strip

An ECG or cardiac rhythm recording may reveal the substrate for a rhythm disturbance, or an actual rhythm disturbance, and is usually obtained when history and physical examination do not reveal a diagnosis. Findings such as complete heart block, supraventricular tachycardia, or ventricular tachycardia may point strongly toward cardiac syncope. However, other ECG abnormalities are common (50% of syncope patients have abnormal ECGs), but the abnormality may not be related to syncope.

Prolonged ECG Monitoring

Holter or patient-activated loop recorders may be useful beyond the initial patient evaluation in excluding an arrhythmic cause for syncope when symptoms are found to occur in the absence of a recorded arrhythmia, or in the rare instance when arrhythmic syncope is frequent enough to occur during monitoring.

Transthoracic Echocardiography

Transthoracic echocardiagraphy has commonly been performed in the further evaluation of syncope patients, but it is seldom useful or positive in evaluation except to confirm what is suggested by history, physical exam, and ECG findings; it is rarely done in the ED.[28]

Electrophysiologic Studies

Electrophysiologic studies may be performed for further evaluation of patients with recurrent syncope and organic heart disease. Such studies are beyond the scope of an acute care evaluation or this text.

Head-Up Tilt Table Testing

Tilt table testing, at times pharmacologically enhanced, may be useful in the further evaluation of patients without heart disease, when initial history and physical are non-revealing, or in patients with heart disease without arrhythmias. Such testing is beyond the scope of the acute care setting or this text.

Electroencephalogram

Electroencephalograms, performed in a search for evidence of seizures, have commonly been performed in patients hospitalized for the evaluation of syncope. They are rarely useful and seldom reveal evidence for a condition that was not suspected clinically.[29]

Carotid Doppler Ultrasound

Carotid Doppler ultrasound is seldom useful in the evaluation of the syncope patient. Transient ischemia of the brainstem, sufficient to cause loss of consciousness, affects other brainstem structures and clinically results in neurologic findings not limited to syncope. If a lesion were found on carotid Doppler ultrasound, it would be difficult to relate it to a true syncopal episode.

Brain Computed Tomography/Magnetic Resonance Imaging

These are rarely needed in the evaluation of the patient with true syncope, except perhaps to look into traumatic consequences of a fall.

REFERENCES

1. Day S, et al. Evaluation and outcome of emergency room patients with transient loss of consciousness. *Am J Med* 1982;73:15–23.
2. Eagle K, et al. Evaluation and prognostic classification for patients with syncope. *Am J Med* 1985;79:455–460.
3. Manolis AS, et al. Syncope: current diagnostic evaluation and management. *Ann Intern Med* 1990;113:994–995.
4. Santini M, et al. The effect of atropine in vasovagal syncope induced by head-up tilt testing. *Eur Heart J* 1999;20:1745–1751.
5. Narkiewicz K, Cooley R, Somers V. Alcohol potentiates orthostatic hypotension. *Circulation* 2000;101:398–402.
6. Lazarus J, Mauro V. Syncope: pathophysiology, diagnosis and pharmacotherapy. *Ann Pharmacother* 1996;30:994–1005.
7. Manolis AS. The clinical spectrum and diagnosis of syncope. *Herz* 1993;18:143–154.
8. Sutton R. Vasodepressor syncope. *Herz* 1993;18:155–163.
9. Linzer M, et al. Psychiatric syncope. *Psychosomatics* 1990;31:181–188.
10. Driscoll DJ, et al. Syncope in children and adolescents, *J Am Coll Cardiol* 1997;29:1039.
11. Camfield PR, Camfield CS. Syncope in childhood: a case control clinical study of the familial tendency to faint. *Can J Neurol Sci* 1990;17:306.
12. Ross B, et al. Abnormal responses to orthostatic testing in children and adolescents with recurrent unexplained syncope. *Am Heart J* 1991;122:748–754.

13. DiMario F. Breath-holding spells in childhood. *Am J Dis Child* 1992;146:125–131.
14. Stephenson JBP. Reflex anoxic seizures ("white breath-holding"): nonepileptic vagal attacks. *Arch Dis Child* 1978;53:193–200.
15. Hilal M, et al. Breath holding spells in 91 children and response to treatment with iron. *Arch Dis Child* 1999;81:261–262.
16. DiMario FJ Jr. Prospective study of children with cyanotic and pallid breath-holding spells. *Pediatrics* 2001;107:265–269.
17. Kapoor WN. Evaluation and outcome of patients with syncope. *Medicine (Baltimore)* 1990;69:160–175.
18. Martin G, et al. Prospective evaluation of syncope. *Ann Emerg Med* 1984;13:499–504.
19. Hoefnagels WA, et al. Transient loss of consciousness: the value of the history for distinguishing seizure from syncope. *J Neurol* 1991;238:39–43.
20. Constantin L, et al. Bradycardia and syncope as manifestations of partial epilepsy. *J Am Coll Cardiol* 1990;15:900–905.
21. Atkins D, et al. Syncope and orthostatic hypotension. *Am J Med* 1991;91:179–185.
22. Koxiol-Mclain J, Lowenstein S, Fuller B. Orthostatic vital signs in emergency department patients. *Ann Emerg Med* 1999;20:606–610.
23. Benbadis SR, et al. Value of tongue biting in the diagnosis of seizures, *Arch Intern Med* 1995;155:2346.
24. Richardson DA, et al. Prevalence of cardioinhibitory carotid sinus hypersensitivity in patients 50 years or over presenting to the accident and emergency department with "unexplained" or "recurrent" falls, *Pace* 1997;20:820.
25. Davies AJ, et al. Frequency of neurologic complications following carotid sinus massage, *Am J Cardiol* 1998;81:1256.
26. Libman MD, et al. Seizure vs. syncope: measuring serum creatine kinase in the emergency department, *J Gen Intern Med* 1991;6:408.
27. Neufeld MY, et al. Sequential serum creatine kinase determination differentiates vasovagal syncope from generalized tonic-clonic seizures. *Acta Neurol Scand* 1997;95:137–139.
28. Recchia D, et al. Echocardiography in the evaluation of patients with syncope, *J Gen Intern Med* 1995;10:649.
29. Davis TL, Freemon FR. Electroencephalography should not be routine in the evaluation of syncope in adults. *Arch Intern Med* 1990;150:2027–2029.

13
THE DIZZY PATIENT

The principal problem in any patient complaining of "dizziness" is defining the problem. Dizziness is not a medical term and must be clarified (through careful history taking) and categorized. into one of four general groups: vertigo, disequilibrium, presyncope, and nonspecified lightheadedness. The key for the clinician is to identify potentially life-threatening conditions, specifically distinguishing a central nervous system process from a peripheral one.

CLASSIFICATION

Vertigo

Vertigo is the feeling or sensation of movement. This may be described by the patient as swaying, spinning, whirling, leaning, or tilting. In general, when there is a definite illusion of movement, the problem lies somewhere along the peripheral or central nervous system pathways related to the vestibular apparatus.

Presyncope

Presyncopal episodes are often described by patients as "dizziness." Unlike the vertiginous patient, however, these patients will describe an impending loss of consciousness. They feel as if they are about to faint and may describe the sensation as lightheadedness or "graying out" (see Chap. 12).

Disequilibrium

Equilibrium depends on a constant stream of sensory information from the vestibular, proprioceptive, and visual systems. This information is integrated by cerebellar centers and influenced by the extrapyramidal pathways to produce confident and rhythmic motion by the patient. Patients with various problems in any of these systems, such as the decreased proprioception as seen in diabetics with peripheral neuropathy or decreased vision, may experience disequilibrium. Most such patients have comorbidities with minor defects in multiple systems, which in combination produce a sense of imbalance, without a sensation of motion, however.

Nonspecified Lightheadedness

The most difficult patients are those who do not fall into any of the three groups mentioned above. These patients generally have extremely vague histories and are unable to pin down any specific symptoms. This group includes patients with hyperventilation syndromes, anxiety neuroses, and other psychiatric disorders. Diagnosing this group represents a considerable challenge to both the patience and the skill of the physician.

The focus of this chapter is to provide a framework for approaching the patient with a chief complaint of "dizziness," primarily in order to distinguish central from peripheral etiologies. Hypoperfusion states causing presyncope, neuropathies causing disequilibrium, and systemic processes causing generalized weakness are presented in other chapters, although they are important conditions that should be considered when approaching these patients.

EPIDEMIOLOGY

"Dizziness" is a common component of many acute medical conditions. The incidence increases with age and is one of the most common chief complaints in patients over 75 years of age.[1] True vertigo accounts for approximately half of patients complaining of "dizziness," whereas near-syncope comprises a significant proportion of the rest.[2] Of those patients with vertigo, vertebrobasilar insufficiency is the most concerning diagnosis to be considered. Even in the absence of posterior circulation disease, dizziness from all causes is associated with disability and injury, especially from falls in the elderly.

PATHOPHYSIOLOGY OF VERTIGO

Vertigo results from dysfunction in the vestibular system from either its peripheral or central components. The peripheral vestibular apparatus includes the labyrinth located in the petrous portion of the temporal bone and the vestibular portion of the eighth cranial nerve, which courses through the cerebellopontine angle connecting the labyrinth to the brainstem. The labyrinth is composed of three semicircular canals, which register head rotation, and the otoliths (utricle and saccule), which sense head position relative to gravity. The central vestibular apparatus consists of vestibular nuclei at the pontomedullary junction in the brainstem; these nuclei are intimately connected to the nuclei controlling eye movement and the cerebellum. Position is registered centrally based on balanced input from the paired labyrinths. Vertigo occurs when input from one labyrinth is interrupted; the resulting unbalanced input from a single labyrinth creates the sensation of movement. In general, acute processes result in vertigo. Chronic processes, such as degenerative disease or expanding tumors, usually result in disequilibrium but not actual vertigo since the brain has time to accommodate to the deficit.

DIFFERENTIAL DIAGNOSIS

Central Vestibular Causes

Although less common than peripheral causes, central causes of vertigo are the most concerning (Table 13-1). Disorders include vertebrobasilar insufficiency, brainstem

---

TABLE 13-1

DIFFERENTIAL DIAGNOSIS OF DIZZINESS

Cardiopulmonary Causes
Arrhythmias
Postural hypotension
Hypovolemia (anemia)
Myocardial ischemia
Structural cardiac or valvular disease
Hypoxia
Vasovagal episode (also neurologic)

Neurologic Causes
Peripheral vestibular causes:
    Benign paroxysmal positional vertigo
    Vestibular neuritis
    Labyrinthitis
    Ménière's disease
    Perilymphatic fistulas
Central vestibular causes:
    CVA
    Vertebrobasilar ischemia
    Cerebellopontine angle mass
    Basilar artery migraine
    Multiple sclerosis
Multisensory deficit syndrome/disequilibrium syndrome

Other
Drug effects
Thyroid disorder
Hyperventilation
Anxiety

and cerebellum infarct, and hemorrhage; basilar artery migraine, cerebellopontine angle (CPA) tumors, and degenerative diseases are other considerations. Table 13-2 summarizes findings that help to distinguish central from peripheral vertigo. In general, when compared with peripheral vertigo, the symptoms of central vertigo are less acute, more persistent, and associated with neurologic deficits. Symptoms associated with brainstem ischemia include diplopia, ataxia, dysarthria, or facial weakness. However, many exceptions exist, and clinicians must always have a high index of suspicion, especially in those patients with cardiovascular risk factors.

Slowly growing lesions such as acoustic neuromas do not generally produce symptoms because compensatory mechanisms have time to evolve. Indeed, it is these compensatory mechanisms that facilitate recovery from acute insults. CPA tumors and posterior fossa masses may produce vertigo, or if their principal involvement is the cerebellum, they may produce only a feeling of unsteadiness. Such disequilibrium is usually unrelenting and progressive and may move to involve multiple cranial nerves and long tract signs.

Benign Paroxysmal Positional Vertigo

Benign paroxysmal positional vertigo (BPPV) is the most common cause of peripheral vertigo. This syndrome is characterized by a rapid onset of vertigo, associated with a change of head position, which lasts less than 30 to 60 seconds (Table 13-3). Often, patients will complain of the acute onset of symptoms after rolling over in

TABLE 13-2
PERIPHERAL VERTIGO VERSUS CENTRAL VERTIGO

Finding	Peripheral	Central
Nausea and vomiting	+++	+ / ++
Nystagmus	Horizontal or rotatory Fatigable Suppressed with fixation	Any direction Classically, vertical No suppression with fixation Does not fatigue
Gait imbalance	0 / +	++ / +++
Hearing loss	Varies: none in BPPV and vestibular neuronitis; present in labyrinthitis and Ménière's disease	Varies
Neurologic deficits other than hearing loss	0	0 / +++

TABLE 13-3 ————————————————————
CHARACTERISTIC FINDINGS IN BENIGN PAROXYSMAL
POSITIONAL VERTIGO

Provoked by head movement
Nystagmus that has delayed onset and short duration
Fatigability of nystagmus on repeat testing
Reversal of nystagmus on returning to an upright position
Surpression of nystagmus with visual fixation

bed, gazing upward, or bending forward. Findings include a. horizontal/rotary nystagmus with associated nausea and/or vomiting. Characteristically, symptoms abate when the patient lies still with the eyes closed. The pathogenesis of this condition is thought to be due to the accumulation of free-floating calcium carbonate particulate debris that forms a plug in the posterior semicircular canal. When the affected canal is down, as when the patient is in a recumbent position, the calcium carbonate plug acts as a plunger and stimulates the labyrinth. The latency reflects the time required for the plug to move in the canal and stimulate the system; fatigue reflects the process of the plug breaking apart. A history of prior head trauma has been linked to the onset of BPPV, presumably due to dislodged endolymphatic debris.

Ménière's Disease

Ménière's disease is a peripheral nervous system disorder resulting from an increase in endolymph volume (endolymphatic hydrops). Distention of the endolymphatic system results in vertigo, and the increased pressure on hair cells results in an associated hearing loss. The duration of the vertigo and. nausea/vomiting in Ménière's disease tends to be hours rather than seconds, as in BPPV. Onset is most frequently in the fifth decade of life. It also differs from BPPV in that it is associated with a sensation of "fullness" in the affected ear with a fluctuating sensorineural hearing loss and tinnitus. Disequilibrium may also be present.

Vestibular Neuronitis

Vestibular neuronitis is a constellation of symptoms that includes acute-onset vertigo, nausea, vomiting, and disequilibrium. It is thought to be viral in etiology, generally occurring in otherwise healthy individuals. Hearing remains unimpaired because only the vestibular apparatus is involved. All audiologic testing is normal. No brainstem findings or other cranial nerve abnormalities are found. The time course of symptoms tends to be over a period of days, with symptoms usually peaking during the first day and then gradually improving over the next few days. As may be seen with all the peripheral causes of vertigo, the patients appear acutely and severely ill.

Labyrinthitis

Labyrinthitis may be differentiated from vestibular neuronitis in that there is both nystagmus and vertigo along with hearing loss. Viral labyrinthitis has been reported in association with multiple-viral illness and is generally short lived and of little consequence. Bacterial labyrinthitis, however, can occur in patients with middle ear disease with fistulas, or mastoid disease, or in association with meningitis. These patients represent a medical emergency and require prompt diagnosis and treatment.

Posttraumatic Vestibular Syndromes

Perilymphatic fistulas between the middle and inner ear may result after trauma, after a forceful Valsalva maneuver, or after acute external pressure changes as in scuba diving. Replication of the patient's symptoms on Valsalva maneuver or pneumatic otoscopy, combined with a suggestive history, is diagnostic. Acute traumatic tympanic membrane rupture can also lead to immediate onset of vertigo, nausea, and/or vomiting associated with hearing loss. A similar constellation of symptoms can be seen in patients with fractures through the petrous portion of the temporal bone.

Disequilibrium Syndromes (Multisensory Deficits Syndromes)

A generalized feeling of unsteadiness in the nonvertiginous elderly patient usually represents a multisensory deficits syndrome. These patients frequently relate that their problem is worse in the evening when they are fatigued and their visual inputs are diminished. Such patients frequently do well in familiar surroundings where only minimal information is necessary for them to make decisions but do poorly in unfamiliar situations. Multisensory deficits can be tremendously exaggerated by medications including those used to treat vertigo.

Other Causes

Other causes of dizziness include drug toxicity, hypoglycemia, anemia, hypothyroidism, and multiple sclerosis; psychiatric causes include anxiety and hyperventilation, although these diagnoses are ones of exclusion and rarely definitively made by emergency physicians. All tranquilizers, antiepileptic drugs, and antipsychotic drugs may through multiple mechanisms cause a combination of disequilibrium, near-syncope, and mild forms of vertigo that the patient may be unable to separate on a historical basis (Table 13-4). Ototoxic drugs that cause a sense of unsteadiness and hearing loss rarely actually cause vertigo since the deficits are bilateral.

EVALUATION

Patients presenting with a complaint of dizziness should have a complete set of vital signs obtained, and triage should include cardiovascular risk factors. Oxygenation and cardiovascular stability should be assessed; if fluid intake has been compro-

TABLE 13-4
DRUGS ASSOCIATED WITH DIZZINESS

Anticonvulsants
Alcohols
Aminoglycosides
Other antibiotics
Heavy metals
Chincona alkaloids
Salicylates
Minor tranquilizers
Major tranquilizers
Diuretics
β-Blockers
α-Blockers
Centrally acting antihypertensives

mised, dehydration needs to be addressed. Patients with vertigo are at risk of vomiting, and thus appropriate precautions should be taken.

Orthostatic hypotension, usually defined as a drop in systolic blood pressure of 20 mmHg or more within 2 minutes of standing upright, is a finding that suggests near-syncope or syncope. Unfortunately, orthostatic changes are neither a specific nor sensitive finding. When identified, further investigation into the causes of orthostatic hypotension are indicated. Possibilities include volume depletion, drug effects, and other causes such as deconditioning and autonomic insufficiency in the elderly.

History

The key to diagnosis of the dizzy patient lies in careful history taking, allowing the patient to describe the symptoms. The correct etiology of dizziness can be made by history alone in over half of patients seen[3] (Table 13-5). If patients report that they have a sense of motion or spinning, follow-up questions regarding relationship of symptoms to position and movement are important. The time course for various causes of vertigo may also be helpful: BPPV usually has an abrupt onset, vertebral basilar insufficiency may develop over minutes or have a stuttering course, Ménière's syndrome has vertigo that may last for hours, and vestibular neuronitis and labyrinthitis have persistent symptoms for days.

Patients with near-syncope as the underlying mechanism of their dizziness will frequently have an increase of symptoms with autonomic stress. Information about the relationship to orthostatic change as well as swallowing, coughing, and urinating should be elicited.

Patients with disequilibrium have particular difficulty when one of their sensory modalities is reduced. In particular, older patients with decreasing vision find

TABLE 13-5

HISTORICAL FEATURES IMPORTANT TO CHARACTERIZE IN A PATIENT WITH A CHIEF COMPLAINT OF DIZZINESS/VERTIGO

- Sensation of motion, whirling, spinning, tilting, leaning
- Relation to change of position, sharp turns, specific positions
- Rate of onset and duration of symptoms
- Relation to autonomic nervous system stress
- Time of day
- Drugs and medications: prescription and nonprescription
- Associated symptoms: nausea, vomiting, blurred vision, loss of vision, motor weakness, hearing loss, tinnitus, headache, difficulty speaking or swallowing, incoordination
- Other medical problems (thyroid disease, diabetes, hypertension, stroke)

that in the evening when rooms are inadequately lighted, they have considerably more difficulty in walking. Also, patients with multisensory deficits have greater difficulty as the day progresses and fatigue affects their system.

A seemingly endless list of drugs may cause not only vertigo but generalized weakness and/or autonomic changes that may be interpreted by the patient as dizziness. Many of the medications that affect blood pressure, electrolytes, or central or peripheral nervous system structures may be the cause of the patient's symptoms. A history of both prescription drugs and over-the-counter medications used should be elicited.

Physical Examination

The physical and neurologic examination should be performed systematically with a focus on the vital signs, cardiovascular system, cranial nerves, posterior column, and sensory functions.

The head exam should assess for evidence of trauma. Examine the tympanic membranes and external auditory canals for the presence of infection or tympanic membrane rupture. Impacted cerumen, foreign body, and acute otitis media are unlikely causes of vertigo but may give a sense of dysequilibrium. The eye exam includes checking for the presence of nystagmus. Peripheral vestibular nystagmus is typically horizontal-rotatory with a slow and fast component. The fast component points away from the affected side. It typically extinguishes with repeated testing or ocular fixation.[4] In peripheral disease the nystagmus is in a constant direction regardless of direction of gaze, although the intensity of the nystagmus may vary. The nystagmus increases in intensity with gaze in the direction of the fast phase (Alexander's law). Visual fixation will reduce the intensity of nystagmus in peripheral disorders, and removal of fixation (e.g., eye closure, Frenzel lenses) will exacerbate peripheral nystagmus and vertigo. Central disorders can produce nystagmus that changes direction with gaze (gaze-evoked nystagmus), although nystagmus can be present in only one direction of gaze. Vertical nystagmus that is spontaneous and nonfatigable represents a central pathology until proven otherwise. Visual fixation does not affect the degree of nystagmus produced by central disorders.

A cardiovascular exam should be done particularly in patients at risk for cardiovascular disease. The carotid arteries should be assessed for bruits. Bruits suggest carotid stenosis, which may suggest cerebrovascular insufficiency as a cause of the patient's symptoms. A systolic murmur suggests aortic stenosis, which may explain near-syncope or syncope also associated with exertion.

Neurologic Examination

A cranial nerve evaluation should be performed and documented, with special attention to cranial nerves VII, VIII, and IX. Cranial nerve VIII deficits may help elucidate the etiology of vertigo. The best general test of cranial nerve VIII is the use of soft whispered speech. The test is performed by having the examiner whisper letters and numbers in one ear while masking sound in the opposite ear. Masking can be accomplished by simply rubbing the fingers or hair in front of the opposite ear. The level at which the patient can then hear is recorded. Soft-whispered speech, whispered-speech, loud-whispered speech, spoken-speech, loud-spoken speech, and finally no response are the levels generally employed for the whispered-speech test. Table 13-6 presents the differential of acute unilateral and bilateral hearing loss.

TABLE 13-6

DIFFERENTIAL DIAGNOSIS OF ACUTE HEARING LOSS

Bilateral central
Meningitis
Systemic infections
Ototoxic drugs
Multiple sclerosis
Congenital syphilis
Idiopathic
Hysterical

Unilateral
Direct head trauma and acoustic trauma
Ménière's disease
Viral illness
Spontaneous rupture of the round-window membrane or inner-ear membrane
Vascular disorders
Post surgical
Post anaesthesia

The Weber test is used to localize sound depending on the area of neurologic involvement. The test is performed placing a vibrating 256-Hz tuning fork on the vertex of the head. If hearing is normal, sound will be heard equally in both ears. In patients with an air conduction disorder (middle ear disease or blockage of the external canal), sound will lateralize to the side with the conduction loss. If the cochlear nerve is involved, the sound will lateralize to the unaffected side.

The Rinne test further confirms whether a hearing loss is conductive or neurosensory. A 500-Hz or higher tuning fork should be struck and held onto the mastoid process behind the ear. The tuning fork is then rapidly removed and held in front of the ear. The patient is asked where the sound was loudest. If the patient feels the sound was loudest while the tuning fork was on the bone, the patient has a conductive hearing loss. If the sound is loudest in front of the ear, which is the normal condition, any hearing loss the patient has must be on a neurosensory basis.

Cerebellar function is assessed using finger-to-nose, finger-to-finger, and rapid alternating movement tests. Ambulation is a key component of the evaluation, although care must be taken to ensure the patient does not fall. Patients with peripheral vertigo are typically able to walk without assistance, whereas patients with an acute cerebellar infarction or hemorrhage are generally unable to ambulate unassisted. Romberg testing is used to distinguish somatosensory deficits from cerebellar processes (see Chap. 2, on the neurologic exam).

Diagnostic Maneuvers

The Dix-Hallpike maneuver (sometimes referred to as the Nylen-Bárány maneuver) is a provocative test designed to precipitate BPPV and thus to help distinguish peripheral from central vertigo. The maneuver involves moving the patient rapidly from a sitting position to a position with the head hanging at a 30-degree angle off the end of the bed with one ear downward and then repeating the test with the other ear down. When positive, the patient will, after a brief (up to 30 seconds) latency period, complain of a sensation of rotational vertigo, accompanied by nystagmus. The nystagmus tends to be horizontal or rotatory, with the superior aspect of the eye bearing toward the dependent ear. The sensitivity of the maneuver for BPPV approaches 90%.[5] Repetition of the maneuver leads to a reduction in the intensity of vestibular symptoms, and thus it is also used in therapeutic management.

Diagnostic Testing

No one panel of tests is indicated for all patients with a complaint of dizziness; instead, testing is tailored to clinical suspicion with a low testing threshold for anemia, hypoglycemia, and pregnancy. Likewise, a single 12-lead ECG is rarely definitive but is indicated along with continuous rhythm monitoring when dysrhythmias are in the differential diagnosis.

Neuroimaging is indicated in patients with signs of a central process, focal neurologic deficits, headache, or risk factors for cerebrovascular disease for which no other explanation of the symptoms can be found. A noncontrast head computed tomography (CT) scan is a good screening test for patients with suspected central lesions causing vertigo, but it has limitations that preclude it from being definitive. Magnetic resonance (MR) brain imaging and angiography are preferred except for detecting acute hemorrhage. MR imaging is more likely to detect subtle brainstem or inferior cerebellar infarction, whereas MR angiography is indicated to assess for vertebrobasilar occlusive disease. Decision making for advanced neuroimaging must take into consideration the patient's presentation, risk factors, and availability for follow-up care.

Special mention needs to be made regarding the patient with sudden onset of headache, severe vertigo, vomiting, and cerebellar incoordination. Such patients should be considered as having an acute cerebellar hemorrhage and are best treated as if they have a life-threatening emergency. An emergent noncontrast head CT is indicated. Along with vertigo, patients with acute cerebellar hemorrhage often present with unilateral ataxia, small pupils, vomiting, and diaphoresis. Paralysis of conjugate lateral gaze or sixth nerve palsies may also be seen.

Specialized Neurologic Testing

Audiometry is used in evaluating dizzy patients with unilateral hearing loss, although it is not indicated as an emergency test in the ED. It is helpful in diagnosing Ménière's disease and acoustic neuromas. Electronystagmography (ENG) is a test of vestibular function that uses electrodes to monitor nystagmus that appears spontaneously or when induced by lateral gaze, positional change, or caloric testing. ENG testing has been proposed as helpful in distinguishing peripheral from central vestibular disorders; however, at this time its benefit is unclear and it is not recommended.[6]

EMERGENCY DEPARTMENT MANAGEMENT

Management of acute peripheral vertigo includes bed rest, fluids, and reassurance. Medications that suppress vestibular signs can be helpful acutely.

Therapeutic Maneuvers

The canalith repositioning maneuver, often called the Epley maneuver, is a noninvasive bedside intervention designed to reposition particulate debris from the semicircular canal to the utricle[7] (Table 13-7) Once the particulate matter is repositioned, abnormal vestibular input is eliminated. This maneuver is reported to have a 50% to 100% success rate in patients with BPPV.[7,8]

Vestibular rehabilitation exercises, which consist of repetitive side-to-side head movements performed while lying down, have been shown to decrease the intensity of vertiginous episodes in BPPV and to facilitate recovery. These exercises should be provided as part of the discharge instructions.[9]

TABLE 13-7

CANALITH REPOSITIONING MANEUVER (EPLEY MANEUVER) FOR TREATING BENIGN PAROXYSMAL POSITIONAL VERTIGO

1. Begin with the patient in a sitting position: calcium carbonate debris settles in the bottom of the posterior canal.
2. Lay patient down with head hanging 30 degrees off the edge of the gurney and left ear toward floor, for 30 seconds.
3. Rotate head clockwise to opposite side so that the other ear is toward the floor, for 30 seconds.
4. Continue rotating the patient clockwise so that face is toward the floor, for 30 seconds: In this position the debris should enter the common crus of the posterior and anterior semicircular canals.
5. Sit the patient up: Clot should enter the utricle.
6. Repeat the maneuver until no nystagmus is precipitated.
7. Instruct the patient to not lie down for 48 hours (wearing a soft collar can help; patient should sleep semi-reclined).

Vestibular Suppressants

Four categories of medications have efficacy in the management of vertigo, regardless of the etiology: antihistamines, anticholinergics, phenothiazines, and benzodiazepines (Table 13-8). Antihistamines and anticholinergics work through inhibiting muscarinic acetylcholine receptors involved in feedback from the brainstem to the vestibular labyrinth, rather than via direct H_1 receptor blockade. Meclizine is probably the most commonly used antihistamine for peripheral ver-

TABLE 13-8

OUTPATIENT VESTIBULAR SUPPRESSANT THERAPY

Class	Medication	Dosage
Antihistamines	Meclizine	25 mg PO q8–12h
	Diphenhydramine	25–50 mg PO q6h
Anticholinergics	Scopolamine	0.5 mg transdermal patch q3–4d
Phenothiazines	Promethazine	25 mg PO/PR q6h
	Prochlorperazine	10 mg PO q6–8h; 25 mg PR q12h
Benzodiazepines	Diazepam	2 mg PO q8–12h

tigo, although dimenhydrinate and diphenhydramine are alternatives. In patients with prominent nausea or vomiting, the phenothiazine antiemetics such as promethazine or prochlorperazine are effective and also work through their anticholinergic mechanisms to treat the vertigo. Benzodiazepines have also been used in the treatment of vertigo; they work through generalized inhibition of neural activity.

It is key to emphasize that all the medications mentioned above may cause drowsiness and indeed may exacerbate symptoms in patients with disequilibrium syndromes, presyncope, or undefined "dizziness." They are only indicated when true vertigo is present. Even in BPPV, vestibular suppressants should be used judiciously since the natural course of the disease is one of fluctuating symptoms with intermittent brief symptomatic episodes separated by asymptomatic periods. Vestibular suppressants have been shown to suppress the intensity of symptoms but not necessarily the frequency of attacks.[10] Long-term use of these medications may also impair vestibular compensation.

DISPOSITION

Patients with suspected posterior circulation disease require hospitalization or consultation with a neurologist. Patients with suspected cerebral vascular ischemia should be started on antiplatelet therapy, although the timing of initiation of these medications is undetermined. Admission may be necessary for patients with severe symptoms accompanied by disequilibrium despite therapy (particularly the elderly at risk for falling).

Patients discharged home should be advised not to drive and to minimize situations in which falling could cause harm. As discussed above, vestibular suppressants are only indicated in cases of true vertigo and are potentially dangerous in patients with other causes of dizziness. Patients with BPPV should be instructed on the importance of vestibular rehabilitation exercises and the possibility of recurrent symptoms.

SUMMARY

Successful ED management of a patient with an acute complaint of dizziness is built on a careful history and physical examination. The history focuses on symptom description and time course. The physical exam investigates abnormal vital signs, the presence of nystagmus (horizontal or vertical, fatiguing or nonfatigable), hearing loss, evidence of head trauma, or neurologic deficits. For patients with peripheral vestibular symptoms, the Dix-Hallpike maneuver may be confirmatory. Patients with peripheral vertigo do not need extensive diagnostic testing but instead require supportive care that includes hydration and vestibular stabilizing medications. Patients who have acute neurologic deficits should have emergent neuroimaging with appropriate neurology or neurosurgical consultation.

REFERENCES

1. Tinetti ME, Williams CS, Gill TM. Dizziness among older adults: a possible geriatric syndrome. *Ann Intern Med* 2000;132:337–344.
2. Herr RD, et al. Immediate electronystagmography in the diagnosis of the dizzy patient. *Ann Emerg Med* 1993;22:1182–1189.
3. Kroenke K, et al. Causes of persistent dizziness. A prospective study of 100 patients in ambulatory care. *Ann Intern Med* 1992;117:898–904.
4. Hotson JR, Baloh RW. Acute vestibular syndrome. *N Engl J Med* 1998;339:680–685.
5. Hoffman RM, Einstadter D, Kroenke K. Evaluating dizziness. *Am J Med* 1999;107: 468–478.
6. American Academy of Neurology. Assessment: electronystagmography. Report of the Therapeutics and Technology Assessment Subcommittee. *Neurology* 1996;46:1763–1766.
7. Epley JM. The canalith repositioning procedure: for treatment of benign paroxysmal positional vertigo. *Otolaryngol Head Neck Surg* 1992;107:399–404.
8. Lynn S, et al. Randomized trial of the canalith repositioning procedure. *Otolaryngol Head Neck Surg* 1995;113:712–720.
9. Yardley L, et al. A randomized controlled trial of exercise therapy for dizziness and vertigo in primary care. *Br J Gen Pract* 1998;48:1136–1140.
10. Furman JM, Cass SP. Benign paroxysmal positional vertigo. *N Engl J Med* 1999;341: 1590–1596.

NECK AND BACK PAIN

Acute and chronic neck and back pains are extremely common presenting complaints in the acute care setting. This chapter focuses on evaluation of the patient who presents with neck or back pain with either no trauma or with minor trauma such as bending, lifting, or minor falls. Issues related to major trauma are covered in Chapter 4. A variety of disease entities from muscle spasm to metastatic cancer can be associated with such complaints. As the vast majority of patients who present to an acute care setting have medically benign conditions that usually resolve with conservative management[1] and rarely are given a specific etiology,[2] an important component of the initial evaluation is to decide whether the patient has signs or symptoms that could represent more serious pathology and risk to the patient's neurologic well-being. Only a few entities can threaten the integrity of the spinal cord/central nervous system (CNS) or nerve roots and thus represent the potential for acute decompensation. These are listed in Table 14-1. Some of the entities, such as epidural abscess, typically progress if untreated, and some, such as herniated nucleus pulposis, infrequently progress. Thus, not all these entities represent equivalent risk to the patient. Although other life-threatening conditions such as acute myocardial infarction, aortic aneurysm, and dissection can present with a component of neck or back pain, they are not covered in this book. The focus of this chapter is the patient with pain caused by a disease process in the spine.

Historical Features

Among the most important diagnostic historical features are the age of the patient, the duration of pain, the location of the pain, the magnitude of forces in cases of trauma, the radiation in specific nerve root patterns, the relation to neck or back movement, the mode of onset, underlying medical conditions, systemic complaints, and atypical features (Table 14-2). Referral of pain from other areas, such as the chest or abdomen, may point toward nonneurologic etiologies. Patients younger

TABLE 14-1

POTENTIAL IMMEDIATE THREATS TO SPINAL
CORD/CNS/NERVE ROOT INTEGRITY

1. Spinal abscess (epidural, subdural)
2. Bony compression: fractures (including pathologic), dislocations
3. Herniated nucleus pulposis
4. Hematoma (epidural, subdural)
5. Subarachnoid hemorrhage (spinal, intracranial)
6. Arterial dissection

than 18 years[3] or over 50 are at increased risk for more serious underlying pathology such as tumor or infection in both age groups, and abdominal aortic aneurysm and cancer in the older population. As most benign causes for back and neck pain resolve or are significantly improved by 6 to 8 weeks, pain lasting longer raises suspicion of more serious pathology. Atypical features such as pain unrelieved by rest and recumbence or night pain raise concern for tumor or infection, as do systemic complaints such as fever, chills, night sweats, or unexplained weight loss. Immunocompromise or IV drug use also represent increased risk for spinal infection. Back pain radiating below the knee raises suspicion for nerve root irritation. Bilateral sciatic pain worsened by activity, prolonged standing, and back extension can point toward lumbar stenosis. Such pain is usually relieved by rest and forward flexion.

Associated Neurologic Symptoms

Concomitant onset of problems with loss of bowel or bladder control and difficulty walking may indicate that an emergency exists. Acute loss of bladder innervation usually results in urinary retention, with possibly subsequent overflow incontinence. Loss of bowel control usually does not occur acutely. Most conditions that pose a potential threat to the patient's neurologic well-being have associated neurologic

TABLE 14-2

HISTORICAL FEATURES OF BACK AND NECK PAIN

1. Localization
2. Radiation of the pain
3. Mechanism of injury; rate of onset
4. Relation to movement
5. Associated neurologic symptoms
6. Urinary control
7. Underlying disease entities (cancer)
8. Weight loss
9. Fever

signs and/or symptoms. The presence of neurologic symptoms strongly directs the extent of the neurologic examination. The results of both the history and the examination form the basis for decisions about the need for additional testing.

Underlying Disease

Spinal column pain with or without associated physical findings may have a different meaning in patients with underlying disease such as severe collagen vascular disease, IV drug use, sickle cell anemia, metabolic bone disease, or (especially) a known history of cancer. A history of a febrile illness may point toward an infectious etiology.

EXAMINATION

General Physical Examination

Observation of patients in standard movements of walking, sitting, and standing may reveal helpful information about their complaints and activity limitations, and splinting to avoid pain exacerbation (Table 14-3).

Vital Signs

Temperature may be useful in the patient with a suspected spinal column disease. A patient with complaints of back pain and an elevated temperature or a history of one may have an acute infectious process that may or may not be revealed on the general physical and neurologic examination. It is uncommon but not rare that patients with an infectious process related to the spine do not have a fever at the time of presentation. A past history of a febrile illness may be the only clue to an infectious etiology.

Spine

Direct inspection and palpation of the spine can be helpful. Point tenderness will help to guide further evaluations and may reveal evidence of direct trauma or

TABLE 14-3 ——————————————————————
EXAMINATION FOR NECK AND BACK PAIN

General physical exam
Temperature
Spine: palpation, range of motion
Abdomen
Neurologic exam
Motor-bulk, strength
Straight leg-raising (back)
Sensation
Reflexes
Spurling's sign (neck)

underlying infection. Areas of redness or warmth may also indicate underlying infection but are nonspecific. Palpation of the musculature in both the neck and lumbar regions may reveal spasm, which may be the result of or contributing to the patient's pain. Noting the range of motion of the spine in flexion, extension, rotation, and side bending may help with a determination of the extent of the painful conditions, but it is not differentially diagnostic.

Abdomen

Abdominal diseases may present with back pain predominant over abdominal pain. Tenderness in the costovertebral angles may suggest renal involvement. Severe low back pain with a tender pulsatile abdominal mass indicates the possibility of an abdominal aortic aneurysm. The focus of this chapter is the patient without abdominal pain.

Rectal Examination

If there is a significant question about spinal cord or cauda equina dysfunction such as with a complaint of urinary retention or perineal numbness, examination for rectal tone is important. Loss of the bulbocavernosus reflex reflects interruption of the S2 to S4 reflex arc, which is active in bladder contractions. This reflex is elicited by placing the examiner's gloved finger in the rectum and squeezing the head of the penis in the male or tugging on a Foley catheter in the female or male. A prompt contraction of the rectal sphincter is the normal response.

Neurologic Examination

The emphasis in the neurologic examination should be related to spinal nerve roots or spinal cord and associated motor and sensory findings. These are tailored to the suspected area of involvement of the spine and any history of neurologic deficit, with emphasis on the upper extremities in neck concerns and lower extremities in back pain.

Motor Examination

Motor examination includes looking at the specific muscles innervated by the lower cervical nerve roots and lumbar and sacral nerve roots (Table 14-4). Motor strength is usually compared bilaterally. In the legs, testing plantar flexion strength is best done by having the patient walk, if he or she is able, on the toes. Patients with mild plantar flexion weakness may be able to overcome the examiner's hand resistance in testing plantar flexion strength.

With the acute back pain patient, motor bulk is rarely affected, and abnormal motor movements are rarely seen. Patients who have such findings should be suspected of having more long-standing neurologic involvement.

TABLE 14-4 —————————————————————————————

NERVE ROOT COMPRESSION SYNDROMES

Nerve root	Pain	Sensory loss	Motor loss	Reflex loss
C5	Neck, shoulder, upper arm	Lateral shoulder	Deltoid, biceps	Biceps
C6	Neck, shoulder, extending down to lateral aspect of arm involving thumb and forefinger	C6 dermatome out to thumb and forefinger	Biceps	Biceps
C7	Neck and lateral aspect of the arm to third and fourth fingers	C7 dermatome third and fourth digits	Tricepts and extensor carpal ulnarius	Triceps
C8	Ulnar aspect at forearm and fifth digit hand	C8 nerve root including fifth digit	Intrinsic muscles of the hand and wrist extensors	None
T1-T12	Isolated dermatome of specific nerve root	Dermatomes; specific nerve root	Essentially untestable	None
L4	Upper thigh Anterior surface of inner thigh	Anterior Medial surface of thigh L4 distribution down to medial aspect of the foot	Quadriceps	Knee jerk
L5	Lateral aspect of the thigh and outer side of calf across dorsum of the foot to great toe	L5 dermatome usually involving the great toe	Extensor hallucis longus	None

(continued)

TABLE 14-4

NERVE ROOT COMPRESSION SYNDROMES (continued)

Nerve root	Pain	Sensory loss	Motor loss	Reflex loss
S1	Pain in back of the thigh and calf involving the toes	S1 distribution usually involving fourth and fifth toes, back of thigh	Gastrocnemius plantar flexion	Ankle jerk
S2–S4	Perineum	Perianal-saddle area	Bladder	Bulbocavernosus and anal wink

Sensory Examination

As with the motor examination, attention should be paid to sensory involvement of the cervical and lumbosacral roots/spinal cord as indicated by the history. The sensory exam is important in patients who are thought to have thoracic spinal root involvement. Since the musculature is essentially impossible to evaluate in this region, sensory findings may be the only clue to thoracic spinal root problems. Sensation is of particular importance in assessing the lower lumbar nerve roots. Loss of sensation around the genitalia and rectal areas is a good indication of involvement of the lower spinal cord (conus medullaris) or cauda equina. Stroking the skin next to the rectum should cause a contraction of the sphincter known as anal wink in patients with an intact S2 to S4 reflex arc.

Reflexes

Reflex analogues of the various indicated nerve roots should be checked (Table 14-4). Pathologic reflexes such as the Babinski sign in the foot or Tromner's sign in the hand may be indicative of long-term upper motor neuron dysfunction and do not occur in cases of isolated nerve root dysfunction.

ANCILLARY TESTING

Laboratory Testing

In the acute evaluation of neck and back pain, very few laboratory tests are of value in assessing the patient. In suspected epidural abscess/vertebral osteomyelitis, the sedimentation rate is usually elevated. A complete blood count with elevated white blood cells may be seen but is not very sensitive or specific.

Metabolic bone disease and cancer generally require evaluation beyond the scope of the acute care setting. In patients in whom there is no definite cause for back pain and in whom there are no focal neurologic findings, symptomatic treatment with repeat evaluation and expanded testing may be an appropriate management strategy.

Radiographic Testing

With most acute presentations of nontraumatic neck and back pain, radiographic evaluation is not usually indicated or helpful.

Cervical Spine Evaluation

Cervical spine x-rays should be considered for patients who complain of posttraumatic neck pain. For consideration of significant neurotrauma, see Chapter 4.

Lumbosacral Spine Evaluation

Indications for plain film x-rays of the lumbosacral spine have been studied extensively. Direct trauma to the lumbar spine with tenderness on physical examination probably indicates the most compelling reason for emergency x-ray evaluation. In patients with lifting, straining, or bending injuries unassociated with direct trauma, there is little evidence to suggest that x-ray evaluation is helpful for initial management. Since this group of patients represents the largest proportion of back pain seen in the acute care setting, careful selection of x-ray ordering is important. Plain L-S spine radiographs may be productive and helpful in altering therapy in those patients with pain unimproved for 1 month, those with a history of cancer, those who are over 50, and those with suspected vertebral infection. Under these circumstances, one is looking to include or exclude signs of vertebral involvement from infection or malignancy, spinal stenosis, spondylolisthesis, and nonpathologic vertebral fractures. There are other imaging modalities that will define any of these entities better.

Computed Tomography

A plain computed tomography (CT) scan may help to define bony abnormalities. It is not particularly sensitive for cord compression or abnormalities or for ligamentous instability. CT myelography may be useful to define cord/cauda equina compression.

Magnetic Resonance Imaging

Magnetic resonance imaging (MRI) is more sensitive for cord abnormalities and compression. It may define a herniated nucleus pulposis well. It is the diagnostic modality of choice, if available, in nontraumatic acute quadra/paraplegia to exclude mass lesions compressing the spinal cord. The presence of ferrous metals in or about the patient, a contraindication to use, may exclude it from being used in selected cases.

Bone Scan

This modality has been largely replaced by MRI, except in screening to localize abnormalities in the known cancer patient.

Specific Disease Entities

The combination of history and the physical examination should allow the examiner to categorize neck and back pain into specific etiologies (Table 14-5).

Myofascial Conditions; Acute Soft-Tissue Injuries

All forms of trauma, but particularly high-speed automobile-type trauma from rapid deceleration, may produce forces that may cause considerable strain on muscular and ligamentous elements supporting the spinal column. Neck muscle tenderness following rapid-deceleration injuries, with or without resultant spasm, represents a common problem. In patients who have normal neurologic examinations and normal cervical spine films, a conservative approach to management with symptomatic relief is advised. In rare instances, ligamentous instability may not be revealed on initial radiography, and follow-up may be indicated for those patients not improving.

Muscular tenderness in the lower back without specific findings on neurologic examination usually entails a conservative approach. In patients with mild to moderate pain, simply avoiding painful activities and receiving analgesics generally suffice. Bed rest, although once popular, is probably not helpful. Pelvic traction appears to offer no advantage.[3]

Nerve Root Syndromes

Specific nerve roots along the spinal column may be compressed by either herniated disks, vertebral spondylosis, or a combination. These disease processes may

TABLE 14-5 ——————————————————————

CAUSES OF BACK AND NECK PAIN

1. Myofascial syndromes
2. Discs, nerve root syndromes
3. Degenerative diseases of the spine: spondylosis, osteoporosis
4. Malignancy
5. Spondylolysis and spondylolisthesis
6. Neurologic complications of underlying disease
7. Acute myelitis
8. Spinal epidural abscess or hematoma
9. Referred pain: gynecologic, urologic, abdominal, vascular
10. Psychiatric

be indistinguishable from each other on a clinical basis and indeed may be distinguished only by spinal imaging. Initial management of both problems is the same, and rarely do patients require surgery.[4] Table 14-4 delineates the common nerve root compression syndromes for both the cervical and lumbosacral regions. In general, patients with nerve root compression syndromes will complain of dull, aching, often intermittent pain, which may become suddenly worse with straining, coughing, or sneezing. Numbness in the appropriate dermatome distribution commonly occurs. Such pain is usually relieved by lying down. It may radiate in specific nerve root distributions. Cervical disc pain can be referred to the subscapular region.

With cervical root compressions, symptomatology is often made worse by pushing down on the patient's head, which puts compressive force on the cervical spine (Spurling's test).

In the lumbar region, aching pain in the buttocks and lateral aspects of the thigh, usually termed sciatica, is the most common presenting complaint. These symptoms can generally be magnified by straight leg raising with the patient lying supine (Lasegue's test). For this test to be done properly, the patient must be relaxed and should not assist in lifting the leg. All lifting should be done by the examiner. The only sign considered reliable for disc herniation is radiating pain in the leg (sciatica) that occurs between 30 and 70 degrees of elevation. Back pain alone is nonspecific. Contralateral straight leg raising, with radiating pain in the leg opposite to the one being lifted, is considered very suspicious for herniated nucleus pulposus.

The vast majority of lumbosacral discs herniate laterally, causing irritation of the nerve root. In a small number of cases, the disk may herniate in the midline, causing compression of the cauda equina. An acute cauda equina compression syndrome is characterized by low back pain with perineal numbness, acute urinary retention, diminished or lost rectal tone, and paralysis in the legs. As the compression may involve the lowest spinal cord (conus medullaris), depending on the spinal level of involvement, in addition to the nerve roots of the cauda equina, a Babinski sign may be found. Such compression with definite neurologic deficits represents an emergency. Neurosurgical decompression may be indicated emergently. Diagnostic imaging such as MRI or, if MRI is not readily available, a CT myelogram can define the lesion best prior to decompression. Midline herniation of a disk in the cervical region with cord compression may cause spasticity in both the arms and the legs and loss of posterior column sensory function below the level of the involvement.

Midline spinal cord compression in the lower thoracic and upper lumbar regions will cause compression of the lower spinal cord or cauda equina. It should be noted that the spinal cord usually ends between the L1 and L2 vertebral bodies. Lesions below this level may affect multiple nerve roots of the cauda equina but will not involve the spinal cord. Lumbosacral lesions may present with loss of sphincter tone, exertional leg pain, and decreasing strength. The vast majority of nerve root compression syndromes can be handled on a more conservative and routine time course. Even for the patient with definite specific nerve root involvement, pain medications and observation with proper neurologic follow-up are the most common management parameters.

Degenerative Disease of the Spine

Degenerative disease of the spine, or spondylosis, is a common problem with elderly patients. The degenerative process is a result of collapse of the nucleus pulposus with resultant bulging of the anulus fibrosus. Calcification of the anulus fibers causes hypertrophic changes, including cervical spurs, or osteophytes. Spinal stenosis may result. Patients with cervical spinal stenosis may develop cord compression with spasticity in the legs. Patients with lumbar spinal stenosis may walk bent forward at the waist. Symptoms caused by spondylolysis may include nerve root compression and spinal cord irritation and compression. Indications for surgery follow those of any suspected compressive mass on a nerve root or spinal cord.

Spondylolysis and Spondylolisthesis

Spondylolysis is a condition in which the posterior portion of the vertebral arch is separated between the superior and inferior articular processes or facets. The underlying etiology is related to fractures of the neural arch, which may not become symptomatic for many years. When spondylolysis is present, spondylolisthesis, which is forward displacement of one vertebral body onto the vertebral body below, can occur. Spondylolysis and spondylolisthesis generally cause low back pain, which may begin gradually or may be associated with an injury. Because spondylolisthesis usually occurs at the L5 to S1 level, the spinal cord is not involved. With severe displacement, however, compression of nerve roots may occur.

Neurologic Complications of Underlying Spinal Disease

A particular problem in the acute care setting is the patient with a known disease of the spine who may have long-standing back pain that has become worse. Patients with ankylosing spondylitis, rheumatoid arthritis, Paget's disease, metastatic cancer, and metabolic bone disease and osteoporotic compression fractures may have back or neck pain. The history and physical examination are used to determine whether there is involvement of the spinal cord or spinal roots. Patients with evidence suggesting spinal cord involvement may require immediate radiologic evaluation. As in other forms of spinal cord or root compression, proper follow-up examinations may be necessary to determine the need for intervention. Patients with rheumatoid arthritis may have neurologic complications from subluxation of the vertebrae. Atlantoaxial subluxation may result in compression of the upper cervical spinal cord.

Transverse Myelitis

Myelitis is a nonspecific term designating inflammation of the spinal cord. Myelopathy is an even more nonspecific term indicating dysfunction of the spinal cord. Transverse myelitis may be partial or complete and refers to a process in which the lesion extends horizontally across the spinal cord, resulting in loss of neurologic function below the level of the lesion. Symptoms and signs such as urinary retention or overflow incontinence, saddle anesthesia, major motor weakness in the arms or legs (paraparesis, quadraparesis), long track signs, and sensory levels raise suspicion for either intrinsic cord abnormalities or extrinsic cord compression. Extrinsic cord compression can be due to tumors (benign or malignant, primary or metastatic), abscess, or hematomas.[5] Inflammatory myelopathies can be extremely variable with respect to the degree of back pain. Symptoms may come on in a matter of hours, days, or weeks and may be impossible to differentiate from structurally compressive lesions of the spinal cord without radiographic imaging, optimally MRI (Table 14-5).

Differential diagnosis of acute spinal cord lesions requires careful attention to the progression of symptoms. Acute myelitis and acute polyneuritis (Guillain-Barré syndrome) may be ascending polyneuropathies. The spinal cord symptomatology caused by epidural abscesses, epidural hematomas, and spinal cord tumors tends to be focal in nature and does not have an ascending quality. Table 14-6 emphasizes the differential diagnosis in acute myelopathy.

Spinal Epidural Abscess and Epidural Hematomas

An extremely rare but potentially dangerous cause of symptomatic back pain is spinal epidural abscess. The spinal epidural abscess is a direct result of vertebral osteomyelitis or discitis,[6] so patients generally have exquisite point tenderness on back examination. Spinal epidural abscess may proceed to compress and/or infarct the spinal cord, giving a cord compression syndrome indistinguishable from that of the midline disk herniation or spondylosis.

Patients may have an acute presentation with rapid progression of symptoms or a chronic course of over 3 months. The pain may be particularly severe, unrelieved by rest, and worse at night. Patients with IV drug abuse, sickle cell anemia, osteomyelitis, recent spinal surgery,[7] or infection elsewhere in the body are more prone to this condition. The patient usually has a history of a febrile illness but may not be febrile on presentation, making consideration of an infectious etiology difficult. Early diagnosis can be very difficult.[8] Rarely does the patient appear septic. Management of a suspected epidural abscess requires radiologic evaluation, optimally MRI, and immediate consideration of surgery combined with long-term antibiotic therapy. The most common organism isolated is *Staphylococcus*, but a wide variety of infectious organisms can be found. An elevated sedimentation rate, although nonspecific, is typically found. The white blood cell count may or may not be elevated, and a normal

TABLE 14-6
CAUSES OF MYELOPATHY

Primary infectious viral syndromes or bacterial, spirochetal, rickettsial, fungal, or parasitic conditions
Postinfectious or parainfectious myelitis
Toxic; metabolic
Irradiation myelitis
Idiopathic
Myelopathy: compression from tumor, abscess, hematoma
Other: vascular occlusion

white blood cell count does not exclude the diagnosis. Blood cultures are frequently positive. Plain radiographic findings lag behind clinical symptoms by several weeks and may take up to 2 months to become positive. Positive findings include bony destruction and less specific vertebral end-plate irregularities and disc space narrowing.

In very rare cases, a spontaneous epidural hematoma may occur with resultant spinal cord compression.[1] This may occur during anticoagulation[9] or thrombolytic therapy[10] or from spontaneous hemorrhage from the posterior internal venous plexus.[11] It cannot be distinguished from other causes of cord compression without radiologic evaluation.

Other Spinal Hemorrhage

Another very rare cause for sudden, severe back or neck pain and possible sciatica with neurologic symptomatology is spinal subarachnoid hemorrhage. A vascular malformation of the spinal cord hemorrhages, with subsequent sudden severe pain and neurologic symptoms and signs related to the spinal cord segments involved. Aortic dissection may mimic this presentation. Intracranial subarachnoid hemorrhage may rapidly migrate to the cervical and lumbar subarachnoid space, with resultant severe neck or back pain. This entity is covered in Chapter 7. Migration of the blood to the intracranial subarachnoid space from spinal subarachnoid hemorrhage may produce a headache. Spontaneous bleeding from intraspinal tumors may present with similar symptoms.

BACK PAIN IN CHILDREN AND ADOLESCENTS

Back pain is an uncommon complaint in children and adolescents. It may, however, indicate significant illness or injury. Whereas in adults the vast majority of cases of low back pain do not represent significant or serious medical illness, and usually resolve with conservative measures, this is not necessarily the case in the child. Minimal back pain may be the result of a significant illness. Herniation of an intervertebral disc, although possible, is very uncommon in the pediatric age group. Other significant causes for consideration include vertebral fracture, if there has been significant injury, overuse injuries, spondylolysis/spondylolisthesis, intervertebral discitis, vertebral osteomyelitis, ankylosis spondylitis, neoplasms, Scheurmann's disease, and juvenile rheumatoid arthritis (Table 14-7). It should be noted that the usual childhood idiopathic scoliosis is rarely painful.

PATIENTS WITH RECURRENT BACK PAIN IN THE EMERGENCY DEPARTMENT

The primary issue with most patients who present to an acute care setting with an exacerbation of an ongoing back or neck problem is symptomatic relief. However, some patients will have progression of an underlying benign process (such as disc disease), whereas others may have a new etiology mimicking prior symptoms. These patients

TABLE 14-7
BACK AND NECK PAIN IN CHILDREN

Benign Bony Tumors
Osteroid osteoma
Benign osteoblastoma

Malignancy
Ewing's tumor
Osteogenic sarcoma
Bone cyst
Neuroblastoma
Wilms' tumor
Lymphoma
Leukemia

Developmental
Spondylolisthesis/spondylolysis
Scheurmann's disease

Inflammatory
Discitis
Vertebral osteomyelitis/epidural abscess
Collagen vascular disease
Ankylosing spondylitis

Mechanical
Fracture
Hip joint disease
Muscle spasm/strain
Herniated nucleus pulposis

are the most problematic. One should consider "red flags" that would indicate the entities covered in Table 14-1. Depending on the findings, and the date and type of prior imaging, repeat imaging such as MRI may be necessary. The findings that tend to push one to more rapid consideration of definitive diagnostic imaging are objective weakness and difficulty with urinary control. The extent of any neurologic deficit and the degree of pain relief obtained in the acute care setting will dictate the location (inpatient versus outpatient) and timing (urgent versus scheduled) for such studies. Contact with prior treating physicians and review of prior imaging studies may be helpful in determining whether repeat or definitive testing may be indicated.

REFERRED PAIN

The scope of this book does not permit a full discussion of each entity that may present with back pain. Note that renal stones, acute pyelonephritis, abdominal aortic aneurysms, and retroperitoneal conditions may all present as back pain. Lower lumbar and sacral back pain may be related to lesions of the genitalia in both males and females. Prostatitis and diverticulitis may also present as back pain. The elderly patient with sudden onset of nontraumatic low back pain with abdominal pain should be considered at risk for having an expanding or rupturing abdominal aortic aneurysm.

Psychiatric Disease

Acute and frequently chronic back pain patients may present for medical treatment as a manifestation of psychiatric disease. Psychogenic neurologic syndromes are covered in Chapter 10.

References

1. Cherkin DC, A comparison of physical therapy, chiropractic manipulation, and provision of an educational booklet for the treatment of patients with low back pain. *N Engl J Med* 1998;339:1021–1029.
2. Atlas SJ, Deyo RA. Evaluating and managing acute low back pain in the primary care setting, *J Gen Intern Med* 2001;16:120–131.
3. Beurskens AJ, et al. Efficiency of traction for nonspecific low back pain. 12-week and 6-month results of a randomized clinical trial, *Spine* 1997;22:2756–2762.
4. Deyo RA, Loeser JD, Bigos SJ. Herniated lumbar intervertebral disk, *Ann Intern Med* 1990;112:598–603.
5. Schmidt RD, Markovchick V. Nontraumatic spinal cord compression. *J Emerg Med* 1992;10:189–199.
6. Mackenzie AR, et al. Spinal epidural abscess: the importance of early diagnosis and treatment. *J Neurol Neurosurg Psychiatry* 1998;65:209–212.
7. Calderone RR, Larsen JM. Overview and classification of spinal infections. *Orthop Clin North Am* 1996;27:1–8.
8. Sampath P, Rigamonti D. Spinal epidural abscess: a review of epidemiology, diagnosis, and treatment. *J Spinal Disord* 1999;12:89–93.
9. Rodriguez y Baena R, et al. Spinal epidural hematoma during anticoagulant therapy. A case report and review of the literature. *J Neurosurg Sci* 1995;39:87–94.
10. Sawin PD, Traynelis VC, Follett KA. Spinal epidural hematoma following coronary thrombolysis with tissue plasminogen activator. Report of two cases. *J Neurosurg* 1995;83:350–353.
11. Groen RJ, Ponssen H. The spontaneous spinal epidural hematoma. A study of the etiology. *J Neurol Sci* 1990;98:121–138.

abdominal epilepsy   Attacks of severe abdominal pain, either as an aura to a seizure or by themselves without a seizure.

abducens nerve   Sixth cranial nerve; provides innervation to lateral rectus muscle of eye, the action of which abducts the eye.

absence attacks   Petit mal epilepsy; consists of sudden fixed vacuous stare without response to environment of short duration (10 to 30 seconds). There may be minor eyelid fluttering.

abulia   Lack of spontaneity or effervescence of personality.

acalculia   Inability to perform mathematical calculations (not simple memory tasks such as $2 + 2 = 4$).

acoustic neuroma (neurinoma)   A benign tumor originating from the eighth cranial nerve.

Adie's pupil   A pupil that responds poorly and slowly to light (and slowly dilates in the dark); responds better in convergence. Usually unilateral, the pupil is dilated in average light and is usually found in females with absent tendon reflexes. The pupil is unusually sensitive to 2.5% methacholine (mecholyl).

AED   An abbreviation frequently used for antiepileptic drug.

agnosia   The loss of ability to recognize the import of sensory stimuli agraphia. The loss of ability to write in the absence of paralysis.

akinetic mutism   Severe deficiency or loss of movement and lack of speech. Patient appears asleep but can be aroused, and eyes will follow. Causative lesions involve reticular activating system in upper pons and midbrain such as basilar artery thrombosis. Also called coma vigil.

alexia   Inability to read.

Alzheimer's disease   A dementing illness with characteristic brain atrophy, senile plaques, and neurofibrillary tangles. Peak onset at age 50 to 60 years but reported in widely varying age groups.

amaurosis fugax   "Fleeting blindness" with temporary monocular visual loss due to ocular vascular insufficiency, commonly embolic in etiology. Amaurosis implies blindness without apparent eye lesion.

amblyopia   Defect in vision resulting from imperfect sensation of the retina without organic eye lesion.

amnestic-confabulatory syndrome (Wernicke-Korsakoff syndrome)   A confusional state characterized by retrograde amnesia and anterograde amnesia. Confabulation need not continually be present, but the patient must be alert and other cognitive functions that do not depend on memory may only be impaired to a minor degree.

analgesia   Loss of ability to perceive painful stimuli.

anesthesia   Loss of ability to perceive all sensory stimuli.

anesthesia dolorosa   An extremely intense, deep-seated pain located cortically and usually caused by severe involvement of thalamic structures.

anisocoria   Unequal pupils.

anomic aphasia   Difficulty naming objects, conditions, or qualities without serious limitations in speaking or writing.

anosognosia   Loss of ability to recognize hemiplegia; more broadly used, lack of ability to recognize any neurologic deficit or other disease or disability.

anterior circulation   Refers to circulation supplied by internal carotid artery. anterior spinal artery (cord) syndrome. See page 237.

Anton's syndrome   Cortical blindness with denial of blindness (anosognosia) caused by bilateral lesions in occipital lobes.

aphasia   Loss of powers of speech without paralysis of muscles required for word production.

aphasia, anomic   A variety of conduction aphasia in which conversational speech is fluent but with lack of substantive words and great difficulty in finding words, at times causing total inability to name objects.

aphasia, Broca's   An expressive aphasia in which the patients know what they wish to say but are unable to say it. Unable to talk, repeat, or read aloud.

aphasia, conduction   A variety of fluent aphasia, similar to Wernicke's aphasia except that the speech is more broken and there are more hesitations for word finding. Many cliches and four- to five-word phrases are interjected. Comprehension is normal; repetition is poor.

aphasia, global   Total loss of language ability with inability to speak or comprehend written or spoken words, read, write, repeat, or name.

aphasia, Wernicke's   A type of fluent aphasia with high volume of word output but no meaningful or substantive words, so that no meaning is conveyed. Frequently one word is substituted for another.

apneustic breathing   A respiratory pattern with a pause at full inspiration. Reflects abnormality at middle or caudal pontine level.

apoplexy   Refers to sudden hemorrhage from any organ or, as in apoplectic stroke, to a sudden vascular lesion of brain marked by coma and paralysis.

apraxia   A disturbance in the performance of skilled acts;

aqueduct of Sylvius   A channel for circulation of spinal fluid through the midbrain and upper pons connecting the third and fourth ventricles.

arachnoiditis   An inflammatory reaction in the arachnoid membrane, which forms the external limit of the cerebrospinal fluid–containing space.

Argyll Robertson pupil   A pupil that does not react to light (directly or consensually) but does constrict on accommodation.

Arnold-Chiari malformation   A congenital malformation of the lower brainstem characterized by displacement of midline cerebellar structures into the spinal canal and a distorted elongated pons and medulla.

aseptic meningeal reaction   Increased white cells in spinal fluid due to a nonbacterial cause, e.g., viral, chemical.

asterixis   See page 146.

ataxia   Failure of coordination of movements.

automatisms   A condition in which an individual is consciously or unconsciously, but involuntarily, compelled to the performance of certain (often purposeless) motor or verbal acts, for example, yawning.

Babinski sign   An extensor toe sign consisting of dorsiflexion of the great toe, fanning of the toes in response to scraping the plantar aspect of the foot from the heel to metatarsophalangeal joints. Indicative of pyramidal (motor) tract dysfunction above age 18 months to 2 years.

basal ganglion   Gray matter located with the thalamus deep in the cerebral hemisphere.

Beevor's sign   Upward movement of the umbilicus on contracting the abdominal muscles due to paralysis of lower abdominal muscles.

Bell's palsy   See pages 114, 115.

Bell's phenomenon   Upward rotation of the eyeball; an attempted eye closure in patients with Bell's palsy.

bitemporal hemianopsia   Visual field loss in both lateral (temporal) areas, usually as a result of disease at the optic chiasm.

Broca's aphasia   See *aphasia.*

Broca's area   An area in the posterior portion of the inferior frontal gyrus of the dominant hemisphere.

Brown-sequard syndrome   See pages 236, 237.

Brudzinski's sign (neck)   Passive flexion of the head on the chest followed by flexion of both thighs and legs so that both lower extremities may be flexed on the pelvis. A sign of meningeal irritation; also found in partial decerebration.

bulbar palsy   Weakness accompanied by atrophy and fasciculations of muscles supplied by motor nuclei of tongue, pharyngeal muscles, palate, and sometimes lips. Characteristically there is dysphagia, dysarthria, and regurgitation of foods with difficulty protruding the tongue.

bulbocavernosus reflex   See page 312.

caloric testing   See page 67.

carotid sinus syndrome   Syncope and bradycardia produced by mechanical stimulation of the carotid sinus. An exaggerated normal response.

carpal tunnel syndrome   Compression of the median nerve at the wrist as it passes through the carpal tunnel. Features include numbness and paresthesias in the first three digits of the hand with weakness and possibly atrophy of the median nerve-supplied muscles. Paresthesias typically worse at night, precipitating shaking of hands.

catalepsy   Sudden loss of voluntary motion of the entire body with diffuse muscular rigidity; similar to catatonia.

cataplexy   Attacks of limb weakness with loss of tone precipitated by emotional stimuli; usually associated with narcolepsy.

cauda equina   Latin for a horse's tail: the bundle of spinal nerve routes arising from the lumbar enlargement and conus medullaris and running through the lower part of the subarachnoid space within the vertebral column.

causalgia   A distressing type of burning pain accompanied by vasomotor and trophic changes; usually secondary to nerve injury.

central cord syndrome   See page 237.

cerebellopontine angle syndrome   Tinnitus with progressive deafness, numbness, and/or pain in the ipsilateral face, ipsilateral facial palsy, vertigo, ipsilateral dysmetria, and ipsilateral sixth nerve palsy; commonly due to acoustic neurinomas.

cerebral palsy   A nonspecific term used to describe a disorder of motor function that begins in infancy; characterized by spasticity and/or involuntary movements; caused by brain dysfunction.

Chaddock's sign   An extensor toe sign with response and significance similar to Babinski's sign; produced by blunt stimulation of the lateral aspect of the foot.

Charcot-Marie-Tooth disease   A familial peripheral neuropathy characterized pathologically by hypertrophic peripheral nerves; commonly affects distal limb musculature, resulting in weakness at ankles, atrophic calf muscles, high arches; occasionally involves hand involvement. The hypertrophied peripheral nerves may be palpable. The expression of this disease is very variable.

chorea   See pages 146, 149, 150.

clonus   A series of rhythmic muscle contractions caused by sudden passive stretching of the muscle.

cluster headache   See page 168.

coma   See Chapter 3.

coma vigile   See page 38.

complicated migraine   A term used when the neurologic deficit, e.g., hemiplegia, persists after the classic or hemiplegic migraine, thus simulating a cerebral infarction.

concussion   See Chapter 9.

conjugate gaze   A condition in which the visual axes of the two eyes are parallel in all positions of gaze.

constructional apraxia   Inability to draw geometric figures or to write with eyes open; figures drawn may have major parts missing or misplaced; usually due to a lesion in the angular gyrus.

conus medullaris   Medullary cone; a tapering lower extremity of the spinal cord.

corneal reflex   Reflex eyelid closure on stimulation of the cornea as by a wisp of cotton; mediated by fifth or seventh cranial nerves.

cortical blindness   A condition in which blindness is due to dysfunction in the occipital cortex and pupillary reflexes are preserved. See *Anton's syndrome.*

cortical denial syndrome   Inability to perceive sensory stimuli contralaterally when the stimuli are applied bilaterally simultaneously with preservation of ability to perceive that stimulus when it alone is applied; referred to as sensory extinction or inattention.

cortical sensation   Functions usually considered to be mediated by the cerebral cortex (parietal lobe), which include stereognosis (perceiving and recognizing form by touch), barognosis (perception of weight), topesthesia (ability to localize a tactile sensation), graphesthesia (recognition of letters or numbers written on the skin), and two-point discrimination.

cremasteric reflex   Contraction of cremaster muscle with elevation of the testicle on stroking the inner upper thigh with a blunt object; innervated by ilioinguinal and genitofemoral nerves via Ll and L2 cord segments.

Creutzfeldt-Jakob disease   A degenerative disease producing rapidly progressive mental deterioration in midlife with pyramidal and extrapyramidal signs including hyperkinesias, abnormal tone, dysphagia, and dysarthria.

Dandy-Walker syndrome   A congenital form of obstructive hydrocephalus with enlargement of the fourth ventricle out of proportion to the other ventricles, caused by atresia of the foramen of Luschka and Magendie. This cystic enlargement of the fourth ventricle is associated with multiple other congenital anomalies. The clinical presentation is extremely variable and is basically similar to other forms of hydrocephalus.

decerebrate rigidity   See page 267.

decorticate rigidity   See page 54.

déjà vu   A sensation of unreality characterized by feeling familiar with what ought to be an unfamiliar situation.

delirium   Acute encephalopathy.

delirium tremens   An alcohol-withdrawal syndrome characterized by confusion, delusions, hallucinations, tremor, agitation, sleeplessness, and autonomic hyperactivity (fever, tachycardia, sweating).

dementia   Deterioration or loss of previously acquired intellectual functions.

demyelinating diseases   Diseases associated with destruction of the myelin sheath surrounding nerve axons, resulting in defective functioning of that neuron. Multiple sclerosis is the most common of the more than two dozen entities considered.

Devic's disease One of the demyelinating diseases, also termed neuromyelitis optica. The clinical features consist of the acute simultaneous occurrence of transverse myelitis and optic neuritis. Most consider it simply a variant of multiple sclerosis.

diplopia Double vision.

dissociated sensory loss Impairment of some sensory modalities with preservation of others.

drop attack Sudden collapse of the legs without loss of consciousness.

dysautonomia Dysfunction of the autonomic nervous system manifested by orthostatic hypotension, impotence, loss of sweating, and urinary and fecal incontinence.

dysdiadochokinesia Inability to perform rapid alternating movements such as pronating and supinating the hand.

dysgraphia Difficulty writing in the absence of paralysis.

dyslexia Difficulty reading.

dysmetria Loss of ability to gauge distance, speed, or power of a movement.

dysphagia Difficulty swallowing.

dysphasia Difficulty with language functions.

Eaton-Lambert syndrome See page 135.

EEG The record obtained by means of an electroencephalogram—an apparatus consisting of amplifiers and write-out systems for recording the electrical potential of the brain that arrive from electrodes attached to the scalp.

EMG Electromyogram—a graphic representation of the electrical currents associated with muscular action.

encephalitis See pages 73, 98, 166.

encephalopathy Acute alteration of higher intellectual function.

end-point nystagmus (end-position nystagmus) A few rapid nystagmoid movements seen on extreme deviation of the eyes; usually seen on lateral deviation.

ENG Electronystagmography—a method of nystagmography based on electro-oculography; skin electrodes are placed at outer canthi to register horizontal nystagmus or above and below each eye for vertical nystagmus.

enopthalmos Inward protrusion of the eye.

essential tremor See page 148.

extinction phenomena See *cortical denial syndrome.*

extrapyramidal signs Motor signs referable to disturbance in tone (usually rigid), movement (hyperkinesia or bradykinesia), and associated movements.

febrile seizures Convulsions associated with fever in children between the ages of 6 months and 3 years of age without focal neurologic findings and normal spinal fluid examination.

fibrinolysis A hydrolysis of fibrin—either as a naturally occurring mechanism of the body or induced by administered fibrinolytic-thrombolytic agents such as streptokinase, urokinase, t-pa.

finger agnosia Inability to recognize, name, or select individual fingers of either the patient or examiner. Usually points to involvement of the angular gyrus.

foot drop Inability to dorsiflex the foot, due to either weakness of the tibialis anterior muscle (peroneus tertius, extensor digitorum longus, and extensor hallucis longus assist) or its nerve supply, or the deep peroneal nerve or its segmental innervation, L4, L5.

Foster Kennedy syndrome Anosmia and optic atrophy on the side of a subfrontal mass with contralateral papilledema.

Friedreich's ataxia A hereditary spinal ataxia, usually manifesting at puberty. Manifestations include ataxia, hyporeflexia, paresthesias, loss of vibration and position sense, dysarthria, skeletal deformities, and other variable nonneurologic findings.

Froment's sign   A sign of weakness of the adductor pollicis, usually caused by ulnar nerve dysfunction. The patient tries to hold a piece of paper, which the examiner tries to pull out between the ulnar side of the extended thumb and the radial side of the second metacarpophalangeal joint by contracting the adductor pollicis. The sign is positive if the patient flexes the thumb at the interphalangeal joint.

gegenhalten   Resistance to changes in posture or position of a limb, resulting in a rigid hypertonicity. Seen in extrapyramidal disorders.

Gerstmann's syndrome   Finger agnosia, left-right disorientation, acalculia, and agraphia; usually due to lesion in dominant parietal lobe.

Gilles de la Tourette's syndrome (Tourette's syndrome)   See page 149.

global aphasia   See *aphasia.*

globus hystericus   A feeling of constriction or foreign body in the throat; of psychogenic origin.

Gowers' sign   Sciatic pain produced by passive dorsiflexion of the foot with patient supine, legs extended.

grand mal seizure   Major motor seizure; tonic-clonic seizure; generalized convulsions associated with loss of consciousness and jerking movements of all extremities. Also associated with increased tone, defecation, urination; often preceded by an aura.

graphesthesia   See *cortical sensation.*

Guillain-Barré syndrome   See page 127, 128, 210.

habit spasms (tics)   See page 145.

Hallpike maneuver   Nylen-Bairainy Test.   See Chapter 13.

hemianopia   Loss of one-half of a visual field.

hemiballismus   See page 146.

hemichorea   Chorea; see page 119. On one side of the body.

hemiplegic migraine   See page 166.

hepatic coma   See page 76.

histamine (cluster) headache   See page 139.

Hoffmann's sign   Sudden brief flexion of the distal phalynx of the patient's long finger, with the wrist and hand supported, produces sudden flexion of the other fingers and flexion and adduction of the thumb. A pyramidal tract sign.

Hoover's sign   See pages 251, 252.

Horner's syndrome   See page 174.

Horton's headache   Cluster headache; see page 139.

Hutchinson's pupil   A unilaterally dilated, fixed pupil.

hypalgesia   Diminished pain sensation.

hyperacusis   Abnormally acute or painful hearing.

hyperpathia   Increased sensitivity to pain and a deep aching painful sensation—generally related to thalamic lesions.

hypesthesia   Diminished tactile sensation.

hypnagogic hallucinations   Hallucinations that occur as one begins to fall asleep.

idiopathic intracranial hypertension   By definition the ideology of idiopathic intracranial hypertension is not known. At this time it should be regarded as any gradual elevation of cerebrospinal fluid pressure without an anatomically or biochemically explainable ideology.

intention tremor   A tremor that occurs or worsens on volitional movement.

interictal   Periods between seizures.

internuclear ophthalmoplegia   See pages 208, 209.

Jacksonian seizure   Involuntary tonic-clonic movements usually starting in one extremity or side of the face; may go on to altered consciousness. When the seizures remain limited to one side of the body, consciousness is usually retained. Localization of the seizure focus is usually to the contralateral motor context.

jake palsy   Acute peripheral neuritis producing weakness.

jamais vu   A feeling of unreality characterized by lack of familiarity with what ought to be a familiar sensation. The opposite of déjà vu.

Kernig's sign   With the patient supine and the thigh flexed at a right angle to the trunk, complete extension of the leg is impossible. This sign indicates meningeal irritation and is seen in many forms of meningitis.

Kernohan's notch   Also called *crus phenomenon.* A syndrome in which supertentorial pressure causes herniation and compression of the third nerve with the various pressure forces pushing the brainstem to the opposite side, causing compression of the contralateral cerebral peduncle and corticospinal tracts against the sharp edge of the tentorium. This results in hemiplegia ipsilateral to the side of the compressed third nerve.

Korsakoff's psychosis   A psychotic state characterized by failure of memory, imaginary reminiscences, and sometimes marked hallucinations with agitation. It is usually seen in association with acute polyneuritis.

lacunar infarction   Infarction of small penetrating arteries of the brain; usually related to severe hypertension. These infarcts may be asymptomatic but can result in such syndromes as (1) pure motor strokes, (2) pure sensory strokes, (3) clumsy hand-dysarthria syndrome, and various other isolated neurologic lesions.

Lasegue's sign   With the patient supine and the hip flexed when the knee is extended, pain or muscular spasm is present, indicating irritation of the sciatic nerve.

lateral medullary syndrome   See *Wallenberg's syndrome.*

lethargy   A morbid drowsiness from which the patient can be aroused and can appear to be awake and cognizant of surroundings but falls back into inattention or sleep as soon as the stimulus is removed.

Lhermitte's sign   Sudden tingling or electric shock-type sensations up and down the spinal cord when the patient's head is flexed or extended. This has been reported to be positive with meningeal irritation, multiple sclerosis, and cervical cord compressions.

locked-in syndrome   Also called *Count of Monte Cristo syndrome.* Vascular lesion involving the motor pathways of the pons, which are destroyed, sparing the reticular system. This results in paralysis of all lower cranial nerves and extremities but with consciousness present. The patient retains vertical eye movements and will be able to look up on command.

low-pressure (normal-pressure) hydrocephalus   A pathologic increase of cerebrospinal fluid within the skull in which there is dilation of cerebral ventricals and neurologic disturbances but spinal fluid pressure is normal.

macula (macula lutea)   A small yellow-orange area on the inner surface of the retina at a point corresponding to the posterior pull of the eyeball, which serves as the central point of focus for the visual axis.

Magendie's foramen   The anatomic opening on the dorsal aspect of the fourth ventrical, which allows cerebrospinal fluid to enter the subarachnoid space. Obstruction of this structure and the accompanying foramen of Luschka results in noncommunicating hydrocephalus.

marche à petit pas   A short-stepped shuffling gait with a lack of associated hip and arm movements; frequently seen in diffuse cerebral and Parkinson's disease.

Marcus Gunn phenomenon (jaw winking)   A partial pstosis of congenital origin in which opening the mouth and chewing in lateral movements of the jaw cause exaggerated reflex elevation of the ptotic lids. This pathologic movement is presumed to be on the basis of abnormal proprioceptive impulses from the pterygoid muscles, which are relayed to the oculomotor nucleus.

Marcus Gunn pupillary sign　A pathologic light reflex indicating decreased stimuli being transmitted from one eye. On testing the involved eye, the central light reflex causes the pupil to dilate. When the light is moved to the affected eye because of the lack of total light reaching the midbrain, the pupil fails to hold and may actually dilate. These changes can be accentuated by rapid alternate stimulation of the eye with a bright light, the swinging flashlight test.

Ménière's disease　A disease of the inner ear characterized clinically by vertigo, tinnitus, nausea and vomiting, and progressive deafness related to increased pressure in the endolymphatic fluid of the inner ear.

meningitis　Any inflammation of the covering membranes of the brain and spinal cord; may be due to various types of infections, chemical irritation, or underlying disease.

meningocele　A protrusion of the protective membranes (meninges) of the brain or spinal cord through a defect in the skull or spinal column.

meralgia paraesthetica　Tingling and burning that progress to numbness in the lateral lower thigh due to compression or irritation of the lateral femoral cutaneous nerve.

micturition syncope　Sudden loss of consciousness due to an acute decrease in cerebral blood flow precipitated by active urination. The mechanism is thought to be increased parasympathetic activity causing bradycardia and hypotension.

migraine with aura　Classic migraine—those migraine headaches accompanied by visual, auditory, or some other sensory episode prior to the onset of the actual head pain.

migraine without aura　Throbbing, pulsatile headaches that meet the criteria for a migraine headache but are not preceded by any auditory, visual, or other sensory experiences prior to the onset of the head pain.

miosis　Decrease in size of the pupillary aperture; contraction of the pupil.

miotic　Relates to contraction of the pupil or an agent that causes the pupil to contract.

Mobius' syndrome　A congenital facial diplegia. The clinical picture includes paralysis or paresis of the ocular muscles together with paralysis or paresis of the facial muscles. The pathologic basis appears to be hypoplasia of the nuclear centers in the brainstem.

mononeuritis multiplex　Inflammation of several nerves simultaneously in anatomically unrelated portions of the body, generally on an inflammatory vasculitis basis. Diabetes mellitus and collagen vascular diseases are the most common causes.

mononeuropathy　Involvement of a single nerve by a disease process.

monoplegia　An isolated paralysis of only one limb.

Moro reflex　A postural and righting reflex seen in infants. A body startle reflex in which a sudden noise or movement directed toward the body of the infant or a blow on the bed next to the infant causes extension on all limbs and the spine. The reflex is normal during the first 4 to 5 months of life.

mydriasis　Dilation of the pupil.

mydriatic　Any agent that dilates the pupil; a cycloplegic.

myelomeningeocele　Protrusion of both the spinal cord and its covering membranes through a defect of the bony spinal column.

myoclonus　Sudden spasm or twitching of a muscle group frequently seen at the moment of sleep.

myokymia　Quivering or fibrillary tremor; twitching of isolated muscle groups usually around the head and neck region; may occur as a benign and transient condition or may be associated with multiple sclerosis or brainstem disease.

myopia　Nearsightedness; trouble viewing distant objects; may be the result of increased infractive error or elongation of the eyeball.

narcolepsy   Uncontrollable and paroxysmal attacks of sleep. Has been associated with lesions of the posterior hypothalmus, but the actual pathologic process is unknown.

nonconvulsive status epilepticus   A continuing state of seizure activity in which the patient does not present with outward manifestations such as tonic clonic motor activity. (See *subtle status epilepticus*.)

normal-pressure hydrocephalus   A hydrocephalic syndrome with anatomic changes in the brain but cerebrospinal fluid pressure within the normal range when measured with standard lumbar puncture technique.

Nylen-Barany maneuver   A test for positional nystagmus in vertigo. Usually referred to as the Hallpike test. See Chapter 13 for complete explanation.

nystagmus   Rhythmic oscillation of the eyeballs. Multiple types associated with various structural and metabolic abnormalities. The unifying factor in all types is brainstem-initiated eye deviation with rapid cortical correction phase.

oculogyric crisis   Uncontrollable rotation movements of the eyeballs.

ophthalmoplegia   Paralysis of one or both eyes in one or more directions of gaze.

opisthotonus   A tetanic contraction with hyperextension of the spine and extremities.

opsoclonus   Erratic, rapid, nonrhythmic movements of the eyes in both horizontal and vertical directions.

palinopsia   The retention of a visual image or its recurrence after the stimulus has been withdrawn. Most often associated with disease of the parietal occipital region.

palmar grasp reflex   A pathological frontal lobe release sign in which stroking of the palm results in an involuntary grasping motion by the patient.

palmomental reflex   Contraction of the ipsilateral mentalis and orbicularis oris muscles in response to stimulation of the thenar area of the hand. A frontal-lobe release sign.

papilledema   Swelling of the optic nerve head, which may be due to increased intercranial pressure, orbital disease, intraocular disease, or systemic disease.

papillitis   Inflammation of the optic nerve head with edema. Appearance may be confused with papilledema.

paracusia   A paradoxic increase in hearing in deaf people in an environment of increased noise.

paralysis   Loss of strength of voluntary movement in a limb or muscle.

paraplegia   Paralysis of both lower extremities involving the lower portion of the trunk.

paresis   Partial or incomplete paralysis.

Parinaud's syndrome   Loss of upward gaze usually due to a lesion in the pineal gland causing pressure on the superior colliculus.

Parkinson's disease (paralysis agitans)   A diffuse degenerative disease of the brain with both early and severe involvement of the basal ganglions. Associated with rigidity and tremor and progressing to include organic brain syndrome.

Patrick's sign   Pain in the hip when the heel of the painful extremity is placed upon the opposite knee and the thigh is depressed downward. Positive Patrick's sign generally indicates hip joint disease, but it is usually absent in disease entities involving the sciatic nerve.

peripheral neuropathy   A general term for any damage to the nervous system that lies outside the brain and spinal cord. *Neuritis* may also be used to denote any type of damage to the peripheral nerves regardless of etiology, although many physicians reserve the term for conditions of infectious origins.

petit mal seizure   Absence spells; attacks occurring mostly in children characterized by short duration (10 to 30 seconds) of altered consciousness. Motor tone is usually preserved.

Phalen's sign In patients with median nerve compression in the carpal tunnel, painful paresthesias reproduced by holding the wrists in extreme flexion for 2 minutes.

phantom limb A sensation of the continued presence of an absent portion of the body, which may manifest as pain, paresthesias, or sensation of movement.

phantom sensation Spontaneous sensations referred to previously denervated and insensitive areas; frequently associated with lesions of the spinal cord or cauda equina.

phrenic neuralgia Dysfunction of the phrenic nerve from any cause. Most common etiologies include infection, surgery, developmental anomalies, tumors, and idiopathic causes. Diaphragmatic spasms and paresthesias in the distribution of the phrenic nerve may come out in advance of the paralysis. Although it is usually unilateral, bilateral cases do exist and are life-threatening.

plantar reflex The normal plantar response, i.e., plantar movement or flexion of the toes upon stroking the sole of the foot.

posterior circulation The arterial supply of the brain derived from the two vertebral arteries and their union, the basilar artery. The areas supplied include sections of the occipital lobe, midbrain, pons, and medulla, as well as portions of the spinal cord.

posterior column signs Physical examination findings indicative of pathology in the posterior columns of the spinal cord. The posterior columns include the fasciculus gracilis and fasciculus cuneatus. Clinically the syndrome is characterized by alteration of vibration and position sense.

postherpetic neuralgia Persistent motor and sensory dysfunction in peripheral nerves affected by herpes zoster after the skin manifestations have resolved. Most common manifestations are dysesthesias and paresthesias.

presbycusis Loss of ability to perceive or discriminate sounds, which is a part of the natural aging process.

presenile dementia A term that may be used interchangeably with Alzheimer's disease. The pathology includes gross atrophy of the brain with widening of the cortical sulci and enlargement of the ventricals. The clinical picture includes onset of dementia in the fifth and sixth decades.

primary lateral sclerosis A general term for idiopathic involvement of the corticospinal tracts.

prion diseases Any of a number of slow viral diseases of the brain including Creutzfeldt-Jakob disease, Gerstmann-Straussler-Scheinker syndrome, and kuru.

proprioception Sensory information derived from the peripheral end organs of the nerves in muscles, tendons, and joints that supply the central nervous system with information regarding position and movement of body parts.

pseudobulbar palsy Diminution of musculature associated with the brainstem (bulb) due to pathology located in supranuclear areas of the brain. In contrast to actual bulbar palsy due to involvement of the cranial nerve nuclei and peripheral nerves, this is an upper motor neuron process with little to no muscular atrophy. Frequently associated with personality changes that include spasmotic laughing or crying or both simultaneously.

pseudotumor cerebri Benign intercranial hypertension. Increased intercranial pressure in the setting of an otherwise normal patient. Diffuse edema of the brain with no identifiable masked lesion or ventricular system abnormality. Along with idiopathic forms, it has been seen in conjunction with infectious disease, toxins, trauma, and generalized diffuse neuritis.

psychomotor seizure A partial seizure with complex symptomatology and impairment of consciousness. Attacks are characterized by repetitive motor acts or activity inappropriate for the patient's situation.

psychogenic seizures   Also known as pseudo seizures or hysterical seizures—seizures produced by physiologic episodes that can be mistaken for seizures or that lead to seizures that are not truly epileptic in nature. Malingering disorders such as Munchausen syndrome and malingering are conscious events and are differentiated from psychogenic seizures by the fact that the patient knows full well what is going on. The patient is not deliberately feigning the attacks and may have no conscious awareness of what is going on. These can be extremely difficult diagnoses and are sometimes made with the combination of simultaneous time-link video recordings and EEG recordings.

quadrantanopia   Loss of a quarter of a visual field as bounded by a vertical and horizontal radius. May be unilateral or bilateral, superior or inferior. Usually homonymous but may occasionally be bitemporal or binasal.

radiculopathy   Any disease process affecting the intradural portion of a spinal nerve route prior to its entrance into the intravertebral foramen or a portion of the foramen and the nerve plexus.

Raeder's (paratrigeminal) syndrome   An inflammation of the anatomic space containing the components of the fifth cranial nerve, the carotid artery and its sympathetic fibers, and the third, fourth, and sixth cranial nerves. The syndrome is characterized by paralysis of oculosympathetic pathways, which may involve sweating along with facial pain and involvement of the third, fourth, and sixth cranial nerves singly or in combination. Etiologies of the syndrome include carotid artery aneurysms, tumors, ophthalmic herpes, and spreading infections from chronic maxillary sinusitis. In rare cases, trauma may be the etiology.

Ramsay Hunt syndrome   Herpes zoster auris with vesicles on the tympanic membrane and on the face between the ear and mastoid regions, often associated with facial paralysis, loss of taste over the anterior two-thirds of the tongue, and deep protracted facial pain.

retrobulbar neuritis   Inflammation of the optic nerve accompanied by defects in vision and no observable change in the funduscopic exam. The term papillitis is used to refer to inflammatory optic neuritis with observable changes in the optic nerve head.

Reye's syndrome   Encephalopathy associated with fatty degeneration of the liver; seen almost exclusively in children. The disease process is characterized by persistent vomiting usually following a viral illness such as influenza or varicella. Generalized seizures and progressive lethargy and coma rapidly follow.

Rinne's test   A tuning-fork test used to delineate the predominance of either bone or air conduction in patients with hearing loss. (See Chap. 13.)

risus sardonicus   A tight or drawn facial appearance seen with facial muscular spasm; often associated with tetanus.

Romberg's sign   A test of both equilibrium and dorsal column sensation. (See Chap. 2.)

saccades   The general term for rapid eye movements such as the fast phase of nystagmus or the rapid eye movements seen in REM sleep.

Saturday night palsy   A colloquial term for compression neuropathy of the radial nerve in the upper arm; usually reserved for patients whose radial neuropathy is the result of their own malpositioning and lack of activity for prolonged periods.

Schilder's disease   A generalized term for diffuse sclerosis characterized by degeneration of white matter in the central nervous system. Has more recently been divided into multiple hereditary and nonhereditary specific disease patterns.

scotoma   A spot of varying size and shape within a visual field in which there is no vision.

seizure   The sudden onset of a disease with alteration in neurologic discharge. A convulsion. See also *febrile seizure, grand mal seizure, Jacksonian seizure, petit mal seizure,* and *psychomotor seizure.*

sleep paralysis   Associated with narcolepsy. Periods of paralysis developing during relaxation or just before going to sleep.

snout reflex   A contraction of both the upper and lower portions of the orbicularis oris and muscles about the nose, causing protrusion of the lips induced by tapping or touching the lower lips. This is a sign of the loss of frontal lobe functions seen in dementia.

spatial agnosia   Disorganization of spatial judgment in which patients cannot find their way in familiar surroundings. Also characterized by inability to perform constructional tasks such as copying and drawing.

spinal ataxia   A group of diseases characterized by gait disturbance and incoordination. Spinal ataxias differ from generalized cerebellar ataxia in that there is also diminished vibration and position sense and altered deep tendon reflexes, pyramidal track signs, or other evidence of involvement of spinal cord or peripheral nerves.

spinal shock   Weakness, decreased reflexes, decreased sensation; seen immediately following injury to the spinal cord.

stereognosis   The ability to understand the form of an object by means of the sense of touch. A parietal lobe function.

stupor   A state of loss of response to the environment in which consciousness may be impaired in varying degrees. The patient is difficult to rouse but can be brought to purposeful response with noxious verbal or physical stimulation. The patient promptly falls back into a nonresponsive mode when not being stimulated.

subarachnoid space   The area between the arachnoid and pia mater layers of the meninges; contains the cerebrospinal fluid.

subdural space   The area between the dura mater and arachnoid layers of the meninges.

subhyaloid hemorrhage   Bleeding into the space between the retina and the vitreous; almost exclusively found in association with subarachnoid hemorrhage from aneurysmal rupture.

supranuclear palsy   Decreased movement of the musculature supplied by the cranial nerves secondary to upper motor neuron disease involving the cortex, subcortical structures, or corticospinal tracts.

supratentorial   The space above the tentorium cerebelli including the anterior and middle fossa of the skull; containing the cerebral cortex, deep cortical structures, and thalamic structures.

swallow syncope   Transient loss of consciousness secondary to bradycardia with resultant inadequate cerebral profusion initiated by the act of swallowing; a response mediated through the vagus nerve.

syringobulbia   A condition of dysfunction of the lower brainstem (bulb) secondary to cavitation and expansion of the primitive central cord of the nervous system. The brainstem analog of syringomyelia.

syringomyelia   A disease of the spinal cord principally in the cervical region; marked by the presence of expansion of fluid-filled cavities in the region of the primitive central cord. Clinically there is pain and temperature loss as well as decreased motor strength in the upper limbs with relative preservation of motor and sensory findings in the lower extremities. As the disease progresses, upper motor neuron findings in the lower extremities, such as hyperreflexia and spasticities, begin to appear.

tabes dorsalis   A sequela of syphilis with a chronic progressive sclerosis of the posterior spinal roots and posterior columns of the spinal cord and peripheral nerves. The clinical picture includes ataxia with lancinating pains in the extremities and markedly decreased position and vibration sense. Optic nerve atrophy and trophic disorders of the joints are not uncommon.

tarsal tunnel syndrome   Entrapment of the posterior tibial nerve in the region of the medial malleolus of the tibia; symptoms consist of pain, tingling, and numbness in the sole of the foot aggravated by standing and walking.

tectum   Any covering or roofing structure in the nervous system referring to the dorsalmost portion of the brainstem.

tegmentum   The portion of the brainstem dorsal to the cerebral peduncles and the pons.

Tensilon test   Edrophonium chloride test; the use of a coinhibiting drug given to diagnose myasthenia gravis. (See Chap. 5.)

thalamic pain   Associated with cerebral hemorrhage or thrombosis involving thalamic structures; symptoms include alteration of sensory stimuli from the contralateral side of the involved portion of the thalamus. All sensory stimuli from the affected areas take on unpleasant sensations and may be accompanied by a brain or deep aching pain (hyperpathia). This may progress to intractable, deep-seated pain (anesthesia dolorosa).

thrombolytics   See *fibrinolysis.*

Tinel's sign   A tingling sensation felt in the nerve when percussion is made over the site of the nerve.

tinnitus   Subjective noises (i.e., ringing, whistling) in the ears as the result of involvement of the cochlear mechanisms.

Todd's paralysis   Postictal motor dysfunction with usually rapid return to normal function. The area of paralysis may correlate with that area of the brain most involved in the seizure focus.

torticollis   Twisting of the neck secondary to either neck muscle irritation from injury or from involuntary contraction of the neck muscles due to drugs or underlying neurologic disease.

transient global amnesia   An amnestic state involving recent memory but not instantaneous memory or passed memory. Thought to be due to decreased blood flow through the hippocampus. A form may come as intermittent episodes causing loss of memory covering days to weeks.

transient ischemic attack (TIA)   Short-term neurologic dysfunction clearing within 14 hours secondary to inadequate central nervous system profusion secondary to multiple causes. To be labeled a TIA, all neurologic symptomatology must be resolved within 14 hours.

Trousseau's sign   Muscular spasm elicited by pressure over the nerves and arteries supplying the area of spasm.

uncinate fit   A type of focal seizure preceded by an aura of disagreeable smells.

vasovagal syncope   Sudden loss of consciousness due to inadequate cerebral profusion secondary to bradycardia on the basis of increased vagas nerve stimulation. (See Chap. 12.)

Wallenberg's syndrome   Vascular occlusion of the posterior inferior cerebellar artery, which supplies the dorsal lateral portion of the medulla. Signs and symptoms include loss of cerebellar function ipsilateral to the lesion with a loss of pain and temperature sensation from the ipsilateral side of the face. This is accompanied by loss of pain and temperature sensation in the limbs and the trunk on the opposite side of the body. Deviation of the eyes or nystagmus may be present from irritation of the vestibular nuclei.

Weber syndrome   A lesion secondary to dysfunction in the basilar portion of the midbrain. Signs and symptoms include spastic paralysis of the contralateral arm and leg combined with external strabismus of the ipsilateral eye and ptosis. Concomitant involvement of the third cranial nerve results in the dilation of the ipsilateral pupil.

Weber's test   A tuning-fork test used to determine whether a hearing loss is primarily on a conductive or neurosensory basis. (See Chap. 13.)

Wernicke's aphasia   A fluent aphasia secondary to lesions involving the auditory cortex of the temporal lobe. It is a fluent aphasia characterized by active, well-articulated speech that makes little to no sense because patients cannot monitor their own speech processes.

INDEX

Note: Page numbers followed by the letter "*t*" indicate tables, those followed by the letter "*f*" indicate figures.